MILWAUKEE COUNTY

THE MEDICAL COLLEGE OF WISCONSIN

UNIVERSITÄT HAMBURG

Psychopathological and Neurological Dysfunctions Following Open-Heart Surgery

Edited by
R. Becker J. Katz M.-J. Polonius H. Speidel

With 71 figures

Springer-Verlag
Berlin Heidelberg New York 1982

Professor Robin Becker, Ph. D., D. Sc.†

Professor Jeremy M. Katz, Ph. D.
Department of Psychiatry
The Medical College of Wisconsin
Milwaukee County Mental Health Complex
9191 Watertown Plank Road
Milwaukee, Wisconsin 53226, USA

Priv.-Doz. Dr. med. Michael-J. Polonius
Abteilung für Herz- und Gefäßchirurgie und
experimentelle Kardiologie
Chirurgische Universitätsklinik Eppendorf
Martinistraße 52
2000 Hamburg 20, FRG

Professor Dr. med. Hubert Speidel
Psychosomatische Abteilung
Universitäts-Krankenhaus Eppendorf
Martinistraße 52
2000 Hamburg 20, FRG

Proceedings of the Second International Symposium
on Psychopathological and Neurological Dysfunctions
Following Open-Heart Surgery, Milwaukee, USA

ISBN-13: 978-3-642-68612-2 e-ISBN-13: 978-3-642-68610-8
DOI: 10.1007/ 978-3-642-68610-8

Softcover reprint of the hardcover 1st edition 1982

Typesetting: Weihrauch, Würzburg
2119/3140-54321

Foreword
The Surgeon as a Humanist

Medicine is the most humane of the sciences and the most scientific of the humanities.

Cardiac surgery today provides a most natural confluence for the high technology of medicine and the humanistic values traditional in the practice of medicine.

The cardiac surgeon must, of necessity, be knowledgeable in physiology and cardiology, and must also possess consummate surgical technical skill. The attainment of these skills over long years of training leads many of these surgeons to believe or perceive this long struggle as an apotheosis of their position in life, rather than as an education in bringing the latest scientific advances to the care of patients.

The problem lies not only with the cardiac surgeon; it is also contributed to by the patients' perception of heart surgery, heart disease, and the mystery of the science and physiology involved. The patient with heart disease expecting surgery may, for the first time, be facing the finiteness of his existence. The low risk of cardiac surgery today not withstanding, the coronary surgery patients, most likely a type A personality, is faced with a perceived threat to his invulnerability, his self-image, his family, his independence, his control of situations, and his very existence.

These considerable threats and these appropriate thoughts, compounded by a modicum of understanding, contribute to the patient's need and desire to perceive his cardiac surgeon as a modern day thaumaturge. The patient wants his surgeon to be more than human, to make him better, and to remove these discomfiting thoughts from his mind as he repairs his heart. These two parties to the patient-physician relationship both derive gratification from their perceptions and in the *appropriate* degree this leads to the faith and confidence in the physician-patient relationship that contributes to a successful outcome. An exuberance or distortion of these perceptions may, however, leave one or both parties unhappy or unhealed when expectations are not met. It is of critical importance for the surgeon to understand what the patient perceives to be the benefits of the proposed operation in all its facets and to explain, as far as is possible considering the individual's culture, knowledge, and education, what are the reasonable goals that should be obtained by the proposed surgical procedure.

Your presence at this conference is the affirmation of your commitment to bringing a humanistic outlook to our technologic successes, which will contribute to a more holistic practice of cardiac surgery.

It was interesting to hear the responses of many cardiac surgeons who declined to attend this meeting. Many said: "It's worthwhile but cardiac surgeons don't like to think about those complications," or "As a cardiac surgeon I can't afford to get emotionally involved with the patients," or "Other parts of the team take care of those complications," or – the worst of all – "My patients don't have psychological or neurological complications". Except for the last group, who obviously do not have a patient-physician relationship, the others are manifesting their immaturity as human beings with rationalizations for their own defense mechanisms and inability to consider their own mortality and finiteness. It is my feeling that they are missing one of the joys of taking care of patients, namely "sharing".

In taking care of patients in all phases of cardiac surgery over the years, but primarily coronary bypass, I have collected some reminiscences that have formed a consistent pattern of behavioral response seen in the cardiac surgical patient. These patients enter the system by many routes: a myocardial infarction, angina, "sudden death" by ventricual fibrillation with successful resuscitation, or a routine physical examination for employment that includes stress testing, even though asymptomatic.

The demonstration of ischemic heart disease by a catheterization is obviously met with varying acceptance, depending on the route by which the patient entered the system by and on his personality. By his personality I mean the totality of his social, psychological, biologic, economic nature, or his humaneness.

All the patients go through a series of stages known to us as the "grief response," but in this case I would like to refer to it as the "*survival coping response*" (Fig. 1). The stages of denial, anger, bargaining, depression, and resolution are influenced by many factors including personality in the broadest sense, familial and cultural influences, and the mode of entrance into this experience.

Approximately 50% of patients undergoing coronary bypass surgery have difficulties in the preoperative or postoperative period with the management of this crisis.

Except for the sudden death-resuscitated group, *denial* is the first defense mechanism. The pronouncement of the verdict of ischemic heart disease that necessitates surgery results in a challenge to the patient's very existence followed by an effect on his/her family, job, self-image, and the philosophical questions of existence and values.

As previously mentioned, the patients all move through what we call the survival coping response with stages, after denial, of anger, bargaining, depression, and then *resolution*. If the cardiac surgeon is aware of these processes in evolution, he can be the best helper to the patient in carrying them through to a successful conclusion.

Some of the worst psychological problems have occurred when emergency surgery is necessary, the patient going directly from the catheterization laboratory to the operating room. With little preoperative explanation the patient awakes with many long

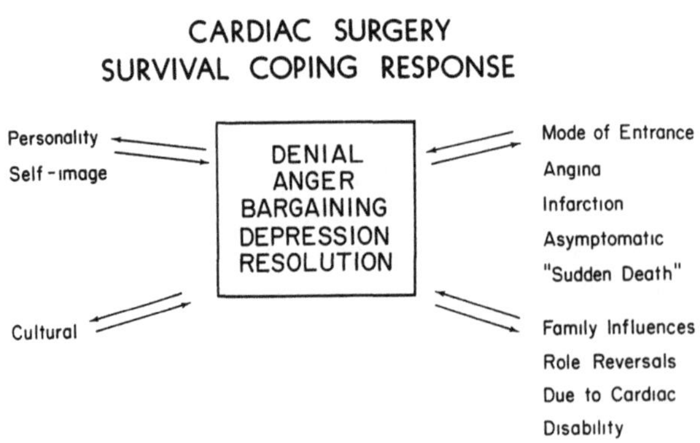

Fig. 1. The survival coping response of patients who must undergo cardiac surgery

scars, discomfort, and instant recognition that his/her world has changed. They have presented many psychological problems all to be dealt with in the postoperative period.

Those who have coped best, I feel, are those who have received a thorough explanation of the entire procedure, indications, risks, benefits, and expected result and who in turn have had time to ask those questions which are germane to their human condition. A waiting period for digestion and assimilation of about 2 weeks, with another chance to ask questions prior to operation, has usually brought them to operation in optimal mental condition. In the early postoperative period there is euphoric period. Between the 2nd and the 5th week there is a "funk" or depressed period and by 6–8 weeks there is resolution of the psychological problems as the patient regains much or all of his/her lost freedom.

Patients do not have exacerbations of angina or seek help in a vacuum. Their life situation *is* frequently the motivating force that prompts them to come forward at a certain time. Quite frequently a family member forces them to seek help as they have not been able to move from the denial phase of dealing with angina. Frequently, job changes or pressures are in the picture. Also, I have noted that marital problems are lurking behind the scene and impotence may be compensated for by the use of angina during intercourse as a defense mechanism. The wife frequently then brings the husband to the cardiologist. Also, a prolonged presence of angina, "cardiac disability," or dependence has led to a role reversal in the family and drastic self-image problems.

The reversal of problems by cardiac surgery with potential re-establishment of self-image and additional family roles has frequently been a new source of familial problems that have to be reworked.

We cannot understand every facet of our patients' existence but we can know what cardiac surgery means to them, their aspirations, their families and thus, in at least this limited sphere of an immensely anxiety provoking experience, learn of their humaneness and let it provide a chance for our humanity to be shared with them. This is what yields the richness of the words patient-physician relationship and *compassion*.

The better the surgeon understands the setting in which the patient seeks help, the better he will be able to deal with the whole patient and his family. Some patients have actually sought cardiac surgery as a way out of this world, their perception being that it was high risk and a socially acceptable way to commit suicide. If one does not wish to be the executioner of such plans, a little talk from the patient revealing helplessness, "I don't care if I die," "I hope I die", "What's there to live for," may suggest to the surgeon that his desired goals for an operation are not consonant with the patient's.

Cardiac surgeons and their technologic advances are constantly portrayed as the most powerful of modern thaumaturges. Their power is associated with mastery of impersonal instruments, machines, procedures, and medications that manipulate physiology usually beyond ordinary lay understanding. However, we must not fall prey to the hubris of Cartesian philosophy suggesting that we can approach cardiac patients as if they were ailing watches. Surrounded on a daily basis by our instrumentation and physiologic and technologic gadgetry, it is often difficult for cardiac surgeons to remember that medicine as a science must deal with the special complexities of man as subject at nexus with man as object of science.

Our own humanism will determine at what level we shall interact with each patient. We therefore have to foster and renew within ourselves that concept of humanism.

I would not attempt to define humanism except to say that I believe as Pellegrine[1] stated, "Humanism encompasses a spirit of sincere concern for the centrality of human values in every aspect of professional activities."

This symposium proved to be exciting and informative as we attempted to clarify the unspoken but recognized confluence of science and humanism in the setting of the cardiac surgical patient.

Robert J. Flemma

[1] Pellegrino E (1979) Humanism and the Physician. University of Tennessee Press, Knoxville

Preface

As early as the mid-1960s, Professor Dr. Georg Rodewald, Director of Cardiovascular Surgery at the University Hospital Hamburg-Eppendorf, Hamburg, West Germany, recognized the importance of psychological and neurological disturbances following cardiac surgery. Despite his attempts to bring about early collaborative work in this area, such work did not begin in Hamburg until the end of the 1960s. At that time members of a psychosomatic research group at the University of Hamburg studied patients with artificial heart valves as part of a larger project on non-heart surgery patients.

However, it was not until the establishment of a Special Research Unit for Psychosomatic Medicine, Clinical Pharmacology and Psychotherapy at the University of Hamburg by the German Research Society (Die Deutsche Forschungsgemeinschaft) in 1974, that this group could begin a major research program. Of major importance to its members was the exchange of results and clinical experience with other individuals studying the same topic.

Taking the initiative, members of the Hamburg group, organized the First International Symposium on Psychopathological and Neurological Dysfunctions following Open-Heart Surgery. The meeting was held March 3–4, 1978 in Hamburg. With the generous financial support of the German Research Society, all known world researchers were invited to participate.

The meeting was most successful. Thirty-six researchers representing five countries attended. Agreement was achieved on three major points: (1) that neurological and psychological problems after heart surgery indeed exist and constitute a significant international medical problem; (2) that members in attendance would work together as a group in confronting these problems (the idea of worldwide cooperation in this area was thus born) and (3) that an international study was necessary but premature without additional world support.

Urged by those present at the first meeting and working closely with Dr. Speidel and members of the Hamburg group, Dr. Jeremy Katz organized the Second International Symposium. The meeting was held March 5–7, 1980 in Milwaukee, Wisconsin, U.S.A. Heart surgery professionals throughout the world were invited to attend.

The meeting was a marked success. Representatives from 18 countries and 24 U.S. states attended. All disciplines involved in cardiac surgery were represented. Three major objectives were achieved: (1) and enlarged and more comprehensive international forum with representation by all disciplines was created; (2) the existence of sufficient world support to begin an international study was demonstrated; and (3) faculty and interested registrants met in special session following the meeting and agreed to actively work together toward an international study.

It is the Editors' hope that this volume, as well as the volume of the first meeting, will bring an increased awareness of psychological and neurological problems after surgery to cardiac surgery professionals. We further hope that their publication encourages even greater mutual sharing of relevant information and clinical experience among world research groups investigating this topic.

We are indebted to many for the volume's final form. To faculty members of the symposium we express our thanks for the quality of their presentations and for their cooperation in submitting manuscripts in a timely fashion. We also acknowledge with great appreciation the efforts of B. Dahme, P. Götze, G. Huse-Kleinstoll and H.-J. Meffert, of the Hamburg group, for reviewing and summarizing a typescript of meeting discussion. Finally, to Ms. Ute Grünthal and Ms. Ursula Kirkerup we express our gratitude for their editing and final preparation of manuscripts for publication.

The Editors[1]

Acknowledgments. The Symposium acknowledges the generosity of the speakers sponsors listed on the following pages. Their support played an important role in the overall success and impact of the meeting.

Opening Remarks were made by Jeremy M. Katz, Ph. D., Symposium Director; Professor Dr. med. Hubert Speidel, Symposium Co-Director; Professor Dr. med. K. H. Hölzer, Director, University Hospital Hamburg-Eppendorf; Leonard W. Cronkhite, Jr., M.D., President, The Medical College of Wisconsin; Bert W. Pyle, Jr., Administrator, Milwaukee County Mental Health Complex; Lawrence I. Bonchek, M.D., Chairman, Department of Cardiothoracic Surgery, The Medical College of Wisconsin; Herzl R. Spiro, M.D., Ph.D., Chairman, Department of Psychiatry and Mental Health Sciences, The Medical College of Wisconsin; Hans H. Brieskorn, M.D., Official Coordinator for U.S.-German Biomedical Research Cooperation.

---

1 Since the Second International Symposium, a Consortium to carry out an international study on psychological and neurological disturbances after heart surgery has been established. The International Consortium on Cerebral and Psychopathological Dysfunctions following Cardiac Surgery was formally created at an organization/planning meeting in April of 1981 in Milwaukee. Dr. Katz will serve as Consortium Director, Dr. Hubert Speidel as International Study Director, and Dr. Richard Blacher as Consortium Newsletter Editor.

Contents

List of Contributors

Torkel Åberg, Doz. Dr., Department of Thoracic Surgery, Akademiska Sjukhuset, Uppsala, Sweden

Robin Becker, Ph. D., D. Sc. †

Donald Bethune, M.D., F.F.A.R.C.S. Consultant Anesthetist, Papworth Hospital, Papworth Everard, Cambridge CB 3 8 RE, Great Britain

Viking Björk, M.D., Professor, Karolinska Sjukhuset, Thoracic Surgery Çlinic, 10401 Stockholm 60, Sweden

Richard S. Blacher, M.D., Department of Psychiatry, New England Medical Center Hospital, 171 Harrison Avenue, Boston, Massachusetts 02111, USA

Henri Boccalon, M.D., Ph. D., Chirurgie Cardiovasculaire, C.H.U Toulouse Rangueil, Chemin du Vallon, 31054 Toulouse Cedex, France

Patricia M. Clarkson, M.B., F.R.A.C.P., Pediatric Cardiologist, Green Lane Hospital, Green Lane West, Auckland 3, New Zealand

Bernd Dahme, Professor Dr. phil., Abteilung für Medizinische Psychologie, Universitätskrankenhaus Eppendorf, Martinistraße 52, 2000 Hamburg 20, FRG

Gisela Dahme, Dr. phil., Annenstr. 12, 2000 Hamburg 4, FRG

Susanne Davies-Osterkamp, Professor Dr. rer. soc., Zentrum für Psychosomatische Medizin, Medizinische Psychologie, Klinikum der Justus-Liebig-Universität, Friedrichstraße 36, 6300 Gießen, FRG

Robert Flemma, M.D., Cardiovascular Surgery Associates, 9800 West Bluemound Road, Milwaukee, Wisconsin 53226, USA

Barbara Flemming, Dr. phil., Dipl.-Psych., Georg-Bonne-Straße 78, 2000 Hamburg 52, FRG

Rita Frantz, R.N., Ph. D., Assistant Professor, College of Nursing, The University of Iowa, Iowa City, Iowa 52242, USA

Helmuth Freyberger, Professor Dr. med., Abteilung für Psychosomatik, Medizinische Hochschule Hannover, Konstanty-Gutschow-Str. 8, 3000 Hannover 61, FRG

Paul Götze, Prof. Dr. med., Psychiatrische und Nervenklinik, Universitätskrankenhaus Eppendorf, Martinistraße 52, 2000 Hamburg 20, FRG

Stanley Heller, M.D., College of Physicians and Surgeons of Columbia University, 722 West 168 Street, New York, New York 10032, USA

Gisela Huse-Kleinstoll, Dr. med., Abteilung für Medizinische Psychologie, Universitätskrankenhaus Eppendorf, Martinistraße 52, 2000 Hamburg 20, FRG

Gudrun Jänsch, Dipl.-Psych., Am Klostergarten 11, 8000 Munich 60, FRG

Jeremy M. Katz, Ph. D., Department of Psychiatry, The Medical College of Wisconsin, Milwaukee County Mental Health Complex, 9191 Watertown Plank Road, Milwaukee, Wisconsin 53226, USA

Chase P. Kimball, M.D., Professor, Department of Psychiatry, University of Chicago, 950 East 59th Street, Chicago, Illinois 60637, USA

Hans-Joachim Krebber, Dr. med., Abteilung für Herz- und Gefäßchirurgie und experimentelle Kardiologie, Chirurgische Universitätsklinik Eppendorf, Martinistraße 52, 2000 Hamburg 20, FRG

Donald Longmore, Dr., F.R.C.S., Department of Clinical Physiology, National Heart Hospital, Westmoreland Street, London WLM 8 BA, Great Britain

Heinz-Jörg Meffert, Dr. phil., Dipl.-Psych., Abteilung für Medizinische Psychologie, Universitätskrankenhaus Eppendorf, Martinistraße 52, 2000 Hamburg 20, FRG

Rudolf Meyendorf, Priv.-Doz. Dr. med., Psychiatrische Klinik und Poliklinik, Nußbaumstraße 7, 8000 Munich 2, FRG

Davinder Mohan, M.D., Chairman, Department of Psychiatry, All-India Institute of Medical Sciences, Ansari Nagar, New Delhi 110 016, India

Klaus Möhlen, Dr. med., Zentrum für Psychosomatische Medizin der Justus-Liebig-Universität Gießen, Friedrichstraße 36, 6300 Gießen, FRG

Abu Nwaefuna, M.D., Professor, Chairman, Department of Psychiatry, A. M. Dogliotti College of Medicine, University of Liberia, Monrovia, West Africa

Renate Paech, Dr. med., Ahornstraße 12, 8032 Lochham, FRG

Hellmut Pokar, Priv. Doz. Dr. med., Abteilung für Herz- und Gefäßchirurgie und experimentelle Kardiologie, Chirurgische Universitätsklinik Eppendorf, Martinistraße 52, 2000 Hamburg 20, FRG

Michael-J. Polonius, Priv.-Doz. Dr. med., Abteilung für Herz- und Gefäßchirurgie und experimentelle Kardiologie, Chirurgische Universitätsklinik Eppendorf, Martinistraße 52, 2000 Hamburg 20, FRG

Charles J. Rabiner, M.D., Professor, School of Medicine, State University of New York at Stony Brook, Department of Psychiatry, Long Island Jewish Medical Center, P.O. Box 38, Glen Oaks, New York 11004, USA

Christian Reimer, Dr. med., Psychiatrische Klinik, Medizinische Hochschule Lübeck, Ratzeburger Allee 160, 2400 Lübeck, FRG

Georg Rodewald, Professor Dr. med., Abteilung für Herz- und Gefäßchirurgie und experimentelle Kardiologie, Chirurgische Universitätsklinik Eppendorf, Martinistraße 52, 2000 Hamburg 20, FRG

Hans Scheld, Dr. med., Zentrum für Chirurgie am Klinikum der Justus-Liebig-Universität Gießen, Kardiovaskuläre Abteilung, Klinikstraße 29, 6300 Gießen, FRG

Wolfgang Spehr, Dr. med., Psychiatrische und Nervenklinik, Universitätskrankenhaus Eppendorf, Martinistraße 52, 2000 Hamburg 20, FRG

Hubert Speidel, Professor Dr. med., II. Medizinische Klinik, Psychosomatische Abteilung, Universitätskrankenhaus Eppendorf, Martinistraße 52, 2000 Hamburg 20, FRG

Herzl R. Spiro, M.D., Ph. D., Chairman, Department of Psychiatry and Mental Health Sciences, The Medical College of Wisconsin, Milwaukee County Mental Health Complex, 9191 Watertown Plank Road, Milwaukee, Wisconsin 53226, USA

Babette-Ann Stanton, Ph. D., Assistant Research Professor of Medicine, Boston University Medical Center, Division of Psychiatry, Department of Behavioral Epidemiology, 720 Harrison Street, Boston, Massachusetts 02118, USA

Su Hong-xi, M.D., Professor of Cardiovascular Surgery, Department of Cardiovascular Surgery, General Hospital of the People's Liberation Army, Peking, Peoples Republic of China

Kenneth M. Taylor, M.D., F.R.C.S., Department of Cardiac Surgery, University of Glasgow, Royal Infirmary, Glasgow G4 OSF C, Scotland

Pekka Tienari, M.D., Professor of Psychiatry, Oulun Yliopisto, Clinic of Psychiatry, 90210 Oulu 21, Finland

Hartmut Träger, Dr. med., Dipl.-Psych., Katholisches Krankenhaus Reinbek, Adolf-Stift, Hamburger Str. 41, 2057 Reinbek, FRG

Juro Wada, M.D., F.A.C.S., Professor, Heart Institute of Japan, Tokyo Women's Medical College, Kawada-cho Shinjuku, Tokyo 162, Japan

Allen E. Willner, Ph. D., Department of Psychiatry, Long Island Jewish Hillside Medical Center, P.O. Box 38, Glen Oaks, New York 11004, USA

Organization of the Meeting

Symposium Director
Jeremy M. Katz, Ph. D.
Department of Psychiatry
The Medical College of Wisconsin
Milwaukee County Mental Health Complex
9191 Watertown Plank Road
Milwaukee, Wisconsin 53226, USA

Symposium Co-Director
Professor Dr. med. Hubert Speidel
II. Medizinische Klinik
Psychosomatische Abteilung
Universitätskrankenhaus Eppendorf
Martinistraße 52
2000 Hamburg 20, FRG

Coordinator of Symposium Development
Ms. Marilyn C. Cheung
Office of Continuing and Allied Professional Education
The Medical College of Wisconsin
8701 Watertown Plank Road
Milwaukee, Wisconsin 53226, USA

Organizing and Editorial Committee
Robin Becker, Ph. D., D. Sc. †, Jerusalem, Israel
Jeremy M. Katz, Ph. D., Milwaukee, Wisconsin, USA
Priv.-Doz. Dr. med. Michael-J. Polonius, Hamburg, West Germany
Professor Dr. med. Hubert Speidel, Hamburg, West Germany

Sponsors

Speakers' Sponsors

Biotronik, Berlin, Germany; The Concerned Hearts Charitable Foundation, Inc., Milwaukee, Wisconsin, U.S.A.; The Concerned Hearts Club of Milwaukee, Milwaukee, Wisconsin, U.S.A.; Die Deutsche Forschungsgemeinschaft, Bonn-Bad Godesberg, West Germany; Fujisawa Pharmaceutical Company Ltd., Osaka, Japan; Laboratoire Travenol – Division Oxygénations, Plaisir, France; Clave's Pharmaceutical Inc., Monrovia, Liberia, West Africa; Medipolar Oy Farmos Group Ltd., Oulu, Finland; Pall Biomedical Products Corporation, Glen Cove, New York, U.S.A.; Polystan, Herlev, Denmark; Shiley Laboratories Inc., Irvine, California; Stöckert Instruments, Munich, West Germany; Telectronics Proprietary Ltd., Sydney, Australia; Wellcome Research Laboratory, Beckenham, Kent, England.

Sponsors

Allen Bradley Foundation, Inc., Milwaukee, Wisconsin; American Family Insurance Group, Madison, Wisconsin; Avco Medical Products, Everett, Massachusetts; Bentley Laboratories, Inc., Irvine, California; Biomedical Specialties, Inc., LaGrange, Illinois; Biomedicus Inc., Minnetonka, Minnesota; Biotronex Laboratories, Kensington, Maryland; Blue Cross-Blue Shield United of Wisconsin, Milwaukee, Wisconsin; Boehringer Ingelheim, Ltd., Ridgefield, Connecticut; Cardiac Pacemakers Inc., St. Paul, Minnesota; Cardiovascular Instrument Corporation, Wakefield, Massachusetts; Critikon, Inc. Raritan, New Jersey; Datascope Corporation, Paramus, New Jersey; Davis + Geck, Wayne, New Jersey; The Eberbach Foundation, Milwaukee, Wisconsin; Extracorporeal Medical Specialties Inc., King of Prussia, Pennsylvania; W.L. Gore & Associates, Inc., Elkton, Maryland; Haemonetics Corporation, Braintree Massachusetts; Hancock Laboratories Inc., Anaheim, California; IBM Corporation, Milwaukee, Wisconsin; Eli Lilly and Company, Indianapolis, Indiana; The Marcus Corporation Foundation, Milwaukee, Wisconsin; Meadox, Oakland, New Jersey; Medical Engineering Corporation, Racine, Wisconsin; Medtronic, Inc., Minneapolis, Minnesota; Midwest Cardiovascular Institute Foundation, Milwaukee, Wisconsin; The Northwestern Mutual Life Insurance Company, Milwaukee, Wisconsin; Pacesetters Systems, Inc., Sylmar, California; Pall Biomedical Products Corporation, Glen Cove, L.I., New York; Pioneer Viggo, Inc., Beaverton, Oregon; Roche Laboratories, Nutley, New Jersey; Roche Medical Electronics Inc., Cranbury, New Jersey; Roerig Pharmaceuticals, New York, New York; Sandoz Pharmaceuticals, East Hanover, New Jersey; Sarns Inc., Ann Arbor,

Michigan; SciMed Life Systems, Inc., Minneapolis, Minnesota; Seecor Inc., Fort Worth, Texas; Shiley Laboratories, Inc., Irvine, California; Smith Kline & French Laboratories, Philadelphia, Pennsylvania; E.R. Squibb & Sons, Inc., Princeton, New Jersey; Sutter Biomedical Inc., San Diego, California; Telectronics Proprietary Ltd., Englewood, Colorado; Travenol Laboratories, Inc., Artificial Organs Division, Deerfield, Illinois; The Upjohn Company, Kalamazoo, Michigan.

I

Incidence and Description of Neurological and Psychiatric Complications Following Cardiac Surgery

Early and Late Neurological Complications After Prosthetic Heart Valve Replacement

V.O. Björk, T. Ivert

Summary

A retrospective study of early neurological complications after heart valve replacement revealed a significant reduction in the incidence (8.4% to 4.1%) and severity when patients operated on during 1969–1975 and 1978–1979 were compared. This was mainly ascribed to the change from continuous coronary perfusion of the beating heart to hypothermic cardioplegia, although contributory effects of changes of disc- to bubble oxygenator, blood- to nonblood-priming and standard to convex-concave Björk-Shiley tilting disc valve were taken into account. A low incidence of early embolism was further reduced during the latter period. Follow-up disclosed favorable prognosis for patients with short periods of postoperative coma and paresis. No sequelae were encountered after postoperative psychosis. The late thromboembolic incidence was, however, unexpectedly high in patients with postoperative neurological complications.

Introduction

Neurological complications after open-heart surgery are major hazards and may contribute to the patient's death or cause permanent disability. Prospective studies, including complete neurological examination before and after operation, revealing even minor cerebral dysfunctions have shown a high incidence of postoperative neurological symptoms. Gilman [8] reported cerebral disorders in 12/35 patients (34%) after heart surgery. Javid et al. [10] found neurological abnormalities in 53 of 100 patients after open-heart surgery. The same diagnostic accuracy is not possible in retrospective studies. Thus, Branthwhite [5] reported a reduction in neurological damage after open-heart surgery from 19.2% to 7.4% following the introduction of filters in the extracorporeal system and precautions to prevent hypotension during the operation.

The purpose of this retrospective study was to analyze the frequency and etiology of gross neurological complications after open-heart surgery with insertion of heart valve prostheses, before and after the introduction of several technical refinements. The summarized effects of changing from disc- to bubble oxygenator, blood- to nonblood-priming solution, continuous coronary perfusion of the beating heart to

Psychopathological and Neurological Dysfunctions
Following Open-Heart Surgery Ed by Becker et al

hypothermic cardioplegia, and from the standard to the convex-concave Björk-Shiley tilting disc valve were related to a significant decrease in postoperative neurological deficits. To assess the fate of patients sustaining neurological complications they were followed for a mean period of 3 years after surgery.

Clinical Material and Methods

Patients undergoing heart valve replacement at the Karolinska Hospital, Stockholm, were compared during two periods. Median sternotomy, arterial cannulation in the ascending aorta and moderate hypothermia (25 °C–30 °C) were routinely used operative procedures.

Group I: This group comprised 901 patients operated on from the introduction of the Björk-Shiley tilting disc valve in 1969 through to December 1975. All patients received the standard valve of delrin or pyrolitic carbon. A disc oxygenator with a filter in the arterial line was used during the operations. Blood was added to the priming solution. Continuous coronary perfusion of the beating heart was employed to protect the myocardium from ischemic injury. Thus, the aorta was not clamped during operations on the mitral or tricuspid valves, except for short periods to facilitate exposure. A side branch from the arterial line with specially devised coronary indwelling cannulas provided blood to the myocardium when the aorta was opened.

Group II: These patients were operated on according to the technical refinements introduced during 1976 and 1977. The study group consisted of 437 patients operated on consecutively between January 1978 and December 1979. The modified convex-concave prosthesis was inserted in all patients. A disposable bubble oxygenator (Shiley) with a filter only in the coronary suction line was used. No blood was added to the priming solution. The aorta was clamped in all operations and hypothermic cardioplegic solution infused through a needle in the aortic root or, if the aorta was opened directly into the coronary ostia, through a cannula. This technique permitted the surgeon to operate on a motionless, bloodless, and flaccid heart.

Patient records were retrospectively reviewed. Early neurological complications were defined as neurological manifestations appearing before discharge from hospital. Impaired consciousness for more than 1 day after surgery, convulsions, extremity paresis, impairment of vision, or psychosis were noted. Operative deaths with neurological signs in the immediate postoperative period were included, but neurological dysfunction secondary to metabolic disturbance or shock before death were excluded as were a few patients sustaining peripheral nerve injuries.

Neurological symptoms apparently of embolic origin occurring after an initially uncomplicated course before the patient's discharge were tabulated separately.

Follow-up results from survivors in Group I were obtained a mean period of 36 months after operation by personal calls, questionnaires or reports from the patient's physician. Autopsy data from all early and late deaths were collected.

Statistical methods. Differences between groups were calculated in fourfold tables with Yates correction or exact probability test. The null hypothesis was rejected if $P < 0.05$.

Results

The hospital mortality and the incidence of neurological complications after various combinations of valve procedures in Group I and II are shown in Tables 1 and 2. The neurological deficits in operative deaths and survivors are tabulated separately. The total incidence of neurological complications was significantly reduced in Group II, the reduction being specially marked in patients having a mitral valve inserted. The gross neurological findings are summarized in Table 3. Patients with postoperative psychosis, but without prolonged postoperative periods of unconsciousness or focal neurological signs, are presented separately. Apparently, neurological damage was less severe in Group II, as the occurrence of coma was significantly reduced. In patients with unilateral paresis left-sided symptoms were significantly more common. Some details from groups and subgroups with neurological complications are given below. Patients with postoperative psychosis and early embolic episodes will be considered separately.

Neurological Complications After Aortic Valve Replacement

Group I: A majority of the patients had calcified valves. Two were explored postoperatively for bleeding. In several patients there was excessive preoperative bleeding with

Table 1. Operative (hospital) mortality, total and with neurological complications after heart valve replacement in two groups of patients

Operative procedure	Group I (operated 1969–1975)			Group II (operated 1978–1979)		
	Number of patients operated	Total operative mortality (%)	Operative mortality with neurological complications (%)	Number of patients operated	Total operative mortality (%)	Operative mortality with neurological complications (%)
AVR	535	31 (5.8)	8 (1.5)	267	9 (3.4)	3 (1.1)
MVR	221	13 (5.9)	2 (0.9)	108	2 (1.9)	0
AVR + MVR	85	5 (5.9)	2 (2.4)	43	2 (4.7)	1 (2.3)
MVR + TVP	45	7 (15.6)	3 (6.7)	12	1 (8.3)	0
Triple-VP	15	2 (13.3)	2 (13.3)	7	2 (28.6)	2 (28.6)
Total	901	58 (6.4)	17 (1.9)	437	16 (3.7)	6 (1.4)

Abbreviations: AVR, aortic valve replacement; MVR, mitral valve replacement; TVP, tricuspid valve procedure (valve replacement or annuloplastic); Triple-VP, triple valve procedure (aortic and mitral valve replacement, valve replacement or annuloplastic of tricuspid valve)

Table 2. The incidence of early neurological complications after heart valve replacement in two groups of patients

Operative procedure	Group I (operated 1969–1975)			Group II (operated 1978–1979)			Significance
	Number of patients operated	Total operative mortality	Number of survivors (%)	Number of patients	Total operative mortality	Number of survivors (%)	
AVR	535	8	20 (5.2)	267	3	8 (4.1)	N.S.
MVR	221	2	18 (9.0)	108	0	3 (2.8)	N.S.
AVR + MVR	85	2	9 (12.9)	43	1	0 (2.3)	N.S.
MVR + TVP	45	3	9 (26.7)	12	0	0 (0)	$P < 0.05^a$
Triple-VP	15	2	3 (33.3)	7	2	1 (42.9)	N.S.
Total	901	17	59 (8.4)	437	6	12 (4.1)	$P < 0.01^a$

Abbreviations: see Table 1
N.S. = not significant
[a] one-sided test

Table 3. Gross neurological symptoms after heart valve replacement in two groups of patients

Operative procedure	Total number of patients with neurological complications	A. Number of patients with focal symptoms and/or coma	Number unconscious after 1 day	Duration of coma in days, median (upper range)	Side of paresis. Number of right	left	bilat.	B. Patients with post-operative psychosis
Group I: (operated 1969–1975)								
AVR	28	22	18	5 (15)	3	8	5	6
MVR	20	19	16	4 (35 months)	3	8	2	1
AVR + MVR	11	9	9	7 (22)	2	4	0	2
MVR + TVP	12	11	10	10 (21)	2	4	1	1
Triple-VP	5	4	2	17 (28)	0	3	0	1
Group II: (operated 1978–1979)								
AVR	11	6	3	4 (7)	0	1	2	5
MVR	3	2	0	0	0	0	1	1
AVR + MVR	1	1	1	18	0	0	0	0
MVR + TVP	0	0	0	0	0	0	0	0
Triple-VP	3	3	3	3 (10)	0	0	0	0
Total					10	28	11	
Significance			P < 0.01	N.S.	P < 0.01			

Abbreviations: see Table 1
N.S., not significant

large blood transfusions. Technical difficulties were common. Two patients had troublesome bleeding from the aortotomy. In one of two patients who had graft replacement of the ascending aorta the circulation was stopped for 47 min at 20 °C body temperature. This patient was unconscious for 9 days and sustained a left-sided paresis, but was essentially free from symptoms and back at work 1 year later. Two patients had short periods of circulatory arrest postoperatively and in one there was accidental air-embolization from the oxygenator through the arterial line. Eight postoperative deaths had neurological damage. Five patients died of severe malacia of the brain. Four of them had had circulatory arrest in the immediate postoperative period and one had air embolization through the left ventricular vent. Two patients never woke up after surgery and died within 2 weeks in myocardial infarction. One patient regained consciousness 5 days after surgery, but died 1 week later of rupture of the left ventricle at the site where the apical vent had been inserted.

Group II: More than half of the patients in this group had calcified valves and three were reexplored for bleeding. Of the survivors, one patient had slight convulsions during the first postoperative night, but an uneventful recovery. One patient had a slight visual disturbance, probably due to preoperative microembolization. One patient encountered a left-sided paresis at reexploration of a fistula of the sinus of valsalve 14 days after aortic valve replacement because of septic endocarditis.

There were three operative deaths with neurological signs. One was in severe heart failure before operation because of septic endocarditiis and in one there were technical difficulties and the aortic balloon pump was used postoperatively to maintain blood pressure. Both patients died in heart failure within 1 week. A third patient died 2 days after aortic valve replacement from the effect of massive preoperative embolization to the brain and abdominal aorta. Autopsy did not disclose the origin of these emboli.

Neurological Complications After Mitral Valve Replacements

Group I: Half of the patients in this group had calcified valves and two were reexplored for bleeding. It is worthy of note that 9/22 patients had moderate aortic insufficiency at preoperative aortography, not enough to indicate valve replacement, but resulting in large regurgitation of blood to the left atrium at the time of operation with frequent coronary suction of the foaming blood. In addition, the left atrial retractor was prone to give aortic insufficiency even when the aortic cusps were intact.

One surviving patient was still comatose on discharge and was treated in a vegetative stage in hospital for 3 years until death due to pulmonary aspiration. Two operative deaths had convulsions after bypass and were comatose. One died in renal and pancreatic failure after 3 weeks. At postmortem examination there was a thrombotic formation in the left atrium, despite adequate anticoagulation treatment. The second patient had malfunction of the liver and renal failure and died in myocardial infarction.

Group II: Both survivors had calcified valves. One patient had a transient weakness of the left side and one had diplopia due to palsy of the oculomotor nerve.

Neurological Complications After Aortic and Mitral Valve Replacement

Group I: Six of the nine patients had calcified valves. One had a left atrial thrombosis removed at operation and another had massive bleeding from a rupture of the inferior caval vein. One patient had a short postoperative period of circulatory arrest and two were reexplored for bleeding.

One patient had a paraplegia due to spinal cord emboli. One patient never regained consciousness and died in septicemia, renal and heart failure after 3 weeks.

Group II: One patient sustained severe brain damage 4 days after initially uncomplicated double valve replacement, when reoperated on for tamponade caused by left ventricular rupture and died of the cerebral injury 2 weeks later.

Neurological Complications After Mitral Valve Replacement and Tricuspid Valve Procedure

Group I: Calcification of the mitral valve was present in 6/12 patients. Two had moderate aortic insufficiency and one excessive operative bleeding. Reoperation for bleeding was necessary in one patient. Two operative deaths had generalized convulsions after bypass, never regained consciousness, and died within 2 weeks in myocardial failure.

Neurological Complications After Triple-Valve Procedures

Group I: Severely calcified valves were present in 1/4 patients. Three patients had massive preoperative transfusions, postoperative impaired clotting, and reoperations. One of them died in renal failure and sepsis after 2 weeks. The fourth patient had 25 min of cardiopulmonary resuscitation before urgently instituted bypass, but died of severe brain damage after 4 weeks.

Group II: In all three patients the indication for surgery was septic endocarditis. One patient had circulatory arrest postoperatively, but regained consciousness within a week and had no sequelae of a right-sided weakness on discharge 1 month after operation. In another patient, a left atrial thrombosis was removed and reoperation for bleeding was necessary. The postoperative course was complicated with coma and low output syndrome until death after 10 days. A third patient was dying of acute sepsis with valve incompetence and heart failure when admitted. There was a short period of circulatory arrest before surgery and postoperative aortic balloon pumping was necessary, but the patient died on the 10th postoperative day. Autopsy disclosed septic infarctions in the heart muscle and brain.

Follow-up Results of Patients with Coma and/or Focal Neurological Deficits After Surgery (Only Patients from Group I)

Follow-up data are shown in the first two columns of Table 4, separating the fate of patients with short and long periods of postoperative unconsciousness. The majority of the patients with moderate disability had some sequelae after extremity paresis, while severe disability included impaired memory and difficulties in reading and speaking. Two of the six patients with histories of late embolic episodes were in the group of three patients in column 1 with moderate disability. It was not possible to rule out whether their complaints originated from the postoperative complications or the embolic events. Two of 12 late deaths were anticoagulant complications. One had a fatal cerebral hemorrhage caused by an overdosage of dicoumarol and one died of a thrombosed prosthesis. All late deaths were examined postmortem. Two patients had intracavitary thrombi, despite anticogulant treatment. Varying degrees of brain infarction were macroscopically visible in all patients with a longer period of coma, while 4/9 patients with short coma periods showed these changes.

Postoperative Psychosis – Early and Late Findings in Group I Patients

The distribution of the patients is shown in Table 3 and the late results in Table 4, column 3. All patients were awake after 1 day and showed no focal neurological symptoms. During the first postoperative week they had transient hallucination, disorientation, or anxiety. One patient operated on with tricuspid valve procedure died of cerebral injury after circulatory arrest during the 2nd week. Late follow-up revealed that all survivors were free from symptoms.

One of these patients had had a late cerebral emboli. One patient had died in heart failure and at autopsy there was infarction in the brain. One of two patients, who died after myocardial infarctions had intracardiac thrombosis at postmortem examination. One patient died 3 months after surgery in severe cerebral damage after a period of circulatory arrest.

Early Embolism: Postoperative Incidence in Group I and II, Late Follow-up Patients from Group I

There were 15 early embolic episodes in 12 patients before discharge from hospital. Only one patient from Group II had an early embolus (Table 5). The time distribution is shown in Fig. 1. All patients except two receiving aspirin and dipyridamol were on dicoumarol treatment. The prothrombin levels were adequately depressed in 8/10 patients at the time of embolism. Five of these patients did not receive heparin during the postoperative period. Cerebral symptoms were encountered in all patients but two, in whom the emboli were localized to the lower leg. One patient had a fatal emboli

Table 4. Follow-up results in patients with early neurological complications and patients sustaining early embolism after heart valve replacement

	Number of patients with paresis or coma less than 7 days	Number of patients with coma 7 days or longer	Number of patients with postoperative psychosis	Number of patients with early emboli
Free from symptoms	25	0	6	8
Moderate disability	3	1	0	1
Severe disability	1	7	0	1
Late deaths	9	3	4	1
Cause of late death	2 sudden death 2 heart failure 2 myocardial infarction 2 rupture of aortic aneurysm 1 valve thrombosis	1 cerebral hemorrhage 1 aspiration 1 heart failure	2 myocardial infarction 1 heart failure 1 cerebral infarction	1 cerebral emboli

Table 5. Incidence of early embolism after various heart valve replacements in two patient groups

Operative procedure	Group I (operated 1969–1975)		Group II (operated 1978–1979)		Significance
	Number of survivors	Number of patients with early emboli (%)	Number of survivors	Number of patients with early emboli (%)	
AVR	527	6 (1.1)	264	1 (0.4)	N.S.
MVR	219	3 (1.3)	108	0 (0)	N.S.
AVR + MVR	83	2 (2.4)	42	0 (0)	N.S.
MVR + TVP	42	0 (0)	12	0 (0)	N.S.
Triple-VP	13	0 (0)	5	0 (0)	
Total	884	11 (1.2)	431	1 (0.2)	N.S.

Abbreviations: see Table 1
N.S., not significant

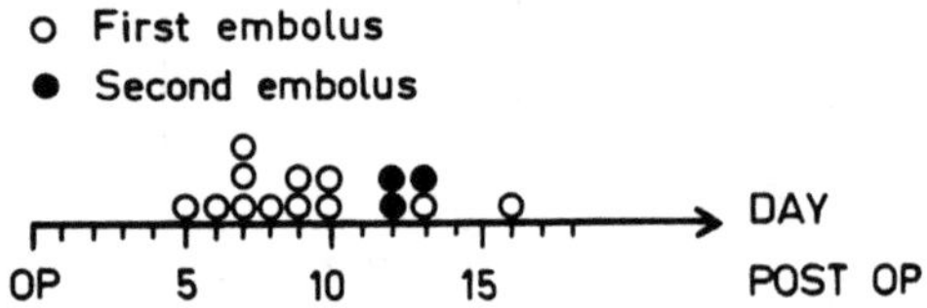

Fig. 1. Time distribution of early emboli after heart valve replacement

and the postmortem examination revealed a thrombosis in the heart and an infarction in the brain.

Until the time of late follow-up, three patients had histories of late emboli occurring after discharge. One of these late emboli were fatal and at necropsy there was a thrombosis at the left atrial suture line. The follow-up results are presented in Table 4, column 4.

Discussion

It is impossible to record in a retrospective study minor neurological dysfunctions [10, 13]. Neurological deficits are easily overlooked when the patient is sedated and treated with a respirator for respiratory insufficiency or myocardial failure. Minor psychological dysfunctions are common after operative interventions, but not acceptable for retrospective studies. They are, however, often better related to environmental factors or psychological variability than to the operative period [15]. We included in the study of postoperative neurological complications patients with transient postoperative neurological complications patients with transient postoperative delirium. These pronounced behavior disturbances probably reflect specific cerebral injury [8, 12]. Patients with such symptoms and gross neurological signs of convulsions, unconsciousness for more than 1 day after surgery, or displaying impaired voluntary movements could be traced from the case reports of our intensive care unit. The true incidence of postoperative neurological deficits was probably underestimated, but as the same study procedure was used for both groups of patients we believe that an unbiased comparison was possible.

Evidently there was no single cause of the cerebral complications. Apparent sources of cerebral emboli were fragments of calcified valves, removed debris from intracavitary thrombosis, or emboli of septic origin. Emboli may enter the circulation *via* the coronary suction or from the extracorporeal equipment *per se* [6, 9]. Neuropathological studies have revealed the presence of fat, fibrin-platelet aggregates and foreign crystalline material in brain after cardiopulmonary bypass procedures [1]. Air trapped in the cardiac chambers and expelled at end of bypass, when the aortic clamp is removed and the left ventricle contracts, is a very major hazard of open-heart procedure. Mastering established techniques to completely evacuate air from the pulmonary veins, left atrium und its appendage, and the trabeculated left ventricle is mandatory.

Table 6. Average age, bypass time, and preoperative blood transfusion in patients with early neurological complications after heart valve replacements

Operative procedure	Group I patients (operated 1969–1975)			
	Number of patients	Mean age (years)	Mean perfusion time (min)	Mean preoperative blood transfusion (ml)
AVR	28	55	127	8800
MVR	20	54	103	5300
AVR + MVR	11	58	161	6900
MVR + TVP	12	50	145	6700
Triple-VP	5	41	192	9300

Abbreviations: see Table 1

Brain ischemia is the second main reason for neurological damage. Advanced age, preoperative hypotension and long perfusion times have been correlated to neurological complications [10]. Pre-existing cerebrovascular disease is assumed to be a contributory factor [8]. In this study the patients concerned were not particularly old. The separate causation of long perfusion times or hypotension could not be validated in these small groups of patients due to concomitant problems, e.g., technical difficulties, bleeding problems or low output postoperatively. Mean age, perfusion time, and amount of preoperative blood transfusion are listed in Table 6. The anterior localization of the innominate artery was probably responsible for the preponderance of left-sided paresis.

Comparison of Groups I and II

The incidence of neurological complications was reduced in Group II patients for all subgroups but the triple-valve procedures. The number of patients undergoing triple valve procedures was small and during recent years patients accepted for this operation were severely deteriorated, namely, all three patients with neurological complications had preoperative histories of sepsis. The overall reduction in complications was achieved by increased experience and vigilance of air-embolization. The relationship of several technical changes to this substantial improvement deserves attention.

Homologous blood in the priming solution can cause serious pulmonary alteration not present when no blood is added [11]. However, the change to total hemodilution was not believed to significantly improve the percentage of neurological complications. The previously used disc oxygenator is frequently reported to generate microaggregates [3]. The microemboli from the bubble oxygenator are of negligible importance and only generated during initial minutes of bypass [14]. The incidence of early embolic episodes was lower in patients receiving the convex-concave modification of the valve, but this difference was not statistically significant.

Undoubtedly, the greatest advance was the introduction of hypothermic cardioplegia. This technique, in addition to providing optimal myocardial protection, facilitated exposure and allowed the surgeon to operate on a motionless, dry and flaccid heart. Operative time and coronary suction were minimized.

Comparison Between Subgroups

In patients undergoing aortic valve replacement many complications were related to preoperative difficulties or postoperative circulatory arrest. The higher incidence of neurological signs in Group I after mitral valve replacement was explained by less than optimal exposure when the aorta was not clamped and the heart was beating. Operation and bypass times were prolonged. The left atrial retractor was prone to make the aortic valve incompetent by deformation of the aortic root and many patients in this group had slight incompetence of the aortic valves as judged by preoperative aortography. The regurgitation of blood further prolonged the operation. The frequent coronary suction increased the trauma to the blood elements and the risk of accumulating, foreign material in the circulation. As the aortic root was not opened, the evacuation of air was not so efficient. Despite suction devices in the aortic root, venting of air can be inefficient [7]. The further increased risk in Group I undergoing combined left and right heart procedures was probably due to inefficient venting of air from the left side before the right heart was opened. Air can lodge in the left ventricle even long after heart action is restored [16]. Hence, extracorporeal circulation must be stopped for several minutes before the aortic vent can be removed, bypass reinstituted, and the right heart opened. A further cause during multiple valve replacements was prolonged perfusion times, as the pump oxygenator traumatizes blood and damages elements of disintegrating platelets, and denatured proteins and fibrin will accumulate. These particles will embolize and result in depressed cerebral function, renal failure, and hypotension [2].

Table 7. Late embolic incidence in patients with early neurological complications and in those subjected to routine follow-up at this clinic after heart valve replacement

Operative procedure	Group I (operated 1969–1975) survivors. Late emboli/ 100 patient years	Patients routinely followed-up. Late emboli/100 patient years	Significance
AVR	3.8	0.7	N.S.
MVR	3.7	4.2	N.S.
AVR + MVR	9.6	2.2	$P < 0.05$
MVR + TVP	3.3	1.5	N.S.
Triple-VP	5.0	0	$P < 0.05$

Abbreviations: see Table 1
N.S., not significant

Follow-up

Apparently there were no sequelae after postoperative delirium and the data indicated favorable prognosis for patients with short durations of unconsciousness or focal neurological deficits.

Seven of 59 survivors with early neurological complications had late embolism. The incidence of late embolism in these patients and in those routinely followed-up at this clinic is shown in Table 7 [4]. Two of the late deaths in patients with early neurological complications were related to unsatisfactory anticoagulant treatment, and in an additional three patients autopsy revealed intracardiac thrombosis. This high thromboembolic incidence may originate from coagulation abnormalities, persisting thrombolic sources for emboli, or the patient's decreased ability to handle prescribed dicoumarol medication.

References

1. Aguilar MJ, Gerbode F, Hill JD (1971) Neuropathologic complications of cardiac surgery. J Thorac Cardiovasc Surg 61:676–685
2. Allardyce DB, Yoshida SH, Ashmore PG (1966) The importance of microembolism in the pathogenesis of organ dysfunction caused by prolonged use of the pump oxygenator. J Thorac Cardiovasc Surg 52:706–715
3. Ashmore PG, Svitek V, Ambrose P (1968) The incidence and effects of particulate aggregation and microembolism in pumpoxygenator systems. J Thorac Cardiovasc Surg 55:691–697
4. Björk VO, Henze A (1979) Ten years experience with the Björk-Shiley tilting disc valve. J Thorac Cardiovasc Surg 78:331–342
5. Branthwhite MA (1975) Prevention of neurological damage during open-heart surgery. Thorax 30:258–261
6. Brennan RW, Patterson RH, Kessler J (1971) Cerebral blood flow and metabolism during cardiopulmonary bypass: Evidence of microembolic encephalopathy. Neurology (Minneap) 21:665–672
7. Brenner WI, Wallsh E, Spencer FC (1971) Aortic vent efficiency. J Thorac Cardiovasc Surg 61:258-264
8. Gilman S (1965) Cerebral disorders after open-heart operations. N Engl J Med 272:489–498
9. Hill JD, Aguilar MJ, Baranco A, Lanerolle P, Gerbode F (1969) Neurological manifestations of cardiac surgery. Ann Thorac Surg 7:409–419
10. Javid H, Tufo HM, Najafi H, Dye WS, Hunter JA, Julian OC (1969) Neurological abnormalities following open-heart surgery. J Thorac Cardiovasc Surg 58:502–509
11. Rabelo RC, Olivera SA, Tanaka H, Weigl DR, Verginelli G, Zerbini EJ (1973) The influence of the nature of the prime on postperfusion pulmonary changes. J Thorac Cardiovasc Surg 66:782–793
12. Sachdev NS, Carter CC, Swank RL, Blachly PH (1967) Relationship between post-cardiotomy delirium, clinical neurological changes, and EEG abnormalities. J Thorac Cardiovasc Surg 54:557–563
13. Silverstein A, Krieger H (1969) Neurologic complication of cardiac surgery. Arch Neurol 5:601–605
14. Solis RT, Noon GP, Beall AC, DeBakey ME (1974) Particulate microembolism during cardiac operation. Ann Thorac Surg 17:332–344
15. Sveinsson IS (1975) Postoperative psychosis after heart surgery. J Thorac Cardiovasc Surg 70:717–726
16. Tsuji HK, Redington IV, Mendez A, Kay JH (1970) The prevention of air embolism during intracardiac surgery. J Thorac Cardiovasc Surg 59:484–488

Visual Disturbances After Open-Heart Surgery

R. Meyendorf

Summary

The visual disturbances of 45 patients after open heart surgery could be divided into disturbances of [1] visual acuity, [2] visual acuracy, and [3] visual realtiy testing. The nonhallucinatory phenomena consisted mainly of loss of color vision, metamorphopsias, visual gnostic disorders, and cortical blindness. The hallucinatory phenomena could be divided into the delirium type of hallucinations with clouding of consciousness and the spectator type of hallucinations with a clear sensorium.

The causes for the visual symptomatology and for cardiac psychoses are seen in microembolization and/or ischemic hypoxia. The basal ganglia and the occipital lobe are areas of predilection for embolic and hypoxic change. Identical psychoses may occur too in cerebral malaria and polycythemia vera, which show the same embolic and anoxic neuropathological changes of vascular occlusion as do many patients who die after open-heart surgery with extra corporal circulation.

Introduction

Cardiac surgery with its use of extracorporal circulation (ECC) and specific problems of vascular surgery still provides an involuntary experimental device for the study of neuropsychiatric phenomena. Various technical improvements, such as the placing of filters in the blood perfusion lines to remove micro debris [1, 27, 50], the reduction in the amount of whole blood transfusion [43], and improvements in operative technique seem to have reduced especially the very obvious complications which were described in the 1950s and early 1960s: *cardiac psychosis* and *cardiac delirium* and the different forms of altered states of consciousness, mainly *stupor* and *coma* [9, 11]. The general incidence of neuropsychiatric disorders from originally 40%–70% to about 20%–50% today is still very high [19, 37].

Besides these syndromes, which are well known due to being obvious, there still exists a neuropsychiatric symptomatology which is revealed only by careful interviewing. One group of symptoms will be discovered only by futher questioning of a minor complaint, which is at first sight not suggestive of a major disorder in patients which appear completely normal. Other patients are reluctant to admit any mental changes due to fear. They are *dissimulating.* Repeated interviews 1–2 weeks after the operation will very often reveal psychotic experiences during the first few days after

Psychopathological and Neurological Dysfunctions
Following Open-Heart Surgery Ed by Becker et al

surgery which the patients would have kept to themselves, had they not been asked again. In 1972 Blacher had already described [8] this type of "hidden psychosis of open-heart surgery". A third group of patients appears to the observer to be alert and not overly disturbed, but in truth is suffering from transient states of *acute mutism* which is related to akinetic mutism, described originally as a pure neurological disorder [15, 16]. Repeated neuropsychiatric assessment 1–2 weeks after surgery will in addition reveal, in certain cases, striking *amnestic syndromes* for psychotic experiences and neuropsychiatric disorders in the first few days after the operation. Some patients can actually remember their experiences of cardiac surgery, including psychotic states, years after the operation. There are others, however, who are later completely amnestic of these episodes or have only indistinct reminiscences. During the first few postoperative days, when they express psychopathological phenomena, the patients appear alert and fully conscious (oriented).

If one keeps in mind the special role of dreaming and allied states of visual experiences in the course of cardiac surgery [31, 41], one is reminded of the mechanism of forgetting or remembering only fragments of dreams, having thus only a vague feeling of what happened. On the other hand, there is the category of vivid impressive dreams which one never forgets throughout life.

Own Investigation. The Material. Incidence of Visual Disturbances After Open-Heart Surgery. The Aim of the Paper

While investigating neuropsychiatric complications after cardiac surgery [37, 39] during two periods – 1972/73 and 1977/78 – I came to realize that besides cardiac psychoses and besides obvious neuro-ophthalmological complications there exists a wide spectrum of hidden neuropsychiatric syndromes which are particularly related to *psychopatho-ophthalmology*.

In the first study of 150 patients, when I was not yet conscious of the problem, there were 15 (10%) which complained spontaneously of some kind of visual disturbances. In the second investigation 120 patients which were questioned systematically – every day postoperatively until the end of the 3rd week – 30 out of 120 (25%) admitted to having or to having had visual symptoms. The total material presented here consists thus of 45 cases, which are listed according to the main or leading symptom, i.e., 1) predominantly disturbances of visual acuity (11 cases); 2) disturbances of visual accuracy (17 cases); 3) disturbances of visual reality testing (17 cases). The aim of this paper is to give a description of the different groups of symptoms and to relate them to other psychopathological phenomena of cardiac surgery and to discuss the main etiological factors: embolization and anoxia.

The Different Groups of Symptoms

Disturbances of Visual Acuity

These disturbances as shown in the following list, were characterized by dimming or blurring of vision, indistinctness of vision and loss of colour vision. The patients complained mostly that they could no longer see as well as before. They asked, for example, whether there was steam or hot air in the intensive care unit because the figures and objects they saw – nurses, doctors, machines – were shadowy or they said that the whole environment was like in a haze. A very common metaphor was seeing "like through a veil" or "through a curtain". It was also said that all things appeared grey and some of the patients actually stated that there was loss of colour vision.

Psychologically the *reactions* of the patients were quite different. A few seemed not to be overtly disturbed at the time of the early period of investigation, 1–5 days after the operation; they would admit later, however, when asked about these symptoms again, that they felt queer and that everything seemed to have been endowed with an intense personal significance and meaning. Others thought from the very beginning, when they complained about their visual symptoms, that things were going wrong with them. Some of them would admit, however, only the visual symptoms at the time of examination and talked freely about their fears only when all was over, 7–14 days after the operation. There were, however, a few patients who were later amnestic for their original symptomatology.

These types of disturbances of visual acuity, including the psychological sequences, had disappeared, generally completely, after 2 weeks.

Disturbances of Visual Accuracy

Under this heading a group of quite different symptoms is listed as follows:

Diplopia
Distortion of objects
- doubling of contours
- edges being displaced or cut off
- surfaces appear bent
- all things appear round
- waviness of linear components

Distortion of faces
- doubling of contours
- parts being displaced or missing
- "monster faces"

Moving phenomena
- horizontal or vertical lines may be seen moving
- objects may be seen rotating
- complex pictures

Micropsia
Macropsia
Upside down vision

Diplopia was a frequent complaint, yet in our investigation only those cases are included which were unrelated to oculomotor palsy or ophthalmoplegia. Very often the patients were not sure whether it was really double vision or whether the second image seemed to grow out of the fixated object.

A next, more complex category of symptoms was apparent **movements of stationary objects**: straight lines, e.g., the frame of a picture, were moving. One patient reported that everything upon which he fixed his eyes, was rotating.

There was **micropsia** and (not as often) **macropsia** and the impression that things were **very far away or very close**. There seemed to be **less of stereoscopic vision.**

Another group of symptoms was **distorsion of objects**: things and persons no longer had their normal size and shape. Typical descriptions were that edges or parts were cut off or displaced, surfaces appeared bent, or everything was round. There was also waviness of linear components.

Distorsion of faces deserves special mention. There was again the complaint of doubling of contours and that parts of a face were missing or also displaced. Heads became very large or extremely small and appeared ugly and sinister such that patients spoke of **monster faces.**

Psychologically these patients reacted similarly to the first group regarding the various phenomena. The images of **metamorphopsias** and **kakopsias** gave rise especially to intense fear which was sometimes expressed and sometimes concealed and only revealed later. There were, however, also some patients who seemed to have a certain insight into the pathological nature of these phenomena as they related them to the adverse effects of the operation, and there were still others for whom they played a role in their paranoid content of thoughts.

Disturbances of Visual Reality Testing

We are faced here with two major groups of symptoms, the agnostic and the hallucinatory type of visual pathology (see following list). Cortical blindness still plays a separate role.

Visual spatial disorientation
– defective localization of objects in space

Visual agnosia
– failure to recognize objects when optic pathways are intact; "mindblindness"

Prosopagnosia
Denial of blindness (Anton's syndrom)

Other "agnostic" syndroms
– denial of operation (anosognosia)
– time agnosia

Enhancement of normal after image
Visual perseveration (paliopsia)
Metamorphopsia

Visual hallucinations
Delirium type (accompanied by mental confusion and disorientation)
– not highly organized: dream-like

Spectator type (accompanied by a clear sensorium)
– highly organized: images of people
complex scenery

Patients of the first group mainly showed **visual spatial disorientation** or **prosopagnosia.** They were noticed to have difficulties in picking up objects from their bed cover or side table as they systematically grasped a few centimeters beside or above the object; or the cup would miss the mouth, though there was no tremor. Four patients showed **prosopagnosia** of a different degree: they were no longer confident about recognized familiar faces or were simply unable to do so; doctors, nurses and even relatives were identified by their voices, though vision was apparently intact, because these patients could see other things.

There were also three cases of **cortical blindness** which presented as **Anton's syndrom**, i.e., denial of blindness. Two were diagnosed at first by the staff as being hysterical.

In this connection the striking phenomena of four cases of **denial of cardiac surgery** as a whole, in patients who did not appear to be grossly mentally disturbed, should be mentioned. These cases of denial of surgery were, however, not associated with visual symptoms.

Psychologically the agnostic group of patients did not give the impression that they were overly disturbed by their symptoms, if they were aware of them at all. There was a strange mental detachment, neglect, or even denial of these defects, which were therefore not always detected by mere questioning for visual disturbances. Only in the context of a very careful clinical examination, which would reveal an organic brain syndrome, were the agnostic patients discovered, by then already 1 week after the operation. Sometimes they went unnoticed by the staff.

Visual hallucinations were the most conspicuous symptoms of the second group of patients. They occurred as hallucinations of the **delirium type** – not highly organized –, accompanied by mental confusion and disorientation, and as hallucinations of the **"spectator type"**, which occurred without clouding of consciousness and without disorientation, which were of a highly organized type, representing complex sceneries: One patient watched a soccer game, another a military parade, and another was amazed to watch a parade of carnival festivities; people with masks and being otherwise disguised in a typical carnival fashion were entering and leaving the recovery room.

Psychologically the delirium type of hallucinations elicited typically fear and anxiety, since they occurred as a rule within a paranoid frame of thinking. The spectator type of hallucinations was never accompanied by delusional ideas and took place in a special affective state of detachment: These patients felt themselves not personally involved, but rather they wondered and marveled and were emotionally detached as they watched the pictures. They insisted, however, that they actually "saw" these phenomena like life scenes and that they were definitely not dreams, imaginations, or illusions. Nevertheless the latter do play an important role in cardiac surgery which will be discussed below.

Discussion

The Nonhallucinatory Phenomena

Cerebral disorders after cardiac surgery are generally divided into neurological and psychiatric syndromes. This is also true for visual symptoms. Hemianoptic defects in the visual fields were described previously in connection with other focal neurological signs – e.g., hemiplegia and facial paralysis – mainly as the result of embolization [48, 56]. Cortical blindness due to anoxia or embolization of the occipital lobe has been reported as well [4]. Visual disturbances after cardiac surgery were, on the other hand, seen in patients who were thought to be suffering from psychogenic or hysterical blindness [18, 20], a diagnosis which was probably false, since two of our own "hysterically blind" patients were actually blind. The "belle indifference" of hysteria proved to be an "Anton's syndrome", i.e., denial of blindness as an expression of anosognosia in organic brain disease.

Patients with visual disturbances have shown, on the other hand, that there indeed exists a great deal of overlapping or interaction of somatogenic and psychogenic causes when it comes to the question of etiology. This is true not only for the visual symptoms but for psychological dysfunctions after cardiac surgery generally. Before psychogenetic factors are considered one has to realize first, however, that open-heart surgery even today implies a global attack on the brain by microembolization and anoxic ischemia [38, 43, 51], which leads to a temporary disintegration of the total cerebral cortex and its motor-sensory systems. The variety of visual symptoms and of neuropsychiatric symptoms as a whole in one and the same patient shows that the total cerebral cortex is involved and not a focal area, e.g., through a single embolus. The breakdowns in the neurophysiological and neuroanatomical systems can be of different severity and types; it is sometimes selective due to phylogenetic and anatomical reasons and to individual predispositions. This is why one can study in cardiac surgery the nature of psychological phenomena and their relationship to organic processes in the brain. The role of organicity is obvious and not questioned in cases where severe focal neurological signs indicate permanent cerebral damage. This is the case when massive air embolism or emboli of larger surgical fragments and longstanding episodes of hypoxia occurred. The majority of neurological symptoms, however, such as extensor responses, disturbances of sensibility and even cases of ophthalmoplegia, aphasia, and other gnostic disorders may be only fleeting and transient. They disappear in the same way as the sometimes very dramatic psychopathological phenomena of hallucinations and delusions disappear.

There are two areas of the brain where specific vulnerability to microemboli and hypoxia can be observed: The area of the basal ganglia [38, 47] and the visual system, especially the occipital lobe [12, 13].

The occipital poles are known to be the cortical area most affected by stagnant hypoxia; they are the terminal areas of vascular supply of the posterior and middle cerebral arteries. Cortical blindness has also been reported after cardiac arrest and myocardial infarction [32, 54]. The failure of recognition of blindness is a common feature of hypoxic cortical blindness, though Anton's syndrome is not specific for cortical blindness. It also occurs with bilateral optic nerve lesions. The only requirement seems to be a general reduction in cerebral function during any kind of blindness [57]. This general reduction of cerebral functioning is probably the main reason for other forms of anosognosia; in our investigation also for the remarkable gnostic defect in four patients who would not or could not accept that the heart operation had already taken place. The agnostic phenomena are particularly striking in the absence of other severe neurological disturbances.

The localization of prosopagnosia is uncertain; it has been recently described in two cases after recovery from cortical blindness – together with disturbances of colour recognition – again incriminating the occipital lobe [7]. But there are cases known with involvement of the corpus callosum [25] and with lesions of the peripheral end organ in connection with confusional states [6]. Since visual hallucinations may also arise at different levels of optical structure [57, 58] we may assume that most visual phenomena may have the nidus of their origin in any part of the visual system, but that modifications – e.g., micropsia and macropsia depend on lesions of associative systems.

Prosopagnosia, which may be conceived as a negative hallucination, is one of the most striking agnostic symptoms and demonstrates well the dissociation of seeing and perceiving, i.e., it illustrates the gnostic aspect of vision.

The relationship of gnostic to visual functions could be seen also in one case of "Gestalt-dissolution". One patient was not sure whether he suffered primarily from a defect of vision or "concentration", as he described the experience of seeing doctors and nurses dissolved into amorphous parts and disappearing as "points" after they were first recognized and completely for a few seconds when they entered the room. Gestalt dissolution can thus be conceived as an extreme lack of visual synthesis demonstrating the integrative function of gnostic faculties of the cerebral cortex. For perceiving our world the optic apparatus is onto- and phylogenetically the oldest. This may explain why optical phenomena play such a central role in the individual regarding orientation in space and time. In man, however, this function of orientation seems always to be dependent on other gnostic functions. Visual spatial disorientation, which is supposed to be related to the parietal lobe [57], appeared to be basically a visual symptom. Since amnestic and gnostic symptoms also played an important role, it was clinically sometimes impossible to decide whether the defective localization of objects in space was due primarily to a defect in vision, in spatial orientation, or the result of an impaired topographic memory, and which role the general change in personality played.

These observations support the hypothesis of Hécaen of two different systems of visual processing, both in anatomy and function, the cortical and mesencephalic systems [30]. The phylogenetic older and common tectal visual center comprises memory, attention, perception, i.e., the visual functions of lower animals which include detection of simple patterns, colours, and of speed. During the process of telencephalization higher, "gnostic" functions take part in visual identification, making seeing more and more an act of perceiving and finally reflective perception. In higher animals and in man, however, normal vision involves an interaction of the two visual systems and both participate in different psychological categories of vision.

It was said before that, besides the occipital pole, the basal ganglia are especially vulnerable to embolic and anoxic complications which occur during cardiac surgery. This explains the evidence of brain stem contribution to visual disturbances of such a variety as could be observed by careful examination of the experiences of the patients in our study. Visual shape identification is supposed to occur over striate and prestriate zones, corresponding to a deficit in "apperceptive agnosia", while there is evidence that the occipital lobes are also necessary for visual imagery and dreams [30]. The principle of localization and association in the C.N.S. seems, however, to be the presupposition for optical cognition. One patient who ascertained that he definitely could see and knew what objects were for, would recognize and identify a cup, a pencil, or a key only as he touched and handled them. By way of tactile identification he seemed to overcome a defect for contour and shape perception. This patient also displayed prosopagnosia and a rather circumscribed defect of time agnosia without other severe memory defects. Besides recognizing persons by their voices he would identify them by other characteristic nonfacial features by way of "scanning" the whole person with his eyes from the feet upwards until he would see a familiar object, e.g., the belt of his son. Trying to look around a person by moving his head or asking him to turn, was another way of identifying the "Gestalt" piece by piece before he grasped it as a whole. This patient underwent an episode of severe hypotension during the course of E.C.C. and later showed scintigraphic evidence of occipital lobe infarction as well as clinical signs of basal ganglia involvement – a moderate akinetic Parkinson syndrome.

Hypoxia and microemboli also explain the variety of the other visual symptoms. Transient diplopia, unrelated to oculomotor palsy, has been observed in intermittent insufficiency of the basilar artery [57] and binocular blurring of vision may be due to embolization of the calcarine cortex by fibrin platelet fragments originating from an atherosclerotic plaque – or in our cases from microemboli generated through the ECC – and propelled into the calcarine branch of the posterial cerebral artery [57]. This explains why funduscopic examination in these patients of blurring of vision was normal. These were not cases with pupiledema. Only when larger emboli or longer episodes of hypoxia occur in the area striata, homonymous visual field defects will be the result. There were three such cases in our material. Not counted among our material of psychopatho-ophthalmology were patients who had mere ophthalmoplegia. One has to realize, however, that ophthalmoplegia may also be a manifestation of vertebral – basilar arterial disease and that it is especially a sign of arterial insufficiency or occlusive vascular disease. The same is true for diplopia.

The Hallucinatory Phenomena

Visual hallucinations can be conceived in the context of our discussion as the extreme opposite of Gestalt dissolution and related phenomena. In both cases gnostic functions are involved. On the one hand, stability of the external world cannot be maintained anymore because of a lack in visual synthesis so that reality becomes nonexistent – and, on the other hand, visual phenomena on the highest level of optical organization appear in the external world as projections of reality. In both cases we meet certain kinds of transitions within one category of phenomena and from one category into the other. In some instances it was, e.g., quite impossible to differentiate between metamorphopsia and hallucinations. Transitions within hallucinatory phenomena developed from elementary, unformed hallucinations as lines, spots, and geometrical figures to those of pictorial nature and sceneries.

Though visual hallucinations may arise as a result of a disorder at any level of the visual pathway, from the peripheral end organ to the area striata, it has long been recognized clinically that structures of the brain stem, especially of the diencephalon, are of utmost importance in the etiology of visual hallucinations [46], thus supporting the evidence of brain stem contribution to visual perception in man [55]. Visual hallucinations, as well as metamorphopsias, may also occur in circumscribed lesions of the visual cortex [30], again supporting in our cases the observation that in cardiac surgery brain stem and visual cortex are areas of special predelection of embolization and hypoxia. It should be mentioned, however, that highly organized visual hallucinations usually also indicate involvement of the temporal lobe [57]. Visual hallucinations may recur during sleep – as in cataract operation – and they have been compared to visual phenomena characterizing nightmares [53]. The hallucinatory nature of dreams and their relationship to delusional ideas are a central theme of psychopathology in cardiac psychosis. After cardiac surgery one can indeed find all kinds and grades of transition from dreaming towards experiencing the dreams as hallucinations. Characteristic of these patients was that they could slip in and out of the hallucinatory state with intervals of insight and lucidity – hence H. Jackson's term "mental diplopia" would be appropriate. The accounts of their experiences varied, but can be summarized as follows: While most of the patients had dreams after cardiac surgery, which could be corrected at the moment of waking up, or within a few seconds afterwards (the usual process), some stated that the dreams experienced during sleeping would go on (as hallucinations!) as they woke up, and that they therefore could no longer distinguish between sleeping and being awake. Insight into the nonveridical nature of their dreams was no longer possible, because there was no point of reference around which critical judgment toward "inside" and "outside" a special state of consciousness could take place. Some patients complained of repetitive vivid dreams or hallucinations as soon as they closed their eyes and would try to stay awake by all means for fear that the "film" would go on if they did not "control their mind". Others insisted that they dreamed with open eyes or "saw things", in the sense of hallucinations, only with their eyes opened, and which disappeared as soon as they closed their eyes. They therefore lay in bed pretending to sleep in order not to watch these pictures. We can see that two totally different states of consciousness must have an influence on dreams and visual hallucinations.

We mentioned before that one could distinguish basically between the "delirium type" and "spectator type" of hallucinations and that a clouded or clear sensorium was the main point of differentiation. The spectator type of hallucinations were not pseudohallucinations in the sense that they lacked corporeality or substantiality, but they were accompanied by insight into their lack of an objective counterpart. Therefore, there was generally no affect due to anxiety and fear connected with these hallucinations.

The insight into the deceptive nature of the hallucinations was, however, not always total, but sometimes partial and very fluctuating. One could indeed observe all kinds of degrees of insight at different times in one and the same person. One criterion of insight seemed to be the question of personal involvement in or detachment from the hallucinatory episodes. This seemed to depend on the affective state and on the degree of impairment of gnostic functions. Some patients would discuss their visual experiences quite frankly, and they reminded one of those which cortical blindness with Anton's syndrome, with a rather euphoric affect which expressed amazement and amusement about the phenomena; others felt rather embarrassed and strange about revealing their symptoms, because they knew that something had happened to them since the operation. The nature of the spectator-type of hallucinations was never frightening – quite unlike those of the delirium type – and the patients insisted that they were true hallucinations, i.e., pictures and complex sceneries, which were not to be confused with dreams and that they occurred only when they were awake.

The delirium types of hallucinations in cardiac surgery are – as with delirium generally – of a frightening and threatening character. They show all shades and grades of transition to similar experiences in dreams. Horror dreams of persecution and of bodily mutilation are typical. A very common motive is the experience of being dissected alive. One patient reported that he saw his head way up the ceiling (a form of autoscopy) as he woke up after the operation. He closed his eyes, yet continued to see his head dangling, and in falling asleep he dreamed of his head which he finally kept on seeing as he woke up again. The delirium type of hallucinations in cardiac surgery illustrates that it is sometimes impossible to decide whether the pathogenesis of a hallucinatory symptom is primarily determined by a disturbance of conciousness, perception, or affect. As anyone may predominate and influence the function of gnostic differentiation, the phenomena themselves seem to change in character. Dreams, illusions, and hallucinations cannot be differentiated any longer.

The intense experience of after images in the intensive care unit (I.C.U.) can be understood to be a type of hallucination in some nondelirious patients. Patients reported that a doctor or a nurse would stay on for a considerable time (since the feeling of time is changed one can also often not rely on guesses "up to minutes") as an after image when they had left the room. Here again one could conceive such an after image as an opposite phenomenon to Gestalt dissolution. On the other hand, one can describe these after images as visual perseverations – in analogy to verbal perseverations which could be observed too in some patients –, or should they be called negative illusions? Metamorphopsias may also be called visual illusions if they mean true perceptual modifications concerning form, contour, size, and movement of objects or people, or also modifications of colour [30] phenomena which all occurred in the I.C.U. On the other hand, not truely perceptual disorders are illusions which are dependent on a particular affective state of mind, mainly fear and anxiety. Affective disturbances influence visual experiences. The visual hallucinations and related phenomena illustrate well the point of contention in psychopathology, whether delusions, which play an equal role in cardiac surgery as perceptual disorders, are primarily a disorder of thought or affect. Cardiac surgery also provides an example of how a changed consciousness of existentiality may depend on a changed consciousness in the sense of an altered sensorium.

The Evidence of the Literature

As already mentioned visual disturbances after cardiac surgery have been reported before primarily as neuro-ophthalmological complications. Whereas the hallucinatory type of visual symptoms is widely known as a main feature of cardiac delirium, the nonhallucinatory, agnostic symptomatology has not been described extensively; it has been hardly recognized as a category of its own. Gilman [24] though, noticed that "gnostic disorders" were the most frequent single clinical type of cerebral complications which varied in degree from "a mild disturbance in the recognition and reproduction of visual patterns to a severe agnosia that is chiefly visual". Freyhan et al. [22] stressed the fact that there exists a high correlation between psychiatric complications and evidence of neurological impairment report, and that besides "changes in visual capacity" one finds "transient aphasias, alexias, agraphias and difficulties with comprehension of spatial relationships".

It was said before that distorsion of faces, which were described under the category of gnostic disturbances as metamorphopsias, led the patients to speak sometimes of monsters which played a role in their paranoid content of thought. On the other hand sometimes one could not differentiate between hallucinations and metamorphopsias. Blacher [8] describes the ambivalent or fluctuating insight into a psychotic thought process of a 43-year-old man with an aortic valve replacement, who knew that the staff were trying to kill him and at the same time knew that this could not be true. "With the same reluctance he described a hallucination of monsters coming through a window. 'It was as if they were coming out of a television screen to hurt me and I was scared'." Transitions and fluctuations of all kinds and grades of psychopathological phenomena and of insight in patients were said to be characteristic of cardiac surgery. A nurse who described her own experience after an A.S.D. repair, when she had, besides other symptoms, visual hallucinations of a bear, stated later: "One part of my mind knew that the symptoms which distressed me were not real, though the periods of awful nameless fear which I suffered were quite beyond my control . . . one part of my mind knew that the bear and the rods were not actually there – but I could see them" [34].

The feeling of depersonalization and derealization which went parallel with "hysterical visual" disturbances was described by Fox et al. [21]. A patient "could not make head or tail of anything . . . everything was like sitting back and watching things on a screen . . . the nurses' movements were mechanical . . . it's almost as though I was dead and watching them". A hypochondrical delusion of actually having died after the operation is reported by Galdstone [23], which reminds one of the "delusion" of four of our patients who were convinced that the operation had not been performed at all. Kovaliov (cited by 3) again pictures a patient who heard human voices and at the same time was "declaring that she had already died . . . that the cells of her body were crying out . . . that her head was being squeezed . . . and another patient "thought that her head was not her own and that her eyes were looking inward". We are reminded of one of our patients who could see his head dangling from the ceiling. Egerton and Kay [20] noticed that visual hallucinations were originating, as many patients remarked, out of the monotony of the ceiling, in manifesting themselves initially by the appearance of patterns on the ceiling or of faces protruding from the small regular holes in the tiling. In the investigation of Heller et al. [31] patients with a "minor delir" had difficulties distinguishing between dreams and reality and those with a "major delir" showed frank hallucinatory episodes with paranoid elaborations. In the interpretation of these phenomena some dismissed them as temporary aberrations attributable to narcotics, poor sleep, or the stress of the operation, while others thought they were "going crazy" or were victims of a paranoid plot, and some actually stated that they were suffering from a "recovery room delirium". This raises the question of which other etiological factors should be discussed in the pathogenesis of cardiac delirium and other psychic phenomena after open-heart surgery.

Causes

The growing literature on the subject of psychological disturbances after cardiac surgery today focuses on preoperative predictions of postoperative complications on the basis of somatic and personality factors, social environment, and on man's relationship to a mechanical and frightening environment in the recovery room or I.C.U. Only the last aspect can be discussed briefly at this point since it relates particularly to the main topic of this paper – the perceptual disorders.

There is no doubt that prolonged sleep deprivation alone, which plays an important role in the I.C.U., may cause severe mental disturbances with pathological changes in perception, and affect cognitive functions which may lead to impairment of reality testing in any or all of these psychic realms and ultimately also toward psychosis. Abnormal sensory input by acoustic and optic overstimulation and sensory deprivation of normal human contact, – i.e., emotional and effective deprivation of human "touch" are other important psychophysiological and psychogenic factors. On the other hand, one has to keep in mind that the majority of patients show no abnormal psychological reactions in the I.C.U. after cardiac surgery; some even feel relieved to be in a "safe" environment! The fact that the I.C.U. plays a role in minor and major psychopathological syndromes depends more on the various degrees of critical psychophysiological conditions as a result of the operation, especially on cerebral dysfunction, than on the technical environment as such. If the C.N.S. is damaged, man is no longer able to cope with the disturbing elements of the I.C.U.

Cardiac delirium and cardiogenic psychoses were known long before cardiac surgery began, when rheumatic heart disease, endocarditis, and acute and chronic heart failure could not be treated as effectively as in our days. The exact study of an extensive literature shows that there is no difference between the psychopathological syndromes of cardiac psychoses in the course of cardiac surgery and those arising independently of cardiac surgery, including the visual disturbances and characteristic perceptual disorders [26, 29, 36, 40]. There are two other systemic diseases which stimulate the pathophysiological conditions of open heart surgery and produce identical neuropsychiatric syndromes: Polycythemia and malaria. Psychoses and visual disturbances may accompany both [5, 14, 28, 42, 49]. The lesions of the brain in polycythemia vera, in cerebral malaria, and in many patients dying after open-heart surgery, especially with E.C.C., are the same. There is evidence of embolic and anoxic changes.

Vascular occlusion and slowing down of the circulation play a role in polycythemia and cerebral malaria. Histopathological changes are those of anoxemia secondary to occlusion of small vessels [5]. The increased viscosity of the red cells in polycythemia and malaria may not always arrest the circulation but may cause a transitory state of ischemia [5]. Similar conditions may prevail in open-heart surgery. In a retrospective investigation of 1360 nonselected patients [44] we found that there exists a significant correlation between use and duration of E.C.C. ($\chi^2 > P = 0.01$) and neuropsychiatric complications, and also between certain priming of the machine, i.e., undiluted blood preserve or whole blood given during E.C.C. ($\chi^2 > P = 0.05$) and the amount of blood transfusion after the operation ($\chi^2 > P = 0.01$).

Other significant ($\chi^2 > P = 0.01$) correlations were

1. *Preoperatively:* (a) A neuropsychiatric history. Forty-two (28.4%) of 148 patients with a previous neuropsychiatric history had cerebral disorders following cardiac surgery compared with 220 (18.2%) of 1212 without such a history, (b) advanced age over 40 and extreme youth under 3 years, (c) low body weight, below 10 kg in children and below 60 kg in adults, (d) acquired heart disease against congenital heart disease, (e) multivalvular lesions, (f) calcified lesions, and (g) increase of NYHA functional class (the last only $\chi^2 > P = 0.05$).
2. *Intraoperatively:* Besides (a) use and (b) duration of E.C.C., (c) duration of operation, and (d) duration of hypothermia beyond 10 min (patients operated without hypothermia exhibited cerebral disorders more often than those operated in hypothermia of less than 10 min. Finally (e) rethoracothomies and (f) repeated defibrillation (the last only $\chi^2 > P = 0.05$).
3. *Postoperatively:* Besides (a) extensive blood transfusion high levels of (b) urea, (c) potassium, and (d) sodium (the last $\chi^2 > P = 0.05$).

The involvement of the basal ganglia in perceptual disorders has been discussed already. There is evidence, however, that the brain stem structures play a major role as well in catatonic and paranoid syndromes. In the early days of cardiac surgery patients were described in the immidiate postoperative period as being quite motionless and without facial expression, showing mask-like, frozen faces, resembling persons with a "catastrophic reaction" [2, 35, 41]. On the other hand, one noticed that the open delusional psychotic syndromes developed later, between the 3rd and 5th postoperative day. In our own investigation we could in fact identify the patients of the early postoperative period as those with a mutistic – catatonic syndrome with a parkinsonian-like facial expression [38]. Many of them had visual disturbances at the same time, as they would reveal later. There is clinical evidence that the states of mute alert-appearing immobility as described in akinetic mutism cannot really be distinguished from psychotic mutism in catatonic schizophrenia and in exogenic akinetic syndromes. Embolization and hypoxic changes of the basal ganglia and temporary disconnection of their neuroanatomical motor systems seem to provide a pathophysiological explanation for these reversible psychomotoric disturbances after cardiac surgery [38]. Paranoid delusions which appear between the 3rd and 5th postoperative day play a role during this period of mutism. These patients behave like catatonic schizophrenics who describe at a later stage of their disease that they were unable to talk and move and could not reveal the delusional content of their thoughts at the time of acute illness with mutism and akinesia. Reversible microembolization and/or transient hypoxic changes in the area of the basal ganglia seem to explain the phenomena of transient mutistic-akinetic syndromes. There is microanatomical evidence that occlusion of capillaries by microemboli of thrombocytes, leucocytes and of silicon, as they occur in E.C.C., may be reversible [44]. This may also explain the different and transient psychopathological syndromes in cerebral malaria, which are identical with those after open-heart surgery, and which were summarized by Arieti as (1) acute deliriums or confusional psychoses, (2) paranoid syndromes or delusional psychoses, (3) typical psychoses such as schizophrenia and manic-depressive psychoses, and (4) organic conditions.

Summary and Conclusions

Fortyfive patients with visual disturbances after open-heart surgery were investigated by analysing their visual experiences. They could be divided into disturbances of (1) visual acuity, (2) visual acuracy, and (3) visual reality testing. Clinically one can distinguish between the nonhallucinatory and hallucinatory phenomena. The most important of the first group were metamorphopsias, loss of colour vision, various gnostic disorders and cortical blindness. The hallucinatory phenomena can be divided into the delirium type of hallucinations, with clouding of consciousness and the spectator type of hallucinations with a clear sensorium. The psychopathology of these disturbances is discussed in relation to cardiac delirium and psychosis.

The main causes for the visual symptomatology and for cardiac psychoses are seen in microembolization and/or ischemic hypoxia. The basal ganglia and the occipital lobe are discussed as areas of predilection for embolic and hypoxic changes in relation to perceptual disorders and psychosis. The same neuro-psychiatric disorders which occur after open-heart surgery could be observed in "cardiogenic psychoses" aside from cardiac surgery when rheumatic heart diseases, endocarditis, and heart failure could not be treated effectively. Identical psychoses may occur too in cerebral malaria and polycythemia vera, which show the same embolic and anoxic neuropathological changes of vascular occlusion as do many patients who die after open-heart surgery with E.C.C.

References

1. Åberg T, Kihlgren M (1977) Cerebral protection during open-heart-surgery. Thorax 32:525–533
2. Abram HS (1965) Adaption to open heart surgery: a psychiatric study of response to the threat of death. Am J Psychiatry 122:659–668
3. Abram HS (1970) The prosthetic man. Compr Psychiatry 11:475–481
4. Alfano JE, Fabritius RE, Garland MA (1957) Visual loss following mitral commissurotomy for mitral stenosis. Am J Ophthalmol 44:213–216
5. Arieti S (1946) Histopathologic changes in cerebral malaria and their relation to psychotic sequels. Arch Neurol Psychiatry 56:79–104
6. Bay E (1950) Agnosie und Funktionswandel. Springer, Berlin Göttingen Heidelberg
7. Beck U, Aschayeri H, Keller H (1978) Prosopagnosie und Farberkennungsstörung bei Rückbildung von Rindenblindheit. Arch Psychiatr Nervenkr 225:55–66

8. Blacher RS (1972) The hidden psychosis of open-heart surgery. JAMA 222:305–308
9. Blachly PH, Starr A (1964) Post-cardiotomy delirium. Am J Psychiatry 121:371–375
10. Blakemore C (1979) Representation of reality in the perceptual world. Ciba Found Symp 69
11. Bliss EL, Rumel WR, Branch CHH (1955) Psychiatric complications of mitral surgery. Arch Neurol Psychiatry 74:249–252
12. Brierley JP (1963) Neuropathological findings in patients dying after open-heart surgery. Thorax 18:291–304
13. Brierley JB (1967) Brain damage complicating open-heart surgery. Proc Soc Med 60:858–860
14. Büssow H (1944) Über Psychose bei Malaria. Allg Z Psychiatr 123:235–272
15. Cairns H (1952) Disturbances of consciousness with lesions of the brain stem and diencephalon. Brain 75:109–146
16. Cairns H, Oldfield RC, Pennymacker JB, Whitteridge D (1941) Akinetic mutism with an epidermoid cyst of the 3rd ventricle. Brain 64:273–290
17. Cullen DJ, Ferrara LC (1975) Fine-screen filtration of pressurized whole blood, packed cells, and fresh-frozen erythrocytes. Anesthesiology 43:578–581
18. Danilowicz DA, Gabriel HP (1971) Postoperative reactions in children: "normal" and abnormal responses after cardiac surgery. Am J Psychiatry 128:185–188
19. Dubin WR, Field HL, Gastfriend DR (1979) Postcardiotomy delirium: A critical review. J Thorac Cardiovasc Surg 77:586–594
20. Egerton N, Kay JH (1964) Psychological disturbances associated with open heart surgery. Br J Psychiatry 110:433–439
21. Fox HM, Rizzo ND, Gifford S (1954) Psychological observations of patients undergoing mitral surgery. Psychosomat Med 16:186–208
22. Freyhan FA, Giannelli S Jr, O'Connell RA, Mayo JA (1971) Psychiatric complications following open heart surgery. Compr Psychiatry 12:181–195
23. Galdston R (1970) Psychotic reactions to the success of cardiac valvotomy: a case report. Psychiatrr Med 1:367–373
24. Gilman S (1965) Cerebral disorders after open-heart operations. N Engl J Med 272:489–498
25. Gloning J, Gloning K, Jellinger K, Quatember R (1970) A case of "prosopagnosia" with necropsy findings. Neuropsychologia 8:199–204
26. Gordon AH, Cohen W (1938) The mental complications of heart disease. Can Med Assoc J 39:517–522
27. Guidoin R, Laperche Y, Martin L, Awad J (1976) Disposable filters for microaggregate removal from extracorporeal circulation. J Thorac Cardiovasc Surg 71:502–516
28. Haber J (1952) Psychosis in Polycythemia vera. J Nerv Ment Dis 115:537–540
29. Head H, (1901) Certain mental changes that accompany visceral disease. Brain 24:345–429
30. Hécaen H, Albert ML (1978) Human neuropsychology. John Wiley & Sons, New York Chichester Brisbane Toronto
31. Heller SS, Frank KA, Malm JR, Bowman FO Jr, Harris PD, Charlton MH, Kornfeld DS (1970) Psychiatric complications of open-heart surgery. N Engl J Med 283:1015–1020
32. Howkins J, McLaughlin CR, Daniel P (1946) Neuronal damage from temporary cardiac arrest. Lancet 250:488–492
33. Hutchinson EC, Stock JPP (1963) Paroxysmal cerebral ischaemia in rheumatic heart disease. Lancet 2:653–656
34. John CA (1964) Hallucinations after cardiac surgery. Nurs Times 60:1347
35. Kimball CP (1972) The experience of open heart surgery. Arch Gen Psychiatry 27:57–63
36. Krinsky CM, Merrit HH (1938) Neurologic manifestations of subacute bacterial endocarditis. N Engl J Med 218:263–266
37. Meyendorf R (1976) Psychische und neurologische Störungen bei Herzoperationen. Fortschr Med 94:315–320
38. Meyendorf R (1976) Hirnembolie und Psychose. J Neurol 213:163–177
39. Meyendorf R (1977) Zur Frage psychischer und neurologischer Störungen bei Herzoperationen. Thoraxchirurgie 25:339–344
40. Meyendorf R (1979) Psychopathology in heart disease aside from cardiac surgery: A historical perspective of cardiac psychosis. Compr Psychiatry 20:326–331
41. Meyer BC, Blacher RS, Brown F (1961) A clinical study of psychiatric and psychological aspects of mitral surgery. Psychosom Med 23:194–218
42. Müller E (1910) Über psychische Störungen bei Polycythämie. Folia Heamatol (Leipz) 9: 233–241
43. Paech R (1979) Cerebrale Störungen als Komplikation von Herzoperationen. Medical dissertation, University of Munich

44. Patterson RH Jr, Twichell JB (1971) Disposable filter for microemboli. JAMA 215:76–80
45. Penry JK, Cordell AR, Johnston FR, Netsky MG (1959) Experimental cerebral embolism with antifoam. J Thorac Cardiovasc Surg 37:342–351
46. Reimer F (1970) Das Syndrom der optischen Halluzinose-Sammlung psychiatrischer und neurologischer Einzeldarstellungen –. Thieme, Stuttgart
47. Schwartz P (1972) Apoplectic lesions of the brain in adults. In: Vinken PJ, Bruyn GW (eds) Handbook of clinical neurology, vol 11. North-Holland American Elsevier, Amsterdam New York
48. Silverstein A, Krieger HP (1960) Neurologic complications of cardiac surgery. Trans Am Neurol Assoc 85:151–154
49. Silverstein A, Gilbert H, Wassermann LR (1962) Neurologic complications of polycythemia. Ann Intern Med 57:909–916
50. Skagseth E, Frøysaker T, Refsum SB (1974) Disposable filter for microemboli in cardiopulmonary bypass. J Cardiovasc Surg 15:318–322
51. Stockard JJ, Blickford RG, Schauble JF (1973) Pressure dependent cerebral ischemia during cardiopulmonary bypass. Neurology (Minneap) 23:521–529
52. Swash M (1970) Transient visual obscurations in chronic rheumatic heart-disease. Lancet 2:323–326
53. Taylor F, Kräupl (1979) Psychopathology. Its causes and symptoms. Quartermaine, Sunbury-on-Thames
54. Towbin A (1955) Recurrent cerebral embolism. Arch Neurol Psychiatry 73:173–192
55. Trevarthen C (1979) The fasks of consciousness: how could the brain do them? Ciba Found Symp 69
56. Tufo HM, Ostfeld AM, Shekelle R (1970) Cerebral nervous system dysfunction following open-heart surgery. JAMA 212:1333–1340
57. Walsh FB, Hoyt WF (ed) (1969) Clinical neuro-ophthalmology, 3rd ed. Williams & Wilkins, Baltimore
58. White NJ (1980) Complex visual hallucinations in partial blindness due to eye disease. Br J Psychiatry 136:284–286

Psychotic Reactions in Patients After Open-Heart Surgery

H.H. Scheld, S. Davies-Osterkamp, K. Möhlen, U. Kalbhenn, M. Kramer,
F.W. Hehrlein

Summary

1. Psychiatric disturbances after open-heart surgery can be classified in two subgroups: first, in one group of patients with predominately delirious symptoms and second, in one group of patients which is determined by anxious paranoid symptoms.
2. The development of postoperative anxious paranoid states is predicted by preoperative psychical and social aspects and cannot be explained by physical factors as shown in this study.
3. Postoperative delirious states were found in patients with pathological EEG alterations.

Introduction

Psychosis and a delirious state develop postoperatively in patients more often after open-heart surgery than in general surgery [5, 12, 14]. The frequency of psychiatric disturbances, as reported in the literature [2, 3, 9, 11] ranges from 10% to 50% (Table 1). Its appearance is of significant risk for the further postoperative period (Polonius et al., this volume).

The problem of postoperative psychiatric reaction cannot only be interpreted in terms of induced morphological and metabolic disturbances. The majority of psychical alterations on the one hand can be detected as predisposition in a patient's history and

Table 1. Psychiatric disturbances following open-heart surgery

Year	Authors	Psychiatric disturbances
1964	Egerton and Kay [2]	41%
1966	Weiss [16]	46%
1967	Gilberstadt and Sako [4]	13%
1969	Kimball [9]	24%
1971	Freyhan et al. [3]	51%
1977	Mervin and Abram [11]	33%
1978	Davies-Osterkamp et al. (this volume)	23%

Psychopathological and Neurological Dysfunctions
Following Open-Heart Surgery Ed by Becker et al

on the other hand it can have a certain meaning for the longer postoperative period [14].

Since it is unknown whether psychological factors determined by physical or preoperative conditions are important for the development of postoperative disturbances, we studied a group of patients with heart diseases during diagnostic procedure, therapy, and rehabilitation.

With respect to this problem investigations were performed by psychologists, psychotherapists, and cardiac surgeons cooperatively. The following questions were studied:

1. Do preoperative psychological and psychosocial aspects influence the direct postoperative reactions?
2. Do physical conditions and surgical procedure determine postoperative psychiatric disturbances?
3. Do immediate postoperative reactions influence further rehabilitations?

Referring to question 1 a study has been reported recently by our group (Davies-Osterkamp et al., this volume). In this presentation we would like to discuss results from investigations which were performed in order to study influences of physical conditions, as well as surgical procedure, on immediate postoperative reactions.

Subjects

This study includes 73 patients who underwent open-heart surgery. Preoperative examination and treatment has been conducted in the same cardiological centre. Age and sex, as well as the type of performed surgical procedure, are shown in Table 2.

Table 2. Surgical management

Surgical treatment	n	Age (x)	Female	Male
1. AVR	24	50	6	18
2. MVR	11	57	6	5
3. ACVB	17	48	–	17
4. AVR + MVR	4	53	2	2
5. ACVP + aneurysmectomy	3	57	1	2
6. ACVB + AVR	2	59	–	2
7. Closure of ASD	4	48	4	–
8. Closure of paravalvular leak	1	51	–	1
9. Removal of left atrial myxoma	1	57	1	–
10. Resection of left ventricular echinococcus cyst	1	34	1	–
11. Pericardiectomy	2	43	1	1
12. Closure of patient ductus arteriosus	1	40	1	–
13. Repair of coarctation of the thoracic aorta	1	23	1	–
14. Closed MV commisurotomy	1	35	1	–
Total sample	73	48	25	48

Postoperative Psychological Reactions

Conspicuous postoperative psychiatric dysfunction was observed in 17 (23%) of the 73 patients after cardiac surgery. Psychiatric disturbances included acute psychotic reactions, paranoid ideations, and delirious states. The 17 patients could definitively be divided into two subgroups (Davies-Osterkamp et al., this volume) (Table 3):

Table 3. Psychic reactions following open-heart surgery

Postoperative reactions	n
A. Severe psychic disturbances:	17
a. delirious state	9
b. anxiety and paranoid state	8
B. Other typical postoperative reactions:	56
a. depressive-distressed	12
b. aggressive-hostile	12
c. inconspicuous	12
d. combinations	22
Total sample	73

Subgroup I: Patients with symptoms of severe anxiety, augmented suspicion, and paranoid ideation. This type of reaction occurred on the 2nd and 3rd postoperative day and lasted for 1–3 days.

Subgroup II: Patients with severe delirious symptoms such as disorientation, memory disturbances, and thinking and consciousness disorders including anxiety and restlessness. These disturbances occurred immediately after operation with a duration of 4 days or longer.

Preoperative Physical Conditions

A significant correlation between the type of heart disease and the development of postoperative psychiatric disturbances could not be established. A higher incidence of postoperative abnormal reactions was observed, however, when a more severe stage of heart disease was established preoperatively. 56% of patients with symptoms of a delirious state and 43% of those belonging to the anxious paranoid subgroup compared to 23% of the remaining patients, were in stage IV according to NYHA classification. This statement is supported by the fact that in patients with delirious symptoms after aortic valve replacement cardiac index is significantly lower than in the paranoid anxious subgroup ($P < 0.01$), or in patients without postoperative psychiatric disturbance ($P < 0.05$) (Table 4).

Sex and age did not differ in both subgroups. In comparison to patients without psychiatric reactions, however, there were significantly more patients with psychiatric disturbances in the age group above 50 ($P < 0.05$).

Table 4. Incidence of psychiatric disturbances according to preoperative cardiac index in patients with AVR

Group	x	s	
Delirious	1.65	0.25	
Anxiety and paranoid	2.78	0.33	$P \leq 0.01$
Without psychiatric disturbances	2.34	0.53	$P \leq 0.05$

Anesthesia

Anesthesia was performed either by neuroleptanalgesia or by electrostimulation in terms of drug-sparing acupuncture analgesia. There was no correlation between the duration of anesthesia and the occurrence of postoperative psychosis. In one-third of the delirious patients, however, electroacupuncture was carried out (Table 5).

Table 5. Relationship between anesthesia and psychiatric disturbances

Group	NLA	CAA
Delirious	6	3
Anxiety and paranoid	8	–
Without psychiatric disturbances	47	9
Total sample	61	12

Abbreviation: NLA, neuroleptanalgesia; CAA, combined electro-acupunctureanalgesia

Surgical Procedure

A significant correlation was not observed between the incidence of psychiatric disturbances and the performed surgical technique (Table 6). It only can be stated that in four cases out of seven, when surgical procedure was expanded, psychiatric disturbances did occur (Table 7).

Surgical Technique

For the purpose of blood oxygenation a bubble oxygenator (Spiraflow BOS 10 from Bentley Company) was used. For the prevention of cerebral microembolism by metal pieces, silicone, sterilization residues, denatured proteins, and insoluble drugs, bloodfilters (PE 427 from Bentley Company) were inserted into the arterial and venous line of the heart-lung machine. All surgical interventions of the initial phase of extracorporeal circulation were carried out during hypothermic perfusion at a body temperature of 32 °C. In each operation protection of the myocardium was performed by injection

Table 6. Incidence of psychiatric disturbances according to operative procedure

Surgical treatment	n	Psychiatric disturbances Delirious	Anxiety and paranoid
AVR	24	2	4
MVR	11	1	1
AVR + MVR	4	2	1
ACVB	17	–	1
ACVB + aneurysmectomy	3	2	–
ACVB + HVR	2	1	–
Closure of paravalvular leak	1	1	–
Closure of patent ductus arterious	1	–	1
Total sample		9	8

Table 7. Relationship between psychiatric disturbances and combined operative procedure

Operative procedure	Group	
	Delirious	Without psychiatric disturbance
AVR + MVR	2	1
ACVB + HVR	1	1
MVR + de Vega plasty	1	–
AVR + closure of VSD	–	1
Total	4	3

of cardioplegic solution at a temperature of 4 °C, as described by Kirsch. In addition the cardiac surface was cooled by icecold saline so that intramyocardial temperature ranged from 22 °C–26 °C.

Extracorporeal Circulation

Bypass Time

The significance of the duration of extracorporeal circulation regarding the origin of postoperative disturbances is still a matter for dispute [1, 2, 6, 7]. In this study absolute value of average bypass time was higher in the group of patients showing psychiatric disturbances postoperatively; differences, however, were statistically not significant (Table 8).

Mean Arterial Pressure

A decreased mean arterial pressure for a longer period of time during cardiac surgery is reported to induce disturbances of the central nervous system [10, 15].

Mean arterial pressure was found to be slightly lower in the delirous subgroup; the difference, however, could not be established statistically (Table 9).

Table 8. Incidence of psychiatric disturbances and bypass time (min)

Group	x	s
Delirious	69.4	16.87
Anxiety and paranoid	68.4	16.76
Without psychiatric disturbances	60.3	25.29

Table 9. Relationship between psychiatric disturbances and mean arterial blood pressure during ECC

Group	x	s
Delirious	91.6	12.65
Anxiety and paranoid	97.7	14.60
Without psychiatric disturbances	96.0	13.60

Mean Flow

The main purpose of extracorporeal circulation is to maintain a sufficient flow of 2.2–2.4 $1/m^2$ min. We found a significantly higher flow rate ($P < 0.01$) in the subgroup of delirious patients (Table 10).

Clinical Parameters After Extracorporeal Circulation

Cardiac Arrhythmia

Cardiac arrhythmias which occur postoperatively are mainly the consequence of altered spontaneous activity due to myocardial damage from extracorporeal circulation. Disturbances in cardiac rhythm as a cause of psychiatric reactions have been reported [1]. We found cardiac arrythmia in 100% of patients of the delirous subgroup, in 65% of those with anxious-paranoid reactions, and in 46% of those patients who had no symptoms of psychiatric disturbances.

Use of Catecholamine

It was generally noticed that in two-thirds of patients in the delirious subgroup catecholamine was given postoperatively because of unstable circulatory conditions, while

Table 10. Incidence of psychiatric disturbances and mean flow (l/m^2/min)

Group	x	s
Delirious	3.4	1.08
Without psychiatric disturbances	2.8	$P \leq 0.01$ 0.52

only 25% of anxious paranoid patients and 13% of patients without psychiatric disturbances needed catecholamine in the postoperative period.

EEG Alterations

In two-thirds of the patients with delirious symptoms minor EEG alterations and transient focus states were observed, as described in 1953 by Jung [8] in localized cerebral tissue damage of single cerebral areas. From such findings it is not possible to differentiate between cerebral embolism and ischemic brain infarcts. It must be concluded that in this group psychosis is due to a reversible brain-organic disturbance. In both other groups alterations of the electroencephalogram were not observed.

References

1. Blachy PH, Starr A (1964) Post-cardiotomy delirium. Am J Psychiatry 121:371
2. Egerton N, Kay JH (1964) Psychological disturbances associated with open-heart surgery. Br J Psychiatry 110:443–439
3. Freyhan FA, Giannelli S Jr, O'Connel RA, et al. (1971) Psychiatric complications following open-heart surgery. Compr Psychiatry 12:181–195
4. Gilberstadt H, Sako Y (1967) Intellectual and personality changes following open-heart surgery. Arch Gen Psychiatry 16:210–214
5. Hazan SJ (1966) Psychiatric complications following cardiac surgery. J Thorac Cardiovasc Surg 51:307
6. Henrichs TF, Mackenzie JW, Almond CH (1971) Psychological adjustment and psychiatric complications following open-heart surgery. J Nerv Ment Dis 152:332
7. Javid H, Tufo HM, Nahati N, Dye WS, Hunter JA, Julian OC (1969) Neurological abnormalities following open-heart surgery. J Thorac Cardiovasc Surg 58:502
8. Jung R (1953) Hirnelektrische Befunde bei Kreislaufstörungen und Hypoxieschäden des Gehirnes. Verh Dtsch Ges Kreislaufforsch 19:170–196
9. Kimball CP (1969) Psychological responses to the experience of open-heart surgery. Am J Psychiatry 126:96–107
10. Lee WH, et al. (1971) Effects of extracorporeal circulation upon behavior, personality and brain function II. Ann Surg 173:1013
11. Mervin SL, Abram HS (1977) Psychologic response to coronary artery bypass. South Med J 70:153–155
12. Meyendorf R (1976) Psychische und neurologische Störungen bei Herzoperationen. Fortschr Med 94:315
13. Morse RM, Litin EM (1971) The anatomy of a delirium. Am J Psychiatry 128:1–143
14. Speidel H, Dahme B, Flemming B, Götze P, Huse-Kleinstoll G, Meffert MJ, Rodewald G, Spehr W (1978) Psychosomatische Probleme in der Herzchirurgie. Therapiewoche 28:8191–8210
15. Tufo HM, Osterfeld AM, Shekelle R (1970) Central nervous system dysfunction following open-heart surgery. JAMA 212:1333
16. Weiss SM (1966) Psychological adjustment following open-heart surgery. J Nerv Ment Dis 143:363–368

Incidence of Psychiatric and Neurological Complications After Cardiac Surgery – Retrospective Versus Prospective Studies

R. Paech, W. Klinner, R. Meyendorf, B. Reichart, E. Kreuzer

Introduction

There are two main disadvantages of retrospective over prospective studies on neuropsychiatric disturbances after cardiac surgery: Neither definition of parameters nor data-recording is standardized beforehand – and developments of symptomatology are often overlooked by an unaware medical staff. Therefore, the incidence of psychopathological dysfunction is always lower in retrospective than in prospective studies and, furthermore, it is impossible to provide an exact description of cerebral disorders in these retrospective studies; so the variety of symptomatology is lost. Systematic and standardized studies, however, generally comprise only a comparatively small number of patients. The advantage of retrospective studies lies in the possibility of covering many cases, an advantage that prompted the present study which, using a large population, examines many currently considered risk factors.

Own Results

Methods and Total Incidence

Records of 1360 non-selected patients of the Department of Cardiac Surgery of the University of Munich, aged 1 year and older, have been examined. Total incidence of psychopathological dysfunction following a heart operation was 19.3% (262 patients). Of these more than half were mild dysfunctions, mainly disturbances of mood and drive. Severe psychiatric symptoms such as cardiac delirious and paranoid and hallucinatory syndromes accounted for 19.5%, 13.3% were primary neurological symptoms such as hemiplegia, lateralizing symptoms, and seizures and 14.5% of the symptoms were coma-like.

Correlating Factors

The following factors correlated significantly with a higher incidence of cerebral disorders ($\chi^2 > P = 0.01$ for all parameters except for NYHA class, priming of extracorporeal circulation, repeated defibrillations, and abnormal sodium level; for these $\chi^2 > P = 0.05$):

Psychopathological and Neurological Dysfunctions Following Open-Heart Surgery Ed by Becker et al

Table 1. Cerebral dysfunction and mortality in correlation with age

Age	n (Total)	Postop. cerebral dysfunction		Deceased	
		n	%	n	%
1– 3	65	10	15.4	10	15.4
4– 7	225	18	8.0	22	9.8
8– 9	95	3	3.2	4	4.2
10–11	67	1	1.5	2	3.0
12–13	44	–	–	3	6.8
14–20	106	15	14.2	4	3.8
21–30	79	17	21.5	3	3.8
31–40	138	36	26.1	15	10.9
41–50	240	63	26.3	22	9.2
51–60	230	75	32.6	22	9.6
61–70	60	19	31.6	12	20.0

1. Preoperative Factors: 28.4% of the 148 patients with previous neurological or psychological disturbance had cerebral disorders following cardiac surgery as compared with 18.2% of those without previous disturbance. Advanced age or youth are other riskfactors: Only 6.5% of the 496 children under 14 years had neuropsychiatric disorders compared with 26.4% of the adults (Table 1). Table 1 shows that children with lower age and adults with higher age had most dysfunctions. Also low body weight seems to heighten the risk as do certain heart lesions:

Patients with acquired disease had an altogether greater incidence of psychopathological disturbances than patients with congenital disease. In cases of acquired disease patients with multivalvular lesion had by far the most disturbances, while in congenital disease those with transpostion of major arteries had the most disturbances (Table 2). In addition, patients with calcified valves demonstrated a significantly greater incidence of cerebral disorders. The severity of clinical symptomatology according to NYHA classification had a significant influence, too. But the incidence of disorders did not

Table 2. Cerebral dysfunction in correlation with type of heart disease

Type of heart disease	n (Total)	Postop. cerebral dysfunction	
		n	%
Multivalv. d.	34	22	64.7
Mitral v. d.	154	47	30.5
Aortic v. d.	216	59	27.3
Coronar h. d.	222	60	27.0
Major art. tr.	28	7	25.0
Coarct. aort.	61	9	14.8
Fallot tetra.	176	18	10.2
ASD	177	18	10.2
Pulm. sten.	51	3	5.9
VSD	113	4	3.5
PDA	45	1	2.2

Table 3. Cerebral dysfunction in correlation with duration of extracorporeal circulation

Duration of ECC (min)	n (Total)	Postop. cerebral dysfunction n	%
1– 30	224	23	9.4
31– 60	549	98	17.9
61– 90	236	73	30.9
91–120	68	29	42.6

Table 4. Cerebral dysfunction in correlation with duration of hypothermia

Duration of hypothermia (min)	n (Total)	Postop. cerebral dysfunction n	%
0	185	28	15.1
1–10	202	21	10.4
11–20	340	68	20.0
21–30	215	47	21.9
31–40	88	30	34.1
41–50	36	15	41.7
51–60	41	16	39.0

Table 5. Cerebral dysfunction in correlation with blood transfusion

Quantity of blood transf. (l)	n (Total)	Postop. cerebral dysfunction n	%
0	219	19	8.7
–0.5	354	37	9.8
0.6–1.0	345	67	19.4
1.1–1.5	225	54	24.0
1.6–2.0	95	29	30.5
2.1–2.5	47	21	44.7
2.6–3.0	26	12	46.2
3.1–3.5	18	6	33.3
3.6–4.0	7	5	71.2

always increase with NYHA class: Although more patients in class IV (35.2%) than in class III (27.9%) had neuropsychiatric disorders, most of these disorders were displayed by patients in class II (41.8%).

2. Intraoperative Factors: 11.2% of the 232 patients were operated on without extracorporeal circulation compared with 21% of the 1128 patients operated on with ECC had psychopathological disturbances. Also, increasing the duration of ECC and certain priming, that is undiluted blood preserve, seems to heighten the risk (Table 3), as also does duration of the operation and of hypothermy: Patients operated on without hypothermia showed more disorders than those operated on in hypothermia of less than 10 min. Beyond the 10-min-limit, however, the incidence of neuropsychiatric disorders increased with duration of hypothermia (Table 4). Also, repeated defibrillations and rethoracotomies seem to be risk factors.

3. Postoperative Factors: Cerebral disturbances were observed following extensive blood transfusion or abnormally high levels of sodium, potassium, creatinine, and urea (Table 5). Of the 1360 patients 9.8% died. Of the 262 patients with cerebral dysfunctions 16.8% died compared with 6.8% of those 1098 without neuropsychiatric complications.

Noncorrelating Factors

No significant correlation could be found between psychopathological and neurological disorders and sex, blood group, duration of symptoms, preoperative cardiac index, previous cardiac surgery, and duration of hypotonia.

Discussion

Concerning almost every factor it is possible to find similar and dissimilar results which have been obtained by other authors. Most authors agree with respect to previous cerebral disturbance, age, certain heart lesions, ECC, duration of operation and hypothermia, and extensive blood transfusion being risk factors [2, 4, 7, 8]. With regard to body weight, rethoracotomy and electrolyte level there are not many articles [3, 6, 11]. Results concerning sex, blood group, calcified valves, duration and severity of symptoms, cardiac index, previous cardiac surgery, and hypotonia are quite inconsistent [1, 5, 7, 9, 10, 12]. The most unexpected result of our own examination was that hypotonia did not seem to have any influence on cerebral disorders. Most authors had found contrary results [7, 8].

Many of the factors described correlate with one another: Patients with multivalvular lesion had the longest duration of operation and ECC. Children with congenital disease had less operations with ECC than adults with acquired disease. Duration of ECC nearly always increases with duration of the operation. Patients who needed repeated defibrillations had a longer duration of ECC. Only 3.9% of the 232 patients operated on without ECC died compared with 9.8% of those 1128 operated on with ECC. Therefore, a clear causality is not implied between each factor described and postoperative cerebral disturbance. Many factors are the manifestation of a basic disorder. One can only be certain that in many cases the symptoms are multietiological. Major influential variables will have to be extracted.

References

1. Åberg T (1974) Effect of open heart surgery on intellectual function. Scand J Thorac Cardiovasc Surg [Suppl] 15
2. Blachly PH, Starr A (1964) Postcardiotomy delirium. Am J Psychiatry 121:371–375
3. Egerton N, Kay JH (1964) Psychological disturbances associated with open heart surgery. Br J Psychiatry 110:433–439
4. Freyhan FA, Gianelli S Jr, O'Connell RA (1971) Psychiatric complications following open heart surgery. Compr Psychiatry 12:181–195
5. Henrichs TF, Waters WF (1972) Psychological adjustment and response to open heart surgery. Some methodological considerations. Br J Psychiatry 120:491–496
6. Huse-Kleinstoll G, Dahme B, Flemming B, et al. (1976) Einige somatische und psychische Prädiktoren für psychopathologische Auffälligkeiten nach Herzoperationen. Thoraxchirurgie 24: 386–389
7. Kimball CP (1972) The experience of open heart surgery. II. Arch Gen Psychiatry 27:57–63
8. Lee WH Jr, Brady MP, Rowe JM, et al. (1971) Effects of extracorporeal circulation upon behavior, personality and brain function. Ann Surg 173:1013–1023
9. Meyendorf R (1974) Die psychischen und neurologischen Störungen bei Herzoperationen. Habilitationsschrift, University of Munich
10. Rubinstein D, Thomas JK (1969) Psychiatric findings in cardiotomy patients. Am J Psychiatry 126:279–291
11. Sorokoumov VA, Voinov VA, Rodin V, et al. (1975) Disorders following operations with extracorporeal circulation. Sov Med 12:59–64
12. Tufo HM, Ostfeld AM, Shekelle R (1970) Central nervous system dysfunctions following open heart surgery. JAMA 212:1333–1340

Sociopsychological Factors in Cardiac Surgery

D. Mohan, N. Gopinath, S. Gupta

Surgical management for some of the cardiac conditions including heart transplantation has gained a momentum in the world during the past 25 years. But in India such facilities are seen mainly in medical teaching institutions. Since the surgical procedure with the heart has morbidity and mortality risk, it has an impact on the emotional life of the individuals undergoing it. Hence it had become rather customary to assess pre- and postoperatively the psychiatric and psychological consequences [1, 2, 4–9, 12, 15, 16] most probably in an effort to prove the efficacy of a given technique. As against the vast literature outside India on the psychiatric and psychological aspects of cardiovascular surgery, the authors are aware of only two studies [13, 14] in India which elicited psychiatric and psychological aspects of surgery for mitral stenosis. None of these studies demonstrated postoperative personality changes in patients. The behavioral concomitants and consequences of cardiac surgery have not been explored in India either by cardiac surgeons or by behavioral scientists. To explore these aspects a study was initiated jointly with the Department of Cardio-thoracic Surgery [10]. The study aims to assess the personality and behavioral changes following open-heart surgery and does not consider the neuropsychological deficits since it has already been suggested [6, 9, 15] that successful cardiac surgery restores severely reduced cerebral blood flow and cerebral hypoxia and brings about subsequent improvement in the cognitive status of individuals so affected.

Cardiac surgery, in fact, is a very complex psychological stimulus and its emotional ramifications extend far beyond the surgical event itself. The study of personality changes following open-heart surgery in Indian context may be of relevance cross culturally.

From the ongoing study on personality changes following open-heart surgery, careful selection was carried out of 11 cases in whom Cattell and Eber's 16 P.F. questionnaire (as adopted by Kapoor in Hindi) was administered immediately before the open-heart surgery and of 11 cases in whom the testing was done 3 years postoperatively. These two groups, even though small, were matched on a one-to-one basis for the variables such as age, sex, education, marital status, and also in relation to the number of stress events occurring during 1 year prior to the onset of cardiac illness. Surprisingly, the intergroup differences in regard to all the 16 P.F. test variables were statistically insignificant and the scores yielded on the variables were generally depressed or low on both occasions.

The observation as to why a positive change in the personality functioning of the patients following open-heart surgery was not seen can be viewed from a number of

Psychopathological and Neurological Dysfunctions
Following Open-Heart Surgery. Ed by Becker et al.

angles. In order to arrive at some conclusion, optimally the personality retesting should have been done on the same series as is taken up preoperatively or, ideally, one more session of personality testing was needed on each patient of the series well before a decision was made regarding the surgical management of the cardiac patients. Cardiac surgery evokes various kinds of reactions in different persons depending upon their premorbid personality status.

As cultural factors have a significant influence on the personality make-up of individuals, it would be worthwhile noting that Indian culture provides a high threshold of toleration of 'dependence' [11] and, therefore, the personality outgrowth in patients following open-heart surgery did not appear to have taken place even 3 years postoperatively. Since the heart is considered to be the locus of feeling and an attribute of character, people in our series regarded a cardiac patient as one subjected to chronic psychological stress both in the remote or recent past. Close relatives of the patient, usually the parents, sibs, wife, or children perceive open-heart surgery as the technique of management of his heart condition with a fear or incapacity or death of the patient. In most of the families extreme changes are then seen. Circumstances leading to the patient's disease are analysed to discover possible causes in his immediate environment. In many instances, parent-son, brother-brother/sister or wife-husband relationships are reported to have been repaired. Often these are interpreted in the context of the past life and the kind of life the individual led (Karma theory) and are seen as punishments for past deeds or sins.

It is not usually the intrafamilial changes that take place which lead to sinking of differences, the patient and doctor or the patient's family and the doctor interaction is also affected. In most cases, it is not always the clinician who may impart instructions to the patient or to his relatives but it is the patient or his relatives who ask for certain "do's" and "do not's" so that the patient remains free from the sickness for the rest of his life. By virtue of this, the clinician in the Indian setting is considered to be the one who fights a battle with Yamaraj (God of Death) and brings back life to the patient. His instructions are carried out literally. The family members of the patient render a great help to the doctor in restoring adequacy and confidence in the patient. They are able to shower love, affection, shelter, protection, security, warmth etc. and appear to be in no hurry to reduce his dependency needs which, in fact, are accentuated at times, leading to undue delay in recovery. To cite an example, a 64-year-old father of a male patient, K.L., 40 years of age now, High School educated, diagnosed as M.V.D., and who also underwent open-heart surgery on 4-8-1976, was able to arrange a light job for him (to write the sales) at a coal depot at Rewari (Haryana) and decided for himself to vend cloth in order to supplement the earnings of the family. The father was a retired school teacher at the time of the operation. He had accompanied the patient from a distance of about 150 km when the patient visited us for a check up and asserted that he would continue to support him till he breathed his last. When asked how things would go after his death, he replied, "God will help him".

Social 'dependence' in the Western cultures, especially in the U.S.A., is considered a defect to be removed (Parens and Saul, cited by 11). 'A common judgement is that for a person to be dependent is less good than for him to be independent: in fact, to call some one dependent in his personal relationships is a condition to be avoided and left behind' (Bowlby, cited by 11). Dependence has an aura of disapproval or disparagement. Even "the birds and beasts after a certain time banish their offspring, disown their acquaintance, and seem to have no knowledge of objects which lately engrossed the attention of their minds and occupied the industry and labour of their bodies," remarked Lord Chancellor of England, Lord Brongham and Vaux in his edition of Palcy's "Natural Theology" published in 1845 [3]. To make one financially and socially independent during and/or after the disease which has caused incapacity in the individual, there is then the emergence of rehabilitation programmes to enable him to strive for his goals. These facts have given a cultural sterotype in the West that 'God helps those who help themselves' and in the East, 'God helps those who seek His refuge'.

Following the great theory of Charles Darwin in the 1860s, and based on the notion of the 'survival of the fittest', distinctness in the discipline of psychology as an aid to establishing individual differences had emerged, particularly in the U.S.A., emphasizing separateness of the individuals and considering later how these individuals can be 'linked together'. In the Indian context – even if the cardiac surgeons have remained content with providing only the survival statistics following open-heart surgery and not adequately documenting the behavioral aspects – they have probably unwittingly promoted dependence in their patients, rightly identifying the 'quantum of dependence which the other significant people in the patient's life can and will be willing to support' [11].

The present to communication helps us to understand that cultural background of an individual is an important variable in determining his threshold, not only for frustration tolerance, but also for accepting the person so affected. In the context of our existing experience, it appears that cross culturally variations may be possible with regard to personality outgrowth following open-heart surgery, or for that matter any debilitating disease leading to a situation of incapacity in individuals. Personality outgrowth in such individuals may have been seen in cultures encouraging 'autonomy' or independence as being advantageous but may not be possible in cultures where dependence is 'eulogized as a virtue which merits great mercies' (Vivekanand, cited by 11).

References

1. Blachly PH, Starr A (1964) Post-cardiotomy delirium. Am J Psychiatry 121:371–375
2. Bliss FL, Rumel WR, Branch CH (1955) Psychiatric complications of mitral surgery. AMA Arch Neurol Psychiatry 74:249–252
3. Brougham and Vaux (1845) Natural theology. Paley's
4. Egerton N, Kay JH (1964) Psychological disturbances associated with open heart surgery. Br J Psychiatry 110:433–441
5. Gilberstadt H, Sako Y (1967) Intellectual and personality changes following open heart surgery. Arch Gen Psychiatry 16:210–214
6. Herbert CT, Movius HJ (1964) Psychological deficits with mitral commissurotomy. JAMA 187:767–767
7. Knox SJ (1963) Psychiatric aspects of mitral valvotomy. Br J Psychiatry 109:656–668
8. Little RB, Pearson MM (1964) Combined insulin coma and ECT following cardiac surgery. Am J Psychiatry 110:786–787
9. Meyer BC, Blacher RS, Brown F (1961) A clinical study of psychiatric and psychological aspects of mitral surgery. Psychosom Med 23:194–218
10. Mohan D, Gopinath N, Gupta S, Mukherjee M, Sandy S, Veenugopal P, Mukherjee Y, Rao IM, Sampathkumer A (to be published) Personality changes following open heart surgery.

11. Neki JS (1976) An examination of the cultural relativism of dependence as a dynamic of social and therapeutic relationships. Br J Med Psychol 49:1–22
12. Priest WS, Zaks MS, Yakorzynski GK, Boshes B (1957) The Neurologic, psychiatric and psychologic aspects of cardiac surgery. Med Clin North Am 41:155–169
13. Raheja HC (1969) A study of psychiatric aspects of cardiac surgery. Thesis, A.I.I.M.S., New Delhi
14. Wahi PN, Wig NN (1969) Neuropsychiatric complications after cardiac surgery. ICMR Inquiry. Report submitted to the Indian Council of Medical Research
15. Willner AE, Rabiner CJ (1979) Psychopathology and cognitive dysfunction five years after open heart surgery. Comp Psychiatry 20:409–418
16. Zaks MS (1959) Disturbances in psychological functions and neuropsychiatric complications in heart surgery – a 4-year follow-up study. In: Luisado AA (ed) Cardiology: An encyclopedia of the cardiovascular system, vol III. McGraw-Hill, New York, pp 162–171.

Psychiatric Complications Following Open-Heart Surgery A Prospective Study

P. Tienari, J. Outakoski, R. Hirvenoja, A. Juolasmaa, I. Takkunen, R. Kampman

Introduction

Open-heart surgery is commonly followed by postoperative psychiatric complications. Most of the investigations so far made have been catamnestic studies which have not distinguished between the predisposing factors and the effects of the operation itself. If the patients are carefully examined prior to the operation and followed up postoperatively and during the rehabilitation period, it should be possible to keep apart the psychic predisposing factors and the organic factors associated with the operation. It is also possible to try to evaluate the predictive capacity of postoperative complications with psychiatric-psychological examination.

We are carrying out a prospective investigation of postoperative complications caused by open-heart surgery. We collected all the successive (adult) cases offered for open-heart surgery (for valvular replacement) in a given district during April 1, 1976 – October 31, 1979. Naturally, not all these patients will be operated on. A thorough psychiatric-psychological examination of each patient is made 3–4 months before the operation. It is repeated 3 or 6 months postoperatively and once more 12 months after the operation. The psychiatric interview is repeated 1 or 2 days before and 1 week after the operation. The postoperative psychic status is recorded every day during the 1st week after the operation. A neurological examination and a quantitative (computer) EEG recording are made both pre- and postoperatively. By January 1980 we had examined preoperatively altogether 160 patients, of whom 81 had been operated on; 67 were re-examined 3–6 months after the operation and 58 had been followed up for a year. The study is still in progress. We shall give some preliminary findings here.

The inter-group differences were analyzed using Student's t-test and the Chi square test. Multiple comparisons between the groups were made using Scheffe's F projection method.

Altogether 81 patients have been operated on so far, 30 of them female and 51 male. The mean age of the women was 47.8 years and that of the men 43.7 years. The mean age of the entire patient population was 45.2 years. The men in this series are younger than the women. Seven patients (8.6%) died during the first postoperative year.

Psychopathological and Neurological Dysfunctions
Following Open-Heart Surgery Ed by Becker et al

Psychiatric Examination

The diagnoses of the immediate postoperative complications were as follows: post-cardiotomy delirium occurred in 22 patients and a functional psychosis in seven, while two had a crisis at the border-line level, four a depressive reaction and seven an hysteric reaction. The total number of psychiatric complications was 42 (51.9%). The remaining 39 (48.1%) patients recovered without psychiatric disturbances.

Altogether 29 patients (35.8%) had a psychotic complication during the immediate postoperative period. Their mean age was 46.8 years. Of the women 43.3% (13/30) and of the men, 31.4% (16/51) had a psychosis. Of the patients aged under 40 31.3% (5/16) had a psychosis, while 36.9% of those aged over 40 (24/65) became psychotic. The total frequency of psychiatric complications was 66.7% among the women (20/30) and 43.1% among the men (22/51). ($X^2 = 4.19 > X^2$ $.05 = 3.84$, df = 1).

The psychic status had been estimated before the operation using a rating scale whereby the healthy subjects were scored with 1, the mildly disturbed ones with 2, the neurotic patients with 3, the patients with character disorders with 4, the border-line patients with 5, and the psychotic patients with 6. Those without psychiatric complications had been rated a bit more healthy (mean 2.2) preoperatively than those having psychiatric complications (mean 2.4). They were also differentiated in our trial to predict the prognosis preoperatively with a scale from 1 (very good) to 5 (very poor). Those without disturbances during the immediate postoperative period had had a mean rating of 1.7 preoperatively, while those with disturbances had had a mean of 2.6.

The men and the women differed from each other in psychic status: the women with postoperative psychic disturbances were preoperatively rated at 2.6 and those without them at 2.1. Among the men there were no differences between the subjects with disturbances and those without them. There was also a clear difference in the estimated prognosis of the women: those with postoperative psychic complications were rated at 3.4 as compared with the subjects without complications, who were rated at 1.9. In the group of men this difference was small (2.2 versus 1.7).

After the postoperative classification of the group with psychic complications into cases of delirium and cases of functional disturbances (functional psychosis, neurotic reactions), we found that the psychic status estimated preoperatively did not differ in the cases with delirium (2.2) from the cases without psychic complications, while a difference compared with the cases of functional disorders was found (2.7 versus 2.2). The differences in the preoperative predictions of prognosis were obvious: the preoperatively predicted rate for the cases without complications was on the average 1.7, being 2.3 in the group with delirium and 2.9 in the group with functional disorders. The cases with delirium or with postoperative functional disorders were even preoperatively predicted to be a risk group.

The preoperative estimate of the prognosis was most successful in the group with no postoperative psychic complications (Table 1). Of the 39 patients who had no postoperative complications, 32 (82%) were estimated to have a good prognosis preoperatively. The estimated prognosis is statistically significant at the 1% risk level.

Table 1. Preoperative prediction of prognosis and postoperative psychic complications

Postoperative complications	Total	Prognosis estimated preoperatively		
		Good	Questionable	Poor
Yes	42	21	11	10
No	39	32	4	3

X^2 9.22 > X^2 0.01 = 9.21, df = 2

The subjects who developed a psychic complication immediately after the operation had been assessed by a psychiatrist 1 or 2 days before the operation to be more anxious than the subjects without complications (difference $P < 0.05$). Hamilton's Anxiety Scale revealed an even clearer difference (Table 2): the patients with postoperative complications were significantly more anxious than the others ($P < 0.001$), the difference being more marked in the group of men ($P < 0.01$) than in the female group (N.S.).

Table 2. Hamilton anxiety scale (1 or 2 days before the operation)

	All	Male	Female
No complication	8.6	8.4	9.2
Psychic complications	15.1	14.5	15.7
	(P < 0.001)	(P < 0.01)	(P < 0.1)
Neurotic reactions	14.8	11.0	18.1
Functional psychosis	20.1	16.7	22.8
Delirium	13.6	15.6	10.7
Mean	12.0	11.0	13.5

According to Beck's Depression Scale, the patients with a postoperative neurotic reaction were significantly more depressive preoperatively than the patients with postoperative delirium ($P < 0.01$). The same observation was made in the group of men ($P < 0.01$), while the group of women displayed smaller difference. In the male group, furthermore, the subjects with a neurotic reaction differed almost significantly from the subjects without postoperative complications ($P < 0.05$).

Age at the time of the operation seemed, on the whole, to be connected with the occurrence of psychic complications immediately after the operation ($P < 0.05$). The same difference was also observable in the male group separately.

Table 3. Psychological tests

1. WAIS:
   - Arithmetic
   - Similarities
   - Digit span
   - Vocabulary
   - Digit symbol
   - Picture completion
   - Block design
   - Picture arrangement
2. Wechsler memory scale:
   - Logical memory
   - Associative learning
3. Benton visual retention test
4. The bender-gestalt test
5. Weckroth's test battery for identification of brain damage [3]:
   - Opposites
   - Sums
   - Pieces
   - Triangles
   - Tapping
6. MMPI
7. Rorschach
8. Beck Depression inventory
9. Hamilton anxiety scale
10. Self-image test
11. Identity diffusion scale (Eriksson)

Preoperative Psychological Examination

The variable measuring psychic performance capacity exhibited a general trend showing that the patients with a postoperative neurotic reaction or functional psychosis were at a lower level compared with the subjects without disorders or with delirium. However, the difference was statistically significant ($P < 0.05$) only in the visual Pieces test.

In the MMPI test the men with postoperative delirium scored lower than the others ($P < 0.05$) on the psychopathy scale (Pd), while the women with delirium scored lower than the other women ($P < 0.05$) on the mania scale. The women with postoperative functional psychosis scored higher than the others ($P < 0.05$) on the mania scale, and in the Rorschach test they appeared more impulsive and affectively labile ($P < 0.05$) preoperatively than the others.

With the exception of the group with postoperative delirium, the other groups had, on an average, a deviating MMPI profile: the T score was above 70 on two scales, and five of the seven patients with functional psychosis had a T score above 70 on three scales.

Follow-up Six Months After the Operation

On the whole, the patients seemed to benefit from the operation even with regard to mental health. Although the results have not been analyzed in detail yet, it seems, for example, that the degree of psychiatric disturbance (based on interview) has declined, as have also depressiveness estimated with Beck's scale and the degree of anxiety estimated by a psychiatrist. According to Beck's depression scale, the patients with postoperative functional psychosis were still more depressed than patients in the other groups, differing most clearly from the group without disorders ($P < 0.001$) and almost significantly from the others ($P < 0.05$). In the group of women the differences were almost significant ($P < 0.05$), while in the male group they were not significant.

The postoperative MMPI profile revealed normalization in the group without complications and the group with a neurotic reaction. The delirium group displayed some impairment, while the group with functional psychosis were clearly impaired on the Pt, Sc and Si scales as well as the MMPI psychosis index ($P < 0.05$).

The neuropsychological tests showed a general trend toward improved performance, too. The most marked improvement was noted in visual tests. However, the subjects with postoperative functional psychosis or delirium improved their performance less than the others. Moreover, the patients with postoperative psychotic symptoms (functional psychosis + delirium) showed impaired test performance significantly more often than the others (Table 3). (The impairment was measured with a global "impairment percentage" obtained by calculating the percentage of test variables in which significant impairment had taken place in each case.) As regards individual tests, the psychotic group showed a significantly greater tendency to impairment than the others in WAIS Block Design, Bender-Gestalt and the Tapping test.

Table 4. Connection of postoperative psychotic disorders with impairment in neuropsychological tests

	Neuropsychological impairment %					
	Over 20		0–20		Total	
	n	%	n	%	n	%
Psychosis[a]	12	54.6	10	45.5	22	100.0
No psychosis	5	13.2	33	86.8	38	100.0
Total	17	28.3	43	71.7	60	100.0

$X^2 = 11.76 > X^2\ .001 = 10.83$, df = 1
[a] Psychosis = functional psychosis + delirium

Summary

We have examined 160 successive patients offered for open heart surgery, of whom 81 have been operated on up until now. Of the subjects operated on, 52% developed psychic complications and 48% recovered without complications. The results of preoperative examinations obtained so far suggest that we may have been most successful in detecting the patients who will recover from the operation without psychic complications. In the light of the findings made so far, it seems that the psychic complications are best predicted by anxiety as estimated by a psychiatrist and as measured using Hamilton's Anxiety Index. The manifestation of complications also seemed to be somewhat connected with age. Furthermore, the association between the changes taking place in psychometric tests and the occurrence of postoperative psychotic reactions suggests that brain dysfunction during the operation has been of crucial significance for the development of those disorders.

References

1. Juolasmaa A, Outakoski R, Hirvenoja R, Tienari P (1979) Neuropsychological disorders in cardiac valvular disease and their relationship to psychiatric complications following open heart surgery.
Unpublished paper presented in the International Neuropsychological Society, Second European Conference, June 27–30, 1979, Nordwijkerout, Holland
2. Juolasmaa A, Outakoski J, Hirvenoja R, Tienari P (1980) The effect of open heart surgery on intellectual performance: A neuropsychological study.
Unpublished paper presented in the Third INS European Conference, June 2–5, 1980, Chianciano-Terme, Italy
3. Weckroth J, Tienari P, Airikkala K (1965) A comparison of the ability structure of two groups of brain injured patients with different locations on the left-right hemisphere dimension. Reports from the Institute of Occupational Health 25, Helsinki

Discussion of Session I

The main part of the discussion involved questions concerning the visual disturbances during the early postoperative period as described by Meyendorf.

Meyendorf stresses that the occipital lobe and basal ganglia are especially vulnerable regarding anoxia, and he thinks that the common effect of microembolism and anoxia is responsible for the visual disturbances in the early postoperative period. He describes them as transient, so that all measures that aim at quantifying these disturbances more accurately must be very short and easily performed, because during this period in the postoperative course the patients are not able to perform very complicated tests.

Willner proposed a test where 6's and 9's are all spread over a paper and where the patients are asked to cross out the 6's and 9's, so that one can mark the gaps in the visual field. He considers this test to be easy enough to use for quantifying visual disturbances.

Compared to other types of surgery Meyendorf says that after looking at 70 patients with kidney transplants he saw these sort of visual disturbances only twice. In his opinion the types of anesthesia and operation used are too different from those used in cardiac surgery to be comparable. However, similar visual disorders can be found in the literature in patients with atrial fibrillation, with microemboli in endocarditis or with malaria, and also after a short cardiac arrest.

Besides the visual disturbances after cardiac surgery there were questions about aphasic episodes in the postoperative period. Meyendorf confirms that there certainly are aphasic episodes in the postoperative period, although in his paper he does not refer to them. He describes them as difficulties in finding words or that people cannot speak as fluently as they did before. He has also seen aphasic or paraphasic tendencies in children.

Concerning questions regarding why the introduction of cardioplegia is thought to be the most important factor in reducing the cerebral damage after open-heart surgery, Björk stresses that air embolism can be much better avoided, especially in mitral valve replacement but also in aortic valve replacement, since cardioplegia is used. There was much more difficulty in avoiding air embolism while operating on the beating heart.

The paper of Paech and co-workers was followed by a discussion of difficulties in using multi-variant statistics to identify predictors of postoperative psychopathology. With the existence of a number of significant correlations between preoperative variables and postoperative psychiatric reactions it is often difficult to differentiate between really significant correlations and those being significant only due to chance.

It has been suggested that if the sample is big enough one can easily divide it into two subgroups to see which of them hold and which do not.

The same presentation directed attention toward preoperative neurological changes. Cohen thinks that neurological damage before the operation seems most likely as patients with cardiac diseases are very susceptible to neurological damage. This is underlined by Hanson. In 421 open-heart cases, all patients with coronary heart disease, he found neurological abnormalities in 21% of the patients prior to surgery.

II

Postoperative Neuropsychiatric Syndromes: Identification and Assessment

The Psychopathology and Cognitive Disorder Syndrome (PCD) in Open-Heart Surgery Patients

A.E. Willner, C.J. Rabiner

Summary

In a follow-up study of 100 patients consecutively scheduled for open-heart surgery, Rabiner and Willner found strikingly different mortality rates during the 5 years after hospital discharge in two groups of patients. Patients who had two different types of abnormality, psychopathology before hospital discharge and devastated scores on the Conceptual Level Analogy Test (CLAT), had a significantly and substantially higher mortality rate than patients who had only one or neither abnormality.

We designate patients with both abnormalities as having the psychopathology and cognitive disorder (PCD) syndrome. The psychopathology of PCD syndrome patients differs from the psychopathology of PCD syndrome patients differs from the psychopathology of patients without cognitive disorder (non-PCD) in several ways:

1. The mortality rate in PCD patients is almost six times as high (63% vs 11%) as it is in patients with non-PCD psychopathology, during the 5 years after hospital discharge.
2. Patients who have either depression and/or organic brain syndrome have more than three as high (82% vs 25%) an incidence of PCD than do patients with neither depressive nor organic psychopathology.

These observations are consistent with a hypothesis that the PCD syndrome is a manifestation of an often unsuspected preoperative organic brain syndrome. We maintain that the PCD syndrome indicates a vulnerability factor which results in many PCD patients developing psychopathology even before the additional stress of open-heart surgery is imposed. The greater incidence of depression and organic brain syndromes in PCD patients than in those having psychopathology but not cognitive disorder is consistent with explanation in terms of hypoxic symptoms in the PCD group. (Cognitive disorder and depression are well recognized symptoms of cerebral hypoxia.) The underlying organic brain syndrome is assumed to be a result of cerebral hypoxia related to reduced cerebral circulation.

The basic approach here is to use scores on a special (CLAT) analogy test as external points of reference in distinguishing two different psychopathological groups.

Several case illustrations will be discussed.

Psychopathological and Neurological Dysfunctions
Following Open-Heart Surgery Ed by Becker et al

Introduction

In a follow-up study of 100 patients consecutively scheduled for open-heart surgery, we found strikingly different mortality rates for two groups of patients during the 5 years after hospital discharge. Patients having two disorders, both psychopathology before hospital discharge and also devastated analogy test scores, had a significantly higher mortality rate than patients with only one or neither disorder.

We designate patients having both abnormalities as having the psychopathology and cognitive disorder (PCD) syndrome. We have not until now described how the psychopathology of PCD syndrome patients differs from the psychopathology seen in other open-heart surgery patients. This paper briefly summarizes our work leading to the identification of the PCD syndrome and then contrasts the psychopathology seen in the two patient groups.

We believe that the PCD syndrome is a manifestation of a usually unsuspected preoperative organic brain syndrome. Moreover, we maintain that the PCD syndrome indicates a vulnerability factor which results in many PCD patients developing psychopathology even before the additional stress of open-heart surgery is imposed. As Meyendorf [12] has shown, the psychopathology currently associated with open-heart surgery has been reported in cardiac patients in the European literature as long ago as 1817. We assume that the underlying organic brain syndrome, which presents as PCD syndrome, is a result of cerebral hypoxia related to reduced cerebral circulation. Cognitive disorder and depression are well recognized symptoms of cerebral hypoxia. One might thus expect to find a significantly higher incidence of depression and organic brain syndromes in PCD patients than in those having psychopathology but not cognitive disorder. Furthermore, one might expect to find a significantly higher incidence of PCD in patients who manifest psychopathology preoperatively than in those who develop symptoms only after the stress of surgery.

Material and Methods

The patients followed are the 69 reported by Willner and Rabiner (1976). Thirty three had coronary bypass surgery, 31 had cardiac valvular surgery, and five had both bypass and vulvular surgery. About 5 years postoperatively all of the patients who could be reached (86% of the overall sample) were interviewed. (The patients had been interviewed preoperatively, postoperatively, and at 18-months follow-up). The clinical interview revealed any evidence of history of psychiatric illness as well as any current psychiatric disorder. A mental status examination inquired about impaired cognitive functions (e.g., defective memory, concentration, thinking, orientation) and psychopathology in general.

Conceptual Level Analogy Test (CLAT)

This test was administered preoperatively, 10 days postoperatively, and at both 18-month and 5-year follow-up examinations. It was scored blind with regard to psychiatric outcome. It is a 42 item multiple choice analogy test which requires vocabulary and information at or below the fourth grade level. The conceptual functioning, however, ranges from being simple to quite complex. Several studies demonstrate a significant relationship between analogy test scores and several other criteria of brain dysfunction: EEG abnormality, neuropsychological test battery scores, neurological soft signa, Bender-Gestalt test findings.

Devastated CLAT Scores

A devastated CLAT score means that the patient obtained no more correct answers than could be expected by chance. Such a devastated score implies extremely poor cognitive functioning and places the patient within the lowest 1% of the normative sample. Yet such patients are very often quite unremarkable on interview, displaying little if any sign of cognitive difficulties or mental slowness.

Results

Table 1 indicates the relationship between preoperative analogy test scores and outcome: in the hospital, and at 18-month and 5-year follow-up. The proportion of patients with devastated preoperative CLAT scores was predicted to rise linearly (in graded series) from good outcome through psychiatric symptoms in the catastrophic outcome group. The Cochran chi-square for linear regression (the component of the total chi-square attributable to a linear relationship between the two variables involved) was used to evaluate the data. Table 1 indicates a highly significant relationship between preoperative CLAT score and postoperative outcome at all intervals. Moreover, the results are quite similar at the three postsurgery time intervals. For example, the proportion of devastated analogy test scores in patients with catastrophic outcome was 77% for in-hospital, 78% for 18-month follow-up, and 80% for 5-year follow-up outcome.

Table 2 indicates a highly significant relationship between preoperative and/or immediately postoperative psychopathology and mortality after hospital discharge.

Since psychopathology and devastated CLAT scores were both significantly related to mortality after hospital discharge, a two-way analysis of variance of proportions evaluated the respective contributions of psychopathology and devastated CLAT scores to mortality. Table 3 shows significant ($P < 0.02$) independent relationships of both variables with mortality. Table 4 shows that the mortality rate of 63% for patients having both disorders (psychopathology and cognitive disorder) was significantly higher ($P < 0.001$) than that of 11% for the remaining patients.

Table 5 divides the 25 patients who had psychopathology into a PCD, and a psychopathology without cognitive disorder group. The incidence of mortality in the PCD group (63%) was significantly higher than that in the non-PCD psychopathology group (11%), $P = 0.017$, Fisher's exact test. Here the presence of a devastated CLAT score was used to divide psychopathological cases into two groups with sharply contrasting mortality rates.

Table 1. Relationship of inhospital CLAT analogy test scores to postoperative outcome for open-heart surgery patients

Preoperative CLAT scores	Good outcome	Psychiatric symptoms	Catastrophic outcome
Inhospital outcome (n = 87)			
Not devastated	38	9	3
Devastated	18 (32%)	9 (50%)	10 (77%)
		Cochran x^2 = 9.07, df = 1, $P < 0.01$	
18-month follow-up outcome (n = 81)			
Not devastated	40	5	2
Devastated	17 (30%)	10 (67%)	7 (78%)
		Cochran x^2 = 11.26, df = 1, $P < 0.001$	
5-year follow-up outcome (n = 63)			
Not devastated	29	5	4
Devastated	12 (29%)	7 (58%)	6 (60%)
		Cochran x^2 = 4.64, df = 1, $P < 0.05$	
5-year follow-up outcome (n = 63) (devastated CLAT score preoperatively or postoperatively)			
Not devastated	27	5	2
Devastated	14 (34%)	7 (58%)	8 (80%)
		Cochran x^2 = 7.70, df = 1, $P < 0.01$	

Table 2. Relationship between inhospital psychiatric diagnosis and mortality during 5 years following hospital discharge

5-year follow-up outcome	Good outcome	Psychiatric symptoms	Preoperative psychiatric symptoms
Alive	39	11	3
Expired	5 (11%)	7 (39%)	4 (57%)

Cochran $x^2 = 10.35$, df = 1, $P < 0.005$

Table 3. Analysis of variance of proportions for relationship between analogy test scores (inhospital and preoperatively) psychopathology, and incidence of mortality during 5 years after hospital discharge

	Psychiatric diagnosis inhospital[a]	
CLAT score preoperative or postoperative	Good outcome	Psychiatric symptoms and preoperative psychiatric symptoms
Not devastated	2/26 (8%)	1/9 (11%)
Devastated	3/18 (17%)	10/16 (63%)

Results of analysis of variance

Source	df	$F_1{}^{\infty}$	P
Psychopathology	1	5.47	$P < 0.02$
CLAT	1	5.57	$P < 0.02$
PxC	1	2.79	NS

[a] In both columns the number and percentage of patients who died are given

Table 6 divides the same 25 patients into two groups, based upon whether or not depression and/or OBS symptomatology was present. Since both depression and organic brain syndromes are frequently seen in hypoxic patients, the patients with depression and/or OBS were predicted to have a significantly higher incidence of PCD than patients with other types of psychopathology. Table 6 indicates that 82% of the depressed and/or OBS patients had PCD as opposed to only 25% of the remaining patients, $P = 0.01$, Fisher's exact test. The PCD patients apparently have a significantly higher incidence of depression and OBS, as well as a significantly higher mortality rate.

Finally, if preoperative psychiatric symptoms represent a significantly greater vulnerability than symptoms occurring only postoperatively, one might expect a significantly higher incidence of PCD in the former than the latter patients. Table 7 indicates a much higher (but not significantly higher) incidence of PCD in patients having preoperative psychopathology.

Table 4. Comparison of mortality rates of patients having both psychopathology and devastated CLAT scores before hospital discharge with patients who did not have both disorders

Condition	5-year mortality	
	Alive	Expired
Patient did not have both disorders	47	6
Patient had both disorders	6	10

$X^2 = 15.31$, df = 1, $P < 0.001$

Table 5. Comparison of mortality rates of PCD patients with those who had psychopathology but not cognitive disorder

5-year mortality			
Condition	Alive	Expired	% Expired
Psychopathology only	8	1	11
PCD	6	10	63

P = 0.017, Fisher's exact test

Table 6. Comparison of incidence of depression and/or OBS in PCD patients with those who had psychopathology but not cognitive disorder

Preoperative and/or postoperative psychopathology	Psychopathological	Group	% PCD
	No cognitive disorder	PCD	
Neither depression nor OBS	6	2	25
OBS and/or depression	3	14	82
% OBS and/or depression	33	88	

P = 0.01, Fisher's exact test

Table 7. Comparison of the incidence of PCD in patients having preoperative psychopathology with those who had psychopathology postoperatively only

Psychopathology	No PCD	PCD	% PCD
Postoperatively only	8	10	56
Preoperative	1	6	86
% Preoperative psychopathology	11	38	

Case Vignettes

Three case vignettes are presented. The first has PCD with preoperative and postoperative psychopathology, the second PCD with postoperative psychopathology only, and the third has non-PCD psychopathology. The first two cases show the combination of depression, organic brain syndrome, and mortality often seen in PCD patients. The third non-PCD case illustrates a more fortunate outcome.

Mr. L.D., a 61-year-old retired electronics worker was quite depressed for several months preoperatively, with sleep disturbance and a substantial weight loss. Before the surgery he had largely recovered from the depression, but was anxious and pessimistic about his chances of survival. He remarked that his first wife had died in the operating room 7 years earlier, after open-heart surgery. In view of his preoperative depressive episode and his devastated CLAT score he was considered to have the PCD syndrome. After an aortic valve replacement he became severely depressed and also showed symptoms of an organic brain syndrome. He was unable to recognize the interviewing psychiatrist, was disoriented with respect to time (he thought it was May when it was actually January), and showed moderate impairment of attention and memory. He also had periods of marked restlessness, agitation, and dysphoric affect. After hospital discharge he had severe organic and depressive episodes, and died 10 months postoperatively.

Mr. R.K., a 67-year-old retired salesman had no preoperative psychopathology. After an aortic valve replacement, he became moderately depressed and showed signs of an organic brain syndrome, including troubles with memory, attention, and concentration. Postoperative retesting was deferred for almost a week because the patient was "mumbling, incoherent, a little deaf." In view of his psychopathology and cognitive disorder, he was considered to have the PCD syndrome. At 18-month follow-up the patient seemed to be doing quite well. However, he said it took a good year to get back to feeling as well as he did preoperatively. At initial contact for 5-year follow-up the patient was moribund, with congestive heart failure, severe liver disorder, and was mentally very slow. Soon thereafter he expired.

Mr. H.K., a 63-year-old executive vice president of a cosmetics firm, with no preoperative psychopathology had a mitral valve replacement. Postoperatively he was delirious, seeing nonexistent "bugs on the walls", "gnats on the window" and a "film of oil" which occasionally interfered with his vision. He had mild difficulties with attention, concentration, and memory. At 18-month follow-up he said "I feel beautiful" and "I would be very encourageing to all patients to go through the operation." He had difficulties due to medical complications during the first 6 to 7 months postoperatively, but when these were resolved he resumed full activity. By 9 months postoperatively he was again working full-time and had started to play golf again. At 5-year follow-up, this 68-year-old man with an eighth grade education was still working full-time as executive vice president of the same large firm. He indicated that he had no problems, and carried out his business responsibilities in fine fashion. In fact he described himself as a workaholic and said that he frequently takes work home. Although he could have retired 5 years earlier, he enjoyed his work. The only difficulty he noted was some sexual potency problems, which perhaps might be expected at the age of 68.

Discussion

These findings seem consistent with the assumption that analogy test scores may be used as an external reference point in distinguishing between two different psychopathological groups, psychopathology of the PCD type and non-PCD psychopathology. Specifically, when PCD syndrome patients and patients whose psychopathology is not PCD are compared:

1. The mortality rate in PCD patients is almost six times as high (63% vs 11%) as it is in patients with non-PCD psychopathology, during the 5 years after hospital discharge.
2. Patients who have either depression and/or organic brain syndrome have more than three times as high (82% vs 25%) an incidence of PCD than do patients with neither depressive nor organic psychopathology.
3. Patients who demonstrate psychopathology preoperatively include a much higher proportion of PCD than non-PCD psychopathology patients (38% vs 11%, not significant).

The PCD syndrome can thus be differentiated from non-PCD psychopathology in terms of a significantly higher mortality rate, a significantly higher incidence of depression and OBS, and a tendency for the psychopathology to occur earlier. These findings are consistent with our hypothesis that the PCD syndrome identifies a usually unsuspected preoperative organic brain syndrome. The case vignettes are presented to contrast the depression and organic brain syndrome often seen in PCD patients and their frequently poor outcome, with the more favorable outcome of patients having non-PCD psychopathology. Presumably the impaired coping ability associated with the cognitive disorder adds significantly to the burden carried by the patient.

There are also major differences in the quality of life of PCD and other open-heart surgery patients. Elsewhere in this symposium, Dr. Rabiner et al. addresses this issue, tracing these differences over a 5-year postoperative period.

References

1. Blachly P, Blachly B (1968) Vocational and emotional status of 263 patients after heart surgery. Circulation 38:524–532
2. Cochran WG (1954) Some methods for strengthening the common chi-square tests. Biometrics 10:417–541
3. Frank K, Heller S, Kornfeld D (1972) A survey of adjustment to cardiac surgery. Arch Intern Med 130:735–738
4. Freyhan FA, Gianelli S Jr, O'Connell RA, et al. (1971) Psychiatric complications following open heart surgery. Compr Psychiatry 12:181–195
5. Heller S, Frank K, Kornfeld D, et al. (1974) Psychological outcome following open heart surgery. Arch Intern Med 134:908–914
6. Heller SS, Frank KA, Malm JR, et al. (1970) Psychiatric complications of open heart surgery: A re-examination. N Engl J Med 283:1015–1020
7. Heller SS, Kornfeld DS, Frank DA, Hoar PF (1979) Postcardiotomy delirium and cardiac output. Am J Psychiatry 135:337–339

8. Kilpatric D, Miller W, Allain A, et al. (1975) The use of psychological test data to predict open heart surgery outcome: a prospective study. Psychosom Med 37:62–73
9. Kimball CP (1969) Psychological responses to the experience of open heart surgery. I. Am J Psychiatry 126:348–359, 1969
10. Kimball CP (1972) The experience of open heart surgery. III. Toward a definition and understanding of postcardiotomy delirium. Arch Gen Psychiatry 27:57–63
11. Kornfeld DS, Heller SS, Frank KA, et al. (1974) Personality and psychological factors in postcardiotomy delirium. Arch Gen Psychiatry 31:249–253
12. Meyendorf R (1980) Psychopathology in heart disease aside from cardiac surgery. In: Speidel H, Rodewald G (eds) Psychopathological and neurological dysfunction following open heart surgery. Thieme, Stuttgart
13. Quinlan DM, Kimball CP, Osborne F (1974) The experience of open heart surgery. IV. Assessment of disorientation and dysphoria following cardiac surgery. Arch Gen Psychiatry 31: 241–244
14. Rabiner CJ, Willner AE (1976) Psychopathology observed on follow-up after coronary bypass surgery. J Nerv Ment Dis 163:295–301
15. Willner AE (1970) Towards development of more sensitive clinical tests of abstraction: The analogy test. Proc Annu Conv Am Psychol Assoc 78:553–554
16. Willner AE (1971) Conceptual level analogy test. Cognitive Testing Service, New York
17. Willner AE, Struve FA (1970) An analogy test that predicts EEG abnormality: Use with hospitalized psychiatric patients. Arch Gen Psychiatry 23:428–437
18. Willner AE, Rabiner CJ, Wisoff BG, et al. (1976) Analogical reasoning and postoperative outcome in patients scheduled for open heart surgery. Arch Gen Psychiatry 33:255–259
19. Willner AE, Rabiner CJ, Wisoff BG, et al. (1976) Analogy tests and psychopathology at followup after open heart surgery. Biol Psychiatry 11:687–696

Brief Psychiatric Inventory for Assessment of Psychopathological Disorders After Open-Heart Surgery*

B. Dahme, P. Götze, M. Wessel

Introduction

In our contribution to the first symposium we pointed out the lack of a standard technique to assess psychiatric disorders after open-heart surgery [2]. Although several well-constructed inventories exist for assessment of psychiatric symptoms, they are nevertheless rarely used even in Anglo-American research. Major reasons for this seem to be the inordinate length of time required to employ the major inventories (e.g., PSE) or the inappropriateness of the short instruments (e.g., BPRS) for measuring psychological changes after open-heart surgery.

In an attempt to rectify this situation, we have constructed a brief inventory to assess psychological changes after open-heart surgery. Classical test theory [5] was employed. It was our hope that the instrument would be as short as possible and easily mastered to permit use by nonpsychiatrists, especially cardiac surgeons and cardiologists. Only a preliminary version of the symptom check test will be presented since development of the instrument is still in progress.

Test construction was based on the assessment of psychological symptoms in a random sample of 99 patients undergoing open-heart surgery. All patients were rated by an experienced psychiatrists 1) 1 week before surgery, 2) at least once a day during the first 4 postoperative days, and 3) 3 weeks after surgery. Each symptom was rated on a four point scale from distinctly present to absent.

Symptoms were measured by the AMDP system (formerly the AMP): Part Two: Psychopathological Status. The system, which comprises 11 scales, includes 110 symptoms, many of which are also part of the PSE (Present State Examination) [5]. The latter is better known and used more in Anglo-American research, while the former is employed to a greater extent in German psychiatric research [1].

Data Reduction Strategy

The short version should be based upon several uncorrelated scales with a minimum of items necessary to assess the relevant postoperative psychopathological symptoms.

*With the aid of the Deutsche Forschungsgemeinschaft, Sonderforschungsbereich 115, Teilprojekt A 3

Psychopathological and Neurological Dysfunctions
Following Open-Heart Surgery Ed by Becker et al

Each scale should be of good internal consistency and homogeneity. The resulting short version should agree closely with the original 110 items form with regard to psychopathological syndromes.

To obtain these goals, methods of item, factor, and cluster analysis have been employed.

Item Analysis

Data reduction was reached by item analysis. Each symptom was examined for frequency of occurrence in the sample. With the exception of the five symptoms comprising the Illusions/Hallucinations Scale and the symptom, self-mutilation and suicide, each symptom was required to be present in 5% of the patients on at least 1 of the 4 postoperative days.

Correlation (^{r}it) of each symptom with the total score of the AMDP scale to which it belongs was subsequently calculated. Finally, coefficient alpha for each symptom scale was computed. Both coefficients are based only upon the items fulfilling the frequency criterion plus the five items mentioned above.

Factor Analysis

Factor analysis was used to regroup symptoms from their original AMDP scales into syndromes of postoperative psychological disturbance. Squared multiple correlations were employed as estimates of the communality with varimax rotation to insure factor orthogonality. All items with a loading of greater than 0.4 were included on a given factor.

Cluster Analysis

Cluster analyses of the 40 item scale, the first short version, were then run for comparison with cluster analyses using the original 11 scale, 110 item form. Analyses were performed on two sets of factor scores. The first set was an unweighted sum of scores for each symptom with a loading greater than 0.4 on a given factor. The second set was the score of the most descriptive symptom on the factor (i.e., the symptom having the highest loading). In each case, scores were included for the 4 postoperative days.

Results

Item Analyses

Item analyses including symptom incidence, item-total correlations (^{r}it) and coefficient Alpha are presented in Table 1. Because of too low internal consistency and homoge-

Table 1. Statistics of the scales and items of the preliminary version of the AMDP brief psychiatric rating scale for assessment of psychopathological disorders after open-heart surgery

Item No.		Symptoms	Percentage of occurrence						Scales of early postoperative disturbances: internal consistency, homogeneity	
			pre-	postoperative				late		
				1	2	3	4		r_{it}	alpha
1	1.	*Reduced consciousness (vigilance)*	00	26	25	17	13	00		
	2.	*Disturbances of orientation*								*0.89*
2		Time	00	12	14	14	09	02	0.77	
3		Place	00	01	04	05	04	00	0.89	
		Situation	00	05	05	06	04	00	0.85	
	3.	*Attention and memory disturbances*								*0.85*
4		Comprehension	29	40	43	30	23	15	0.75	
5		Concentration	46	64	70	61	60	42	0.72	
6		Short term memory	47	39	33	29	27	21	0.73	
7		Recent memory	13	08	09	08	12	07	0.62	
	4.	*Thinking disorders*								*0.43*
8		Slowed thinking	32	58	52	51	43	32	0.37	
9		Narrowed thinking	37	67	66	60	52	17	0.27	
10		Tangential thinking	19	12	14	14	15	13	0.14	
11		Perseverative thinking	02	06	05	04	07	05	0.28	
12	5.	*Secondary hypochondriasis*	00	05	06	02	03	01		
	6.	*Paranoia*								*0.94*
13		Paranoid ideas	00	02	07	05	06	00	0.91	
		Paranoid delusions	00	01	03	03	04	00	0.90	
		Paranoid moods	00	02	06	04	04	00	0.89	
	7.	*Sense misperceptions*								*0.84*
14		Visual illusions	00	03	08	05	05	01	0.69	
15		Auditory illusions	00	04	04	04	02	00	0.63	
16		Visual hallucinations	00	02	04	04	04	00	0.82	
17		Auditory hallucinations	00	01	02	03	03	00	0.75	
18	8.	*Derealization*	00	07	08	04	04	00		
	9.	*Affect disturbances*								*0.90*
	9.1	Depression								

Table 1 (continued)

Item No.		Symptoms	Percentage of occurrence						Scales of early postoperative disturbances: internal consistency, homogeneity	
			pre-	postoperative				late		
				1	2	3	4		r_{it}	alpha
19		Internally restless	66	50	62	56	47	24	0.89	
		Tense	63	50	62	50	43	15	0.86	
20		Anxious	67	43	58	50	35	12	0.80	
21		Depressed, sad	29	20	34	39	26	18	0.59	
22		Hopeless	12	08	19	13	07	01	0.65	
	9.2	Reduced affectivity								*0.74*
23		Blunted affect	04	07	10	09	05	03	0.46	
24		Affective inflexibility	04	09	11	06	05	05	0.73	
25		Feeling of inadequacy	32	09	16	13	11	21	0.59	
	9.3	Other symptoms of affect disturbances								*0.25*
26		Sullen, irritated	07	06	18	17	14	12	0.18	
27		Suspicious, hostile	09	02	10	06	04	01	0.44	
28		Helpless	05	13	16	09	14	02	0.0	
29		Lability of mood	22	08	09	12	11	13	0.03	
30		Euphoric mood	04	08	04	04	03	06	–0.10	
	10.	*Impulse and psychomotoric disturbances*								*–0.75*
31		Restlessness	04	09	17	18	10	01	–0.29	
32		Apathy	14	14	25	35	27	27		
	11.	*Social dysfunction*								*0.49*
33		Social withdrawal	03	07	13	11	07	01	0.36	
34		Aggressive ideas & behavior	00	01	07	04	05	00	0.57	
35		Tendencies toward self harm	00	00	01	02	01	00	–0.03	
36		Suicidal ideas or behavior	00	00	02	00	00	00	0.05	

neity of the correspondent original scales some have been subdivided into subscales. Item-total correlations and coefficient Alpha are referred either to the original or subdivided AMDP scales.

Examination reveals:

1. Frequency analysis has reduced the number of symptoms from 110 to 40.
2. For the 40 items, the number of relevant symptoms per scale ranges from 1 to 5.
3. Some symptom scales have high internal consistency (r_{it}) and homogeneity (coefficient Alpha):
   Disturbances of Orientation, Attention and Memory Disturbances, Paranoid Delusions, Illusions/Hallucinations and Depression. The scale Reduced Affectivity, has moderate reliability. Finally, the remaining scales generally have poor reliabilities.
4. Several original AMDP scales were subdivided using exploratory factor analysis:
   The original scale, Affective Disorders, was subdivided into three subscales: Depression, Reduced Affectivity, and Other Symptoms. The original scale, Impulse and Psychomotoric Disorders, was subdivided into Psychomotoric Restlessness and Apathy.
5. Some symptom scales or item groups have at least two items with $r_{it} \geqslant 0.85$. – These are so highly correlated that they could be considered to measure essentially the same (latent) disturbance. This is given for the symptom patterns:
- disturbances of orientation in place and situation ($r = 0.92$),
- paranoid ideas, delusions, and moods ($0.86 \leqslant r \leqslant 0.89$),
- internally restless and tense feeling ($r = 0.93$).

So it is justified to condense these to three items.
By item analysis the number of items has been further reduced to 36 and this will be the preliminary and version of a rather short symptom check list. The selected 36 items are marked by the respective numbers in the first column of Table 1.

Factor Analysis

Eight factors resulted from factor analysis. The first seven were rather homogeneous whereas the last one had lower internal consistency. Factors are named after those symptoms loading most highly on the factor and include:

1. *General Disorientation:* disorientation, deficits in remembering recent events, motoric restlessness, and some auditory illusions accompanied by subjective helplessness.
2. *Impaired Thinking/Concentration:* impaired attention, concentration and short term memory, clouded vigilance and slowed thinking.
3. *Paranoid-Hallucinatory Syndrome:* delusions, illusions, hallucinations, and derealization.
4. *Worry/Anxiety:* accompanied by narrowed thinking and secondary hypochondriasis.
5. *Sullen Inadequacy:* affective inflexibility, feeling of insufficiency, loss of affect and drive, depressive mood, accompanied by slowed thinking.

Table 2. "Syndromes" of psychopathological symptoms after open-heart surgery assessed by a short version of the AMDP system: psychopathological status. Results of a common factor analysis

Factor I: Disorientation		Factor II: Impaired thinking/concentration		Factor III: Paranoid-hallucinatory syndrome	
Disorientation in		Impaired concentration	0.80	Paranoid	
– time	0.73	Slowed thinking	0.72	– delusions	0.87
– place	0.89	Impaired attention	0.64	– ideas	0.87
– situation	0.87	Reduced consciousness	0.67	– moods	0.85
Restlessness	0.57	Impaired short-term memory	0.54	Visual hallucinations	0.81
Helplessness	0.54	Apathy	0.43	Auditory illusions	0.70
Impaired recent memory	0.48			Hearing voices	0.69
Auditory illusion	0.40			Derealization	0.60
alpha = 0.79		*alpha = 0.81*		*alpha = 0.92*	

Table 2 (continued)

Factor IV: Worry/Anxiety		Factor V: Gloomy inadequacy		Factor VI: Hostility		Factor VII: Loss of control	
Anxious	0.89	Affective inflexibility	0.77	Hostile	0.88	Perseverative thinking	0.82
Feeling of restlessness	0.85	Feeling of inadequacy	0.72	Aggressive		Euphoric mood	0.70
Tense	0.78	Depressed	0.64	– ideas	0.88	Suicide ideas	0.66
Narrowed thinking	0.57	Lack of affect	0.58	– behavior	0.75	Impaired recent memory	0.56
Hopelessness	0.52	Apathy	0.55	Sullen	0.72	Tangential thinking	0.55
Depressed	0.46	Slowed thinking	0.47	Social withdrawal	0.41		
Secondary hypochondriasis	0.46						
alpha = 0.89		*alpha = 0.81*		*alpha = 0.80*		*alpha = 0.74*	

6. *Hostility:* accompanied by a tendency of withdrawal.
7. *Loss of Control:* perseverative (and intricate) thinking, elevated mood, thoughts of suicide, and impaired remembering.
8. *Given up:* characterized by self-mutilation and deep hopelessness.

On the basis of factor analysis one could thus conclude that symptomatology following open-heart surgery can be reduced to the above eight core symptoms.

Cluster Analysis

Results of the cluster analyses are presented in Tables 3 and 4 for composite factor scores.

Cluster analysis of the long version of the AMDP reported previously by Götze [3] and Götze and Dahme [4] yielded five clusters of patients (Table 3): Unremarkable, Slight Psycho-organic Syndrome with Affective-Emotional and Psychomotoric Disturbances, Severe Psycho-organic Syndrome with Disturbances of Perception and Psychomotility, Paranoid Hallucinatory Syndrome with affective-emotional and psychomotoric disturbances, and Delirious Syndrome.

Table 3. Results of cluster analysis: 11 original AMDP scales [3]

	Clusters of the original scales (110 items)
G1:	"Unremarkable" (n = 49)
G2:	"Slight psycho-organic syndrome with affective-emotional and psychomotoric disturbances" (n = 33)
G3:	"Severe psycho-organic syndrome with disturbances of perception and psychomotility" (n = 4)
G4:	"Paranoid-hallucinatory syndrome with affective-emotional and psychomotoric disturbances" (n = 9)
G5:	"Delirious syndrome" (n = 4)

Table 4. Clusters of the short version (4 items)

SV1:	"Unremarkable" (n = 28)
SV2:	"Slight psycho-organic syndrome with anxious-subdepressive moods" (n = 23)
SV3:	"Severe psycho-organic syndrome with disturbances of orientation, concentration, reduced vigilance and lack of selfcontrol" (n = 4)
SV4:	"Delirious syndrome" (n = 4; identical to G5)
SV5:	"Rather unremarkable, very slight symptoms of anxious and tense depression, derealization; maximum of symptoms: 2nd day" (n = 32)
SV6:	"Hostility associated with paranoid-hallucinatory symptoms and anxious, tense depression; maximum of disturbances: 2nd day" (n = 8)

Cluster analysis of this short form yielded six clusters (Table 4): Unremarkable, Slight Psycho-organic Syndrome with Disturbances of Orientation, Concentration, Reduced Vigilance and Lack of Self Control, Delirious Syndrome, Rather Unremarkable, and Hostility. Maximum disturbance for the last two clusters appears to occur on the 2nd day.

Comparison of the two analyses suggests the following observations:

1. The original "Unremarkable" Cluster (G1) has split into two clusters: Unremarkable (SV 1) and Rather Unremarkable (SV 5). However the new Rather Unremarkable cluster (SV 5) also includes patients originally part of the Slight Psycho-organic Syndrome cluster (G2) and the Paranoid-Hallucinatory cluster (G4).
2. Overall contingency of both cluster analyses is significant but not very high (phi = 0.55). Three clusters of the new analyses correspond well to clusters on the original form: G2 with SV2, Slight Psycho-organic Syndrome; G3 with SV3, Severe Psycho-organic Syndrome; and G5 with SV4, Delirious Syndrome. If one omits SV 5 and SV6 from the contingency analysis, an improvement in phi to 0.76 is noted (Table 5).
3. Use of the short form will generally convey information similar to the longer form. This is especially true for assessment of Slight and Severe Psycho-organic Syndromes and Delirium. Greater differences are likely to occur in the assessment of Unremarkable outcomes and outcomes with paranoid-hallucinatory symptomatology.

Conclusion and Summary

In summary, the 11 scale, 110 item AMDP, Part II; Psychopathological status was reduced to a brief 8 scale, 36 item rating questionnaire using item and factor analysis. Subsequent first validation attempt through cluster analysis demonstrated the use-

Table 5. Contingency of cluster analyses of the postoperative psychopathological status assessed by:
1. The 11 original AMDP-scales (clusters G1, ..., G5)
2. The eight new scales derived from the short version (clusters SV1, ..., SV6)

	G1	G2	G3	G4	G5	Σ
SV1	*28*	0	0	0	0	28
SV2	0	*20*	1	2	0	23
SV3	0	1	*3*	0	0	4
SV4	0	0	0	0	*4*	4
SV5	20	8	0	4	0	32
SV6	1	4	0	3	0	8
Σ	49	33	4	9	4	

Contingency of the whole table: phi = 0.5; χ^2 = 119.6, df = 20; $P < 0.001$
Contingency of the upper part [(G1 ... G5) × (SV1 ... SV4)]: phi = 0.76; χ^2 = 102.59, df = 12; $P < 0.001$

fulness of the short form. It is hoped that the short form might serve as a standard assessment instrument both for clinical practice and research. Plans exist for its translation into other languages.

Acknowledgment: The authors are very grateful to Dr. Jeremy Katz for his aid in translation and his essential improvements of the manuscript.

References

1. Arbeitsgemeinschaft für Methodik und Dokumentation in der Psychiatrie (1979) Das AMDP-System. Manual zur Dokumentation psychiatrischer Befunde, 3rd edn. Springer, Berlin Heidelberg New York
2. Dahme B, Götze P (1980) Objective classification of psychopathological symptoms after open heart surgery. In: Speidel H, Rodewald G (eds) Psychic and neurological dysfunctions after open-heart surgery. Thieme, Stuttgart
3. Götze P (1980) Psychopathologie der Herzoperierten. Enke, Stuttgart
4. Götze P, Dahme B (1980) Psychopathological syndromes and neurological disturbances after open-heart surgery. In: Speidel H, Rodewald G (eds) Psychic and neurological dysfunctions after open-heart surgery. Thieme, Stuttgart
5. Lord FM, Novick MR (1968) Statistical theories of mental test scores. Addison-Wesley, Reading/Mass
6. Wing JK, Cooper JE, Sartorius N (1974) The measurement and classification of psychiatric symptoms. University Press, Cambridge

Hamburg Rating Scale for Psychic Disturbances – HRPD*

A Brief Psychiatric Rating Scale for the Assessment of Psychic Disturbances After Open-Heart Surgery (Preliminary Version: August 1980)

Editors: P. Götze, B. Dahme

Co-workers: B. Dahme, B. Flemming, P. Götze, G. Huse-Kleinstoll, H.-J. Meffert, H. Speidel, M. Wessel

Introduction

The Hamburg Rating Scale has been established in a stepwise test construction of several years in order to get easier and more standardized assessment, description, and classification of psychopathological disorders after open-heart surgery.

The actual Scale is based on a former version of the AMP or present day AMDP Scales for assessment of psychopathological symptoms. These Scales have been developed in cooperation with a large section of psychiatric clinics in the German speaking countries. These Scales have been used in USA as well by Freyhan et al. [1] for studying postcardiotomic psychiatric symptoms.

In our first research project we have already omitted 12 irrelevant items from the original version of 110 items. But this 98 item version was very difficult to handle and is not appropriate for research and clinical routine in a nonprimarily psychiatric area such as heart surgery. So we developed a (preliminary) reduced version of only 36 items that – according to our present results – nearly has the same discriminative and classificatory validity as the original 98 item version. Details of the methods employed and results of the test construction are outlined in Dahme et al. (this volume).

Use of Rating Scale

This "manual" is divided into two parts:

- list of 36 items each associated with four rating categories.
- instructions for assessment of the psychopathological symptoms.

It is very important that the observer and rater of the psychic disorders should pay some attention to these instructions in order to obtain an unequivocal assessment and a high interrater concordance.

Conceptually the 36 items belong to 11 general psychopathological categories generally accepted in psychiatry: disturbances of 1) consciousness (vigilance), 2) orientation, 3) attention and memory, 4) thinking, 5) secondary hypochondriasis, 6) paranoia,

*With the aid of the Deutsche Forschungsgemeinschaft, Sonderforschungsbereich 115, Teilprojekt A3

7) sense of misperceptions, disturbances of 8) ego, 9) affect and mood, 10) impulse and psychomotoric abilities, 11) social dysfunction.

The empirical analysis of psychopathological symptoms after open-heart surgery by means of factoranalytical statistical techniques resulted in eight mutually independent symptom groups or syndromes essentially based on these 36 items:

1. General disorientation
2. Impaired thinking/concentration
3. Paranoid-hallucinatory syndrome
4. Worry/Anxiety
5. Sullen inadequency
6. Hostility
7. Loss of control
8. Given up.

These symptom groups can be regarded as rather uncorrelated *subscales* of the whole rating Scale. (For further details look at Dahme et al., this volume).

In applying the rating Scale for research or clinical aims the rating values of each item should be summed up within each subscale to obtain a quantitative raw value for each of the eight subscales (cf. Table 3, see also Table 2 in Dahme et al., this volume).

Technically these eight subscales are of the Likert type. Because homogeneity of items within each subscale has been maximized by factor analysis it is justified to simply sum up the rating values of items within a subscale.

Up to now (March 1981) a crossvalidation of the Hamburg rating Scale is missing. We hope to realize a cross-validation by a multicentric research program.

Table 1. Hamburg Rating Scale for Psychic Disturbances – HRPD.
A brief psychiatric rating scale for the assessment of psychic disturbances after open-heart surgery.
List of 36 items each associated with four rating categories

Name of patient . . . . Code . . . .
Age (in years) . . . . male . . . . female . . . .
Diagnosis. . . . .
Date and time of investigation. . . . .
Date of operation. . . . .
Rater . . . .

		Absent	Present		
			Severity of symptom		
No.	Symptom	0	Moderate 1	Distinct 2	Severe 3
1.	Reduced vigilance				
2.	Disturbances of orientation: Time				
3.	Disturbances of orientation: Place/Situation				
4.	Attention & memory disturbances: Comprehension				
5.	Attention & memory disturbances: Concentration				
6.	Attention & memory disturbances: Short-term memory				
7.	Attention & memory disturbances: Recent memory				
8.	Thinking disorders: Slowed thinking				
9.	Thinking disorders: Narrowed thinking				
10.	Thinking disorders: Tangential thinking				
11.	Thinking disorders: Perseverative thinking				
12.	Secondary hypochondriasis/Phobias				
13.	Paranoia				
14.	Sense misperceptions: Visual illusions				
15.	Sense misperceptions: Auditory illusions				
16.	Sense misperceptions: visual hallucinations				
17.	Sense misperceptions: auditory hallucinations				
18.	Derealization				
19.	Affect disturbances – depression: internally restless, tense				
20.	Affect disturbances – depression: anxious				
21.	Affect disturbances – depression: depressed, sad				
22.	Affect disturbances – depression: hopeless				

Table 1 (continued)

No.	Symptom	Absent	Present		
			Severity of symptom		
			Moderate	Distinct	Severe
		0	1	2	3
23.	Affect disturbances – reduced affectivity: blunted affect				
24.	Affect disturbances – reduced affectivity: affective inflexibility				
25.	Affect disturbances – reduced affectivity: feeling of inadequacy				
26.	Other aspects of affect disturbances: sullen, irritated, dysphoric				
27.	Other aspects of affect disturbances: suspicious, hostile				
28.	Other aspects of affect disturbances: helpless				
29.	Other aspects of affect disturbances: lability of mood				
30.	Other aspects of affect disturbances: euphoric mood				
31.	Impulse & psychomot. disturbances: restlessness				
32.	Impulse & psychomot. disturbances: apathy				
33.	Social dysfunction: social withdrawal				
34.	Social dysfunction: aggressive ideas or behavior				
35.	Social dysfunction: tendencies toward self harm				
36.	Social dysfunction: suicidal ideas or behavior				

Remarks:

Table 2. Instructions for use of the Hamburg Rating Scale for Psychic Disturbances (HRPD)

1. Disturbances of Consciousness

Item

(1) *Reduced Consciousness (Reduced Vigilance):*
In the sense of somnolence or drowsiness. (Do not rate if patient is soporific or comatose).

2. Disturbances of Orientation

(2) *In Time:* The patient does not know the day/month, year or season.
(The day of surgery may be presented as a help in orientation.)

(3) *Place/Situation:* The patient does not know that he is in the intensive care unit (moderate); in the hospital (distinct); or has no idea where he is (severe).
The patient does not clearly recognize the present situation but accepts after explanation (moderate); despite explanation he cannot accept his present situation (distinct); beyond this the patient does not know that he has had surgery (severe).

3. Attention and Memory Disturbances

(4) *Disturbances of Comprehension:* The patient cannot sufficiently grasp the meaning of verbal remarks.

(5) *Disturbances of Concentration:* The patient's attention is easily diverted, for example in conversation, by inner or outer stimuli.

(6) *Short-term Memory Disturbances:* The patient cannot completely repeat from short-term memory the name (e.g., of the researcher), characteristics, two digit numbers, or visual impressions after a period of 5 min.

(7) *Recent Memory Disturbances:* The ability to remember is reduced or practically absent. The patient is unable to remember important recently occurring events (visit of the physician who is treating him or relatives). Associated with this is retrograde, anterograde, and partial amnesias.

4. Thinking Disorders

(8) *Slowed Thinking:* Thought processes are slowed and are perceived as disturbed by the patient himself.

(9) *Narrowed Thinking:* The patient is extraordinarily situationally limited with regard to content of his thinking and especially to everything concerning the operation or aftercare. He can scarcely be diverted to other topics for any length of time.

(10) *Tangential Thinking:* Essential aspects are explained with too much tangential material.

(11) *Perseverative Thinking:* The same facts of a situation are frequently senselessly repeated without the patient noticing it.

5. Secondary Hypochondriasis

(12) *Secondary Hypochondriasis:* The patient tends to scrutinize, more intensively than desirable, his bodily functions as well as the treatment of medical and nursing personnel.

6. Paranoia

(13) *Paranoid Moods/Paranoid Delusions/Paranoid Ideas:*

Paranoid Moods: The patient conveys verbally or nonverbally that he experiences himself or his surroundings as changed and as a consequence is alarmed.

Paranoid Delusions: Objective sense perceptions take on an imaginary new meaning mostly in terms of ideas of reference.

Paranoid Ideas: Imaginary thought, feeling and behavior patterns, not correctable by the patient or those around him. The patterns range from anxiety-arousing (for example, ideas of reference) to terrifying (for example, fears of persecution, or intent to kill).

7. Sense Misperceptions

---

(14) *Visual Illusions:* Actually present persons or objects are falsely identified. Above all, objects can be perceived as changed in their form, color, or function.
(15) *Auditory Illusions:* Actually present voices and sounds are falsely identified.
(16) *Visual Hallucinations:* Subjective visual perceptions without the actual presence of real persons or objects.
(17) *Auditory Hallucinations:* Subjective hearing of voices, sounds or noise without the objective presence of corresponding voices, sounds or noise.

8. Ego Disturbances

---

(18) *Derealization:* The surroundings appear unreal, strange, disconcerting, and thus anxiety arousing.

9. Affect Disturbances

Depression
(19) *Internally restless/tense:* The patient appears mentally troubled and tense in his composure, is most visibly anxious but generally only talks about his mental condition upon questioning.
(20) *Anxious:* The patient expresses anxiety in his mood and behavior or speaks directly about his anxieties.
(21) *Depressed/Sad:* The mood is continuously low. The patient appears defeated, scarcely speaks, and even cries quietly to himself.
(22) *Hopeless:* The patient no longer believes in a positive future or his survival.

Reduced Affectivity
(23) *Blunted Affect:* The patient shows inappropriately little emotion.
(24) *Affective Inflexibility:* Independent of a change in situation, the patient remains bound to the same emotional expression.
(25) *Feeling of Inadequacy:* Confidence in one's own capacities is diminished.

Other Symptoms of Affect Disturbances
(26) *Sullen/Irritated/Dysphoric:* An unharmonious mood colored with tinges of aggression.
(27) *Suspicious/Hostile:* The patient tends to impute to his surroundings negative intentions directed toward him and to behave in a correspondingly rejecting fashion.
(28) *Helpless:* The patient experiences his own incapacity to help himself as very unpleasant. He feels as though he has succumbed.
(29) *Lability of Mood:* A condition of rapid mood changes in which it is discernible that the patient has succumbed to his mood experience.
(30) *Euphoric Mood:* The patient finds himself in an inappropriately elevated mood.

10. Impulse and Psychomotoric Disturbances

---

(31) *Restless:* Constant, frequently undirected motoric activity.
(32) *Apathetic:* The patient scarcely moves himself, appears flaccid without tension, has no interest in his surroundings, speaks little.

11. Social Dysfunction

---

(33) *Social Withdrawal:* The patient is capable of and wants to establish or maintain an appropriate relationship with nursing and medical personnel but will not make the effort to do so.

(34) *Aggressive Ideas and Behavior:* Inappropriate aggressive ideas or behavior, expressed spontaneously or upon inquiry, which are directed at nursing or medical personnel. Aggressive behavior is observed, if it occurs, almost entirely with psychotic patients.

(35) *Tendencies Toward Self-Harm:* The patient hinders or makes impossible nursing or medical treatment due to current ill temper or moods. Active self-damaging tendencies such as the ripping out of arterial catheters or jumping out of bed with all tubes in place occurs only with psychotic patients.

(36) *Suicidal Ideas or Behavior:* Suicidal thoughts or behavior, expressed spontaneously or upon inquiry.

Table 3. Hamburg rating scale for psychic disorders (HRPD). Construction of subscales of the 36 items

No.	Subscale	No. of items forming the subscale
1	General disorientation	(2) + (3) + (6) + (15) + (28) + (31)
2	Impaired thinking/concentration	(1) + (4) + (5) + (6) + (8) + (32)
3	Paranoid-hallucinatory syndrome	(13) + (15) + (16) + (17) + (18)
4	Worry/anxiety	(9) + (11) + (19) + (20) + (21) + (22)
5	Gloomy inadequacy	(8) + (21) + (23) + (24) + (25) + (32)
6	Hostility	(26) + (27) + (33) + (34)
7	Loss of control	(7) + (10) + (11) + (30) + (36)
8	Given up	(22) + (35)

Acknowledgment. The authors are very grateful to Dr. Jeremy Katz for his aid in translation and his essential improvements of the manuscript.

Reference

1. Freyhan FA, Gianelli S Jr, O'Connell RA, et al. (1971) Psychiatric complications following open-heart surgery. Compr Psychiatry 12:181–195

Relationship Between Psychopathological Syndromes Before and After Open-Heart Surgery*, **

P. Götze, B. Flemming, G. Huse-Kleinstoll, H.-J. Meffert, Ch. Reimer, H. Speidel

Introduction

Generally most descriptions of psychopathological syndromes before and after open-heart surgery rely on clinical observation and the ability of the observer to record his findings in a skillful and accurate fashion. Within the Hamburg group [2,4] an objective technique for rating psychopathology after open-heart surgery has been developed. As a consequence such syndromes, as well as their interrelationships, can be described in a fashion which is less subjective and is consonant with the highest standards of measurement in the social sciences.

The present investigation was carried out on 100 patients of both sexes, ages 20–59, who underwent open-heart surgery from 1975–1977 in the Department of Cardiovascular Surgery and Experimental Cardiology, University Hospital Hamburg-Eppendorf. Exept for age, no other selection criteria were used.

The type of heart disease according to age and sex is presented in Table 1. On the whole, the breakdown corresponds very closely to that for the Department of Cardiovascular Surgery of the Hamburg University Clinic during the period mentioned.

A modified standard assessment scale, the AMDP (AMDP = *A*rbeitsgemeinschaft für *M*ethodik und *D*okumentation in der *P*sychiatrie) [1] was used to document psychopathological findings. The 11 AMDP main scales, composed of differing numbers of items (or symptoms), are presented in Table 2. Each item was rated by a qualified ex-

Table 1. Distribution of heart disease by age and sex

Heart-disease	n	♂	♀	Age (x)
Congenital	12	6	6	34
Valvular	57	33	24	48
Coronary	26	22	4	53
Combined	5	4	1	48
Total	100	65	35	48

* Data processing was carried out by M. Wessel

** With the aid of the Deutsche Forschungsgemeinschaft, Sonderforschungsbereich 115, Teilprojekt A3

Psychopathological and Neurological Dysfunctions Following Open-Heart Surgery Ed by Becker et al

Table 2. AMDP scales: Areas of psychopathological disturbances

1.	Vigilance
2.	Orientation
3.	Attention/memory
4.	Formal thinking
5.	Hypochondriac moods/phobia
6.	Paranoia
7.	Perception (illusions, hallucinations)
8.	Derealization
9.	Mood
10.	Psychomotility
11.	Social behavior

pert on a four point scale from present to absent. Ratings were made during the following four time periods.

1. The last preoperative week
2. Each of the first 4 postoperative days
3. The 3rd – 4th postoperative week
4. Three to four years after the operation.

With the aid of cluster analysis (classification algorithm K-means) [5], a multivariate statistical technique, groups or clusters of those patients were formed whose 11 AMDP symptom characteristic profiles were similar in type, intensity and course of illness (Table 2) [2, 4].

Results

Cluster analysis yielded four groups (clusters) in the preoperative phase, five groups in the early postoperative phase, and four pathological groups in the late postoperative phase (Table 3). Each syndrome is named descriptively after the main symptoms characterizing it (in capitals).

Detailed account of the psychopathological syndromes and the individual symptoms comprising them have been given elsewhere [3, 4]. In the present paper the most important relationships between psychopathological syndromes of different phases will be presented and discussed.

Relationship Between Clusters

Relationship Between Preoperative and Early Postoperative Clusters

1. In the preoperative phase 69% of the patients were classified as psychopathologically symptom free, 31% as symptomatic. In the early postoperative phase the figures were 49.5% and 50.5%, respectively.

Table 3. Psychopathological syndromes in the preoperative, early and late postoperative phase

No.	Cluster (psychopathological syndrome)		n	Age (x)
	Preoperative phase			
1.	Symptom-free		69	46
2.	Affective-emotional syndrome with contact disturbances		7	48
3.	Slight psycho-organic syndrome with affective-emotional and psychomotor disturbances		19	49
4.	Phobic moods syndrome		5	53
		Total	100	48
	Early postoperative phase			
1.	Symptom-free		49	45
2.	Slight psycho-organic syndrome with affective-emotional and psychomotor disturbances		33	39
3.	Severe psycho-organic syndrome with disturbances of perception and psychomotility		4	54
4.	Paranoid-hallucinatory syndrome with affective-emotional and psychomotor disturbances		9	48
5.	Delirious syndrome		4	53
		Total	99	48
	Late postoperative phase			
1.	Symptom-free		54	46
2.	Psychomotor moods syndrome		24	45
3.	Slight psycho-organic syndrome with affective-emotional and psychomotor disturbances		14	53
4.	Moderately-severe psycho-organic syndrome with fleeting sensory illusions		4	58
		Total	96	48

2. Overall, 73.3% of the preoperatively symptomatic and 40.6% of the preoperatively symptom-free patients were assessed as disturbed in the early postoperative phase.
3. Thus, although 59.4% of preoperatively symptom-free patients were also symptom free in the early postoperative phase, 11 of the 17 psychotic patients came from this group. Psychotic patients were those falling within the third – fifth early postoperative clusters.
4. Of the 19 patients in the third preoperative cluster, the "Slight Psycho-Organic Syndrome," with one exception, *all* patients were symptomatic postoperatively, and five patients were psychotic!
5. Eight of the nine patients in the fourth early postoperative cluster, the "Paranoid-Hallucinatory Syndrome," showed no preoperative psychopathology.

Relationship Between Early and Late Postoperative Clusters

1. Sixty-four percent of all psychopathologically symptomatic patients in the early postoperative phase were assessed in the late phase as symptom free.
2. Similarly, 64.7% of psychotic patients, which includes those in the third – fifth clusters of the early postoperative phase, were also symptom free. The results suggest that psychosis holds no worse prognosis for the later postoperative period than general psychopathology occurring during the early postoperative period.

Relationship Between Preoperative and Late Postoperative Clusters

1. Almost 72.4% of all psychopathologically symptomatic patients in the preoperative phase were still symptomatic in the late postoperative phase.

Relationship Between Preoperative, Early Postoperative, and Late Postoperative Clusters

1. Only 33% of the patients displayed no psychopathological symptomatology across all three periods. Sixty-seven percent of the patients thus experienced some psychopathology during at least one of these phases.

Relationship of Age, Sex and Type of Heart Disease to Cluster Analytical Syndromes

Preoperative Phase

1. In this phase men are somewhat more frequently symptomatic than women and also older.
2. Patients with multiple valve disease are the most frequently symptomatic; those with congenital disorders the least (Table 4).

Early Postoperative Phase

1. In this phase, no sex differences in frequency of disturbance are noted.
2. The average age of men and women, respectively, is 5 and 4 years higher in symptomatic than symptom-free patients.

Table 4. Incidence of psychopathological disorders by type of heart disease (rel.% of patients)

	Heart disease	n	Age (x)	Rel.% (totally disturbed)	Psychotic (rel.%)
Pre-operative	Multiple valve	14	51	42.9	
	Coronary	26	53	38.5	
	Mitral valve	20	48	30.0	
	Aortic valve	23	45	26.1	
	Combined	5	48	20.0	
	Congenital	12	34	16.7	
	n = 100				
Early post-operative	Multiple valve	13	51	69.2	23.1
	Coronary	26	53	57.5	19.2
	Aortic valve	23	45	47.8	8.7
	Mitral valve	20	48	45.0	25.0
	Combined	5	48	40.0	20.0
	Congenital	12	34	33.3	8.3
	n = 99				
Late post-operative	Multiple valve	12	51	58.3	
	Mitral valve	19	53	52.6	
	Coronary	26	53	46.2	
	Combined	5	48	40.0	
	Aortic valve	22	45	31.8	
	Congenital	12	34	33.3	
	n = 96				

3. Incidence of symptomatology by type of heart disease follows a similar pattern as in the preoperative phase. However, patients with aortic valve diseases are more frequent than mitral valve patients (Table 4).
4. Most noteworthy is that patients with valvular diseases more frequently become psychotic than patients with coronary heart disease, with the exception of aortic valve patients (Table 4).
5. It is also noteworthy that all four patients with a delirious syndrome have valvular diseases (Table 4).

Late Postoperative Phase
1. In this phase relatively more men have psychotic symptoms than women.
2. For both men and women greater age is associated with more frequent disturbance.
3. Patients with mitral valve and coronary disease now lead patients with multiple valvular disease in terms of frequency of occurrence.

Late Follow-up Phase: 3–4 Years Later

Within the scope of a rehabilitation study, we are currently attempting to examine the postoperative course of the 100 patients included in the present study for the period 3–4 years after surgery. The rehabilitation study includes assessment of psychosocial, psychodynamic, psychiatric, neurological and cardiological status.

We are, at present, in contact with 54 of the 100 patients. Of the remaining 46, 35 patients could not be traced, lived too far from Hamburg, could not be induced to participate, or were unable to do so because of illness. Eleven patients died. Interestingly enough, all deceased patients had valvular disease.

The 54 surviving patients clustered into the four groups presented in Table 5. Of these patients, 48.1% were classified as symptom free and 51.9% as psychopathologically symptomatic. Of the 28 patients with psychopathological disorders, 17 were classified under "Slight Psycho-organic Syndrome," seven under "Phobic-Hypochondriacal Moods Syndrome" and four under "Affective-Emotional Syndrome." Twenty-one (80.8%) of the 26 patients who were classified as symptom free in the rehabilitation phase were also symptom free preoperatively.

Table 5. Psychopathological syndromes 3–4 years after cardiac surgery

No.	Cluster	n	Age (x)	♂	♀
1.	Symptom-free	26	45	14	12
2.	Slight psycho-organic syndrome	17	50	14	3
3.	Phobic-hypochondrical moods syndrome	7	51	3	4
4.	Affective-emotional syndrome with psycho-organic disturbances	4	51	4	0
	Total	54	48	25	19

Table 6. Incidence of patients with psychopathological disorders by cardiac diagnoses (3–4 years after surgery)

Heart disease	n	Symptom free	Psychopathological disorders
Congenital	9	5	4
Valvular	23	13	10
Coronary	18	6	12
Combined	4	2	2
Total	54	26	28

Symptomatic patients in the rehabilitation phase appear to distribute themselves over pre- and postoperative clusters without noteworthy patterns. Of these patients 57.1% were symptom free preoperatively.

Relating sex, age, and type of heart disease to clusters, we obtained the following results: Psychopathologically symptomatic patients are on the average 5–6 years older than symptom-free patients. While in the preoperative phase men and women are distributed almost equally between the symptom-free and symptomatic groups, men are more frequently symptomatic in the rehabilitation phase (Table 5). No noteworthy pattern is discernible in the incidence of disturbance by type of heart disease. However, in the larger rehabilitation study, during the rehabilitation phase (Table 6), those patients with coronary disease become psychopathologically symptomatic more frequently than patients with valvular disease.

Discussion/Summary

Distillation of findings presented the following picture. The incidence of some type of psychopathology before or after open-heart surgery appears relatively high, from approximately 30%–50%. Incidence is lowest before surgery but remains consistently near 50% even 3–4 years after. Patients who are symptom free or display a slight psycho-organic brain syndrome preoperatively contribute most frequently to postoperative psychosis observed in the early postoperative period. However, whether the patient becomes psychotic or displays slight psycho-organic symptoms during this phase, the remission rate as assessed during the late postoperative period is relatively high and is about equal for both groups. In addition, preoperative symptomatology makes it likely that psychopathology in the late postoperative period will be observed. Finally, although the incidence of psychopathology generally ranges from 30%–50% within a given period, 66% of all patients experience some symptomatology during at least one phase.

No consistent incidence pattern by age or sex across all phases is observed. However, men tend to be more symptomatic than women for most phases and older patients tend to be more frequently symptomatic than younger.

Patients undergoing multiple valve procedures consistently have a greater incidence of psychopathology than patients with congenital disease across all phases. However, no consistent pattern emerges among patients with various kinds of simple valve or coronary artery disease.

In general, psychometric assessment using the AMDP and cluster analysis confirm the observation of many researchers that open-heart surgery is a procedure which produces much psychopathology. However, the advantage of these techniques is that they permit the elaboration of complex patterns and interrelationships often missed by more subjective methods of assessment.

Acknowledgment. The authors are very grateful to Dr. Jeremy Katz for his aid in translation and his essential improvements of the manuscript.

References

1. Angst J, Battegay R, Bente D, Berner P, Broeren W, Cornu F, Dick P, Engelmeier M-P, Heimann H, Heinrich K, Helmchen H, Hippius H, Pöldinger W, Schmidlin P, Schmitt W, Weis P (1969) Das Dokumentationssystem der Arbeitsgemeinschaft für Methodik und Dokumentation in der Psychiatrie (AMDP). Arzneim Forsch 19:399–405
2. Dahme B, Götze P (1980) Objective classification of psychopathological symptoms after open-heart surgery. In: Speidel H, Rodewald G (eds) Psychic and neurological dysfunctions after open-heart surgery. Thieme, Stuttgart, pp 41–47
3. Götze P (1980) Psychopathologie der Herzoperierten. Enke, Stuttgart
4. Götze P, Dahme B (1980) Psychopathological syndromes and neurological disturbances before and after open-heart surgery. In: Speidel H, Rodewald G (eds) Psychic and neurological dysfunctions after open-heart surgery. Thieme, Stuttgart, pp 48–67
5. Spaeth L (1975) Cluster-Analyse Algorithmen. Oldenbourg, Munich

Discussion of Session II

Dr. Richard Blacher, Moderator: I think that both of these papers considered together provide us with a focus for some interesting discussion. I was very struck by the figures which are so often in keeping with each other. I just happened to look at some of my own statistics using methods quite different from both the Hamburg group and Dr. Willner's group.

I noticed that compared to Dr. Willner's group with his devastated CLAT scores, my patients, with around 30% preoperative organic difficulties, can be included in the same sphere using different testing. I also found, in keeping with the Hamburg results, a 19% depression group, which is very close to their figures, almost all of these patients having the type of depression illustrated by Dr. Willner's case of a survivor – people who live through surgery that may have killed other members of the family or where other members of the family have died from heart disease. All along the syndromes were very much alike, and this provides us, I think, with an opportunity now to have a discussion and questions about the figures and studies. Who would like to start the discussion?

A colleague from Scandinavia: I would like to ask both speakers the same question: that is, you both have a nonhomogeneous patient population; I mean, they have had the same kind of processes but some are valve disease, congenital disease, coronary operation. I think there must be a different population also, every one of these thinking in terms of problems that you have investigated. Would you comment on that problem?

Dr. Willner: It so happens I have a little table on that subject. We had just about equal numbers of patients who had coronary bypass surgery and cardiac valvular surgery. Now the incidence of mortality in the coronary bypass patients was much lower than in the valvular surgery patients, again bearing in mind that I am not talking about mortality in the hospital but during the 5 years following hospital discharge. However, there is an interesting similarity. Of 13 patients with cardiac valvular surgery who had PCD 62% died. Of three patients who had coronary bypass surgery and who had PCD, two died; 67% mortality versus 62% mortality. There is a more notable difference between the outcomes of the people with both disorders who did not have PCD. Of 30 patients with coronary bypass surgery who did not have PCD only one died. So for the coronary bypass patients we have a 3% mortality without PCD and a 67% mortality with PCD. For the cardiac valvular patients, of 23 patients who did not have PCD the mortality rate is 22%, and with PCD 62%. So the mortality for the patients who had PCD is about the same for the cardiac valvular as well as for the coronary bypass surgery. However, the patients with bypass surgery who do not have PCD seem to be considerably better than the valvular surgery patients without PCD.

Dr. Huse-Kleinstoll: I'll answer for the Hamburg group. What we can say is that preoperatively we found psycho-organic symptoms relatively often in patients with coronary disease, and only the patients with double valve disease surmounted the coronary patient. After the operation, during the early postoperative period, the valve patient showed more outstanding psycho-organic symptoms than the coronary patient, so that we have the impression that the coronary patients were not affected so much by the operation itself. But in the later period Dr. Götze noticed from three-year follow-up interviews the coronary patients also had more psychoorganic symptoms, but the symptoms were not so severe as immediately after the operation. However, we must take into account that after the operation those symptoms might be aggravated by sedative drugs.

Dr. Shanahan from Sydney, Australia: I'd like to ask each of the speakers if they have any information concerning the incidence of these various disorders in patients from the community at large who do not have heart disease but who are regarded as normal, or who have some other life-threatening disease. Have similar studies been done, and if so, how do they compare?

Dr. Willner: As for the first part, I would assume that the incidence of organic disorders in the normal population would be quite a bit less than in my sample, and I think perhaps both samples. I also think that the incidence of depression would be quite a bit less in a normal sample, especially the severity of the depression. I perhaps failed to indicate it, but we are dealing with instances of the depression, where people attempted suicide, and in one case successfully carried it out. So the depressions can be quite severe. In terms of the incidence of depression and organic brain syndrome in other kinds of illness, I think that would probably depend on the kind of illness. I would think that there are some types of illness where you would have a considerable amount of depression and brain syndrome and others not. However, I have not done those kinds of comparisons.

Dr. Huse-Kleinstoll: I know of no comparitive studies involving normal people. What we found is that age plays an important role. From our EEG studies we know that age is very much correlated to EEG changes, and that if you try to look at which weighs more, age or the EEG changes, we found that the EEG changes are more important, which might be a hint that in cardiac surgery you find more psycho-organic symptoms preoperatively than in normal people.

Dr. Willner: I would like to speak on that issue also. We obtained the same finding, namely, that although there was a relationship with age, in this instance the PCD disorders seemed to be a good deal more important. One might wonder whether as people get older they might also have a higher incidence of this kind of PCD trouble, and to what extent might the results, for example, be just a side effect of age. In fact, what we did was to divide our sample at the median age, into people who were 56 and younger, and 57 and older. We found that while the incidence of mortality in the younger people was much lower, the PCD variable was actually a much better predictor in the younger people than in the older ones. Let me give you a feel of some more details about this and then explain, what it might mean. In the younger group of patients there were 31 patients who did not have PCD and only three who did. Of the 31 younger patients, only one died, i.e., a mortality rate of 3%. Of the three patients who had PCD, all three died, i.e., a mortality rate of 100%. With the older group of patients, for those who did not have PCD there was a 23% mortality rate, and for those who did have PCD there was a 54% mortality rate. What might this mean? It seems to me that if you are younger and you develop enough kinds of organic troubles to show PCD, that in spite of your youth it is pretty bad that it occurs that early. Our results would seem to indicate that there is a general relationship with age; but, as has just been stated with regard to the EEG findings, the same would apply with the PCD findings, namely, that the organic variables that we are talking about seem to be considerably more important than the age variable.

Dr. Blacher: If I might add something to this, it certainly strikes me that people with PCD perhaps show a more generalized vascular difficulty, which would indicate a more generalized condition. This is very striking to me and I was stimulated by the work of Drs. Willner and Rabiner to test my patients preoperatively because I found an extraordinarily high percentage of patients postoperatively who had organic difficulties. I use a much simpler cognitive measurement, and I was very struck by the fact that patients who would appear normally in doing simple computations to have absolutely no difficulty, and who were quite functional, would have remarkable difficulty in doing simple computations in the preoperative period. These patients included statisticians who were unable to do a simple mathematical computation. Now the problem, of course, is that we have no statistics on the general population, because these people are not suspected at all of having any problem. I also wonder whether or not the depressions that Dr. Willner describes may really be reactions to the awareness on the part of the patients of the loss of their brain function. I have noticed in quite a number of people that those who develop some organic difficulty did not just ignore this; they really become quite anxious and some of them developed what seemed to be a depression. I wonder if you would like to say something about that?

Dr. Willner: Well, I think part of the depression is in people who are aware of their cognitive losses, but a great deal of the depression does not seem to work that way. For example, there are many people who show a great deal of cognitive loss and are not depressed, then several months later they show a great deal of depression but the cognitive losses seem to ameliorate. So there are many people who, when they have organic difficulties, seem to lose the awareness and insight into their troubles. There is a good deal of denial as is seen in other organic conditions. So in part, I think, the depression is because of the recognition of the losses the person has, but in part the depression is the kind that has been reported for patients with anoxic difficulties, ever since the early studies, before airline pressurization was perfected, when airline pilots suffered a good deal with anoxic troubles. At that point one of the major symptoms noted was depression as well as the cognitive disorder. So I think that the depression has multiple causes. One other thing I would like to say is that when we talked about the depression in the hospital we excluded one category, and that was the clear reactive depression. The patient looked depressed and if you asked him why, he said, well, he had a great deal of pain, or he decided that he would have to give up spicy foods which he had always enjoyed. If the patient gave a clear explanation for his depression, one that was convincing, we considered that a reactive depression and did not label it as a pathogenic depression. It was when the patient was quite depressed and you could not get any feeling for why he was depressed, than we labeled it as a specific depression.

A colleague from Sweden: I would like to ask Dr. Willner a couple of questions. Firstly, what were the causes of death, and would they be hidden behind several pure medical causes? Also, are you using this kind of assistance at the moment routinely, and if so, does a PCD syndrome disqualify a patient from surgery in an otherwise marginal situation? And what do you think is the pathophysiological cause of this correlation?

Dr. Willner: Could you mention the questions again to me in order and I will take them one at a time.

The colleague from Sweden: Cause of death, first.

Dr. Willner: The cause of death was often something like congestive heart failure or stroke. We had no postmortem evidence so we do not have a clear picture of what the actual cause of death is. We are going to try to get that clarified as much as we can from a detailed chart review, but the fact is that we have no really precise information on the cause of death that we might have had from postmortems. The second question?

The colleague from Sweden: What do you think is the pathophysiological mechanism?

Dr. Willner: Well, two mechanisms. First of all, with the cardiac valvular patients, if your heart is not able to pump enough blood, then you may have a shortage of blood supply to the brain, and we know that the brain can pay a heavy penalty. So one possibility then would be hypoxemia. A second possibility is that I have noticed that people have mentioned that there is more trouble with mitral valve patients than with other kinds of valve surgery. That was also our experience. We also noted that in the hospital people who had mitral valve surgery and rheumatic heart disease plus a devastated CLAT score had a very poor outcome, and there are several reasons why this might be. First of all, it may be that having mitral valve troubles is more likely to lead to having microemboli, and we quite agree with Dr. Meyendorf's impression that hypoxemia and microemboli are the two major causes of brain dysfunction and are also causes of a great deal of the psychopathology. Secondly, it may well be that these patients are somewhat more vulnerable to getting subacute bacterial endocarditis, which again can lead to microemboli. And thirdly, there is a good deal of work going back to Broich, many years ago, who felt that when you had rheumatic heart disease, as was true of the majority of mitral valve patients then, there could also be rheumatic lesions in the cerebral circulatory system. I can mention several studies of Broich where he took people at the state mental hospital, divided them into three categories: schizophrenic, manic depressive, and not psychotic, and then checked for incidence of rheumatic heart disease in these patients. He found for the schizophrenic patients an incidence of 10%, for the manic depressive patients an incidence of 4%, and for the nonpsychotic patients an incidence of 1%, which at that point was the population incidence. When he then used detailed necropsy data, he found lesions in the cerebral arterials which were quite similar to the lesions found on the heart valves. So I would think again as a summary to this rather long answer that the problems are probably both hypoxemia and microemboli. I think these are especially likely to happen in mitral valve patients, and if the mitral valve patients have severe enough disorders that you have severe cognitive troubles as well, they seem to have a rather difficult time. The third question you asked was if we used the PCD evaluation routinely in patients who are going to be having surgery at our medical center, what are the indications, and whether that might have an influence on postponing the surgery. I will answer the second part of that question first. I would not think that whether or not the patient has a PCD syndrome would lead to canceling the surgery because the mortality rate by now is extremely low. You have many patients whose life might be in jeopardy right now, whereas after surgery, maybe several years in the future, there might be some problems. Another way of looking at this is that Dr. Meyendorf in his talk at the symposium 2 years ago mentioned that surgery will tend to be like an experimental device producing symptom patterns and difficulties that were already there. You might wonder whether, without the surgery, the likelihood exists that the same kind of thing would happen either a bit sooner or a bit later? I think it would not make a lot of difference. If you have a situation where the mortality rate is below about 4% or 5% for both valvular and coronary bypass surgery, having the PCD syndrome would not seem like a good reason for postponing the surgery. If the mortality rate were quite a bit higher, which of course it would be in various centers and various places in the United States and around the world, then it could well be something to consider seriously. The other part of the question is that we have not for some time, either given the patients routine clinical interviews or PCD testing before surgery, because essentially it would make no difference in a decision about surgery in the hospital. We are currently going to be changing that. Dr. Rabiner and I are arranging a study which will first of all replicate the study you have been hearing about, and secondly will identify PCD patients while they are still in hospital. We then want to set up an experimental group and a control group by random assignment of PCD patients and provide behavioral psychotherapy to the experimental group over a 3-year period, in an attempt to see if we can reduce that 63% mortality rate. The idea is that patients who have open-heart surgery have, after surgery, the effects of the surgical stress; they usually have major changes in their employment; they often have a good deal of change in their family role – that's for all the patients. Patients with PCD are extremely likely, while all this is going on, to get quite depressed, which does not help anyone to cope. Also, the cognitive disorder means their ability to cope, their raw ability to work out problems, is reduced very sharply. Essentially what you have is a device for producing enormous stress in people, and we know what the implications of grave stress can be for cardiac surgery patients. So what we have in mind to do, and are arranging to have set up, is a study to identify another group of such patients, and to see if we can reduce the mortality rate by using behavioral psychotherapy aimed at specific stress problems that the patients have that they are unable to deal with. In that instance we will be able to resume both the psychiatric interviews and the testing. The issue has been trying to find, in a particular situation, the concrete benefit which would result. Unfortunately in many centers once the patient leaves the medical center he tends to get lost. We followed one group, we found there that are severe troubles, and now we want to come back and do something about it.

Dr. Becker from Jerusalem: I'd like to address this question to Dr. Blacher, as a psychiatrist who is working uniquely in the department of cardiothoracic surgery and not psychiatry. Could you respond to the question that we have been hearing a lot about, namely, depression, and about psychiatric disturbance preoperatively and postoperatively. What are the effects of life extension at the price of augmentation of life support with a foreign body implant. When we are talking about life extension by virtue of valvular exchange and replacement, we are talking about an altered state of self-awareness with respect to the issue of that life being maintained either by pacemaker, very often conduction, and not infrequently following multiple bypass surgeries, and multiple complex surgical procedures including multiple replacements of more than a single valve at a single moment in time. Where is the area of speculation about the role that existential, phenomenological issues may play in altering the perceptions of a person with respect to unsolicited dependancy on mechanical life-extending devices, and where is the reality of that kind of condition imposing itself on the discussion which we have heard here which largely sits in my brain somewhere at the fourth ventricle, hearing about organicity, but without really understanding that the cognitive price that is paid for survival – cognitive, not in the terms that we're hearing it discussed now – may be very, very exacting and very comprising. But life continues at a very special price under these conditions; the quality of the survival may be comprised.

Dr. Blacher: To answer that I could either give my 3-hour talk, or I could sum it up in 1 min. I think when I disagreed with Dr. Willner about things happening, like depressions, what I mean is that I think everything that goes on with our patients has a meaning. I think patients who do get depressed get depressed for a reason. I do not quite understand a depression in the true psychological terms resulting from an organic insult. It has a meaning to the person and when a patient has something wrong with him organically, he has a psychological reaction. We are used to thinking in terms of, is it organic or is it psychological? However, any of us waking up tomorrow and being unable to remember the date would become terrified. I have seen patients who have presented as pure organic deliria, in whom the upshot in investigating this was that they had mild degrees of organic difficulty following a heart-lung machine procedure, and became so panicky as a result of this that there was an increased anxiety. An increased anxiety made their mental functioning worse; the mental functioning further increased their anxiety, and so forth. The whole business of the valves is interesting. The heart is the most highly perfected organ of the body. It is the central organ of the body, and I will talk more about this when I present my own paper later this week. On the other hand, valves themselves are really completely unknown parts of the heart to everyone but people like ourselves and medical people in general. Patients do not know what valves are; they often think of them in terms of automobiles. I have heard of people coming in who need a valve job. One man, who is a chauffer, said that he thought his valve must have too much carbon in it. One hears things like this, the idea that somehow whatever is wrong with you is able to be fixed up by a good mechanic. However, people do not know about these things. Pacemakers are something different. We have described studies about this. Pacemakers are, after all, the only prosthesis that do something to you rather than that you do something with, and patients who have had a choice between a valve and a pacemaker would rather have a valve, strangely enough. To us one operation is so major and the other is so minor that the emotional investment may be really quite different. It is a great, important area. The thing I would emphasize is that all of these things have meanings to the patients, including all of the results that have been presented by Drs. Willner and Rabiner and by the Hamburg group. What has struck me is that they have been asking the patients questions beforehand about what things mean. We have taken for granted in the past that the only things that have occurred are things that have grossly hit us. Until I began to ask my coronary patients a great many questions preoperatively, I ran a series of about 50 patients in which I was struck by the fact that compared to the valve, the early coronaries had no psychological disturbances. I was struck by that. I remember when people were talking about the fact that the time on the heart-lung machine was the important factor in causing psychic disturbances, my patients having coronaries were running 50% or longer on the heart-lung machine and yet they were having no disturbances. This had to do, I think, with the way in which it was presented to them how their hearts were opened. I think that these factors that have been touched on, regarding the statistical studies of these patients, have added enormously to our understanding when one rounds them off with the interviews and the individual studies of all the patients. I hope that answers your question in a rather wordy way.

Dr. Longmore, London: Have any of you, I wondered, studied heart transplant patients, who have the biggest implant of all and who are quite remarkably euphoric postoperatively. I have never seen or heard of any heart transplant patient who has shown any disturbances which we have heard so eloquently described this afternoon.

Dr. Blacher: I do not know anyone here who has had first-hand experience with heart transplants. The heart transplant is an interesting kind of a problem. I have had people who have discussed it with me with great anxiety, and the question is who survives? Is it the person who receives the heart, who has a new pump now pumping the blood around, or is it the person whose heart is transplanted into a new shell, a new recipient? Because the heart is so filled with fantasies about itself, it hardly is for most people an organ, but rather a rather magical kind of business. I think that patients with heart transplants do get rather severe psychic reactions, though, from what I've heard.

Dr. Shanahan, Sydney: I apologize for getting up twice, but that last question is related to the question that I intended to ask. I actually have quite a close association with the transplant program, as I have been involved in two myself, and the patients do get psychological problems, quite considerably. But they are kept under tremendous surveillance and their compliance with their medical treatment is 100%. Now I was going to ask the panel a question. Each of them has referred to mortality in patients with recognizable psycho-organic disease, and in each case the late mortality was highest in those patients who are most in need of postoperative medical treatment. The multiple valves were the top, the mitral valves were second, the coronary disease third, aortic valve fourth, and congenital heart disease last. That is the order of significance of medical treatment following surgery. So the question is what is the influence of noncompliance with medical treatment in this late mortality, and how many of us here are aware and look into the problem of compliance of medical treatment of our patients? I think a lot of our medical treatment goes down the bathroom sink.

Dr. Willner: We found a heavy mortality for mitral valve patients in the hospital where there was careful attention to compliance. By the time the patients left the hospital the mortality rate for mitral valve was about the same as for the aortic valve patients, perhaps a bit lower. I think there were only about one or two multiple valve patients in the study. I think there was one and that patient also expired in the hospital, so that the issues about differential mortality after hospital discharge in the mitral valve patients and in the multiple valve patients, especially if it's a three-valve situation, would not apply in our case.

Dr. Huse-Kleinstoll: I am unable to answer your question for the late period 3 or 4 years after the operation. The only hint I can give you is that we find a relationship between psychopathology and patients who could not keep to the doctor's orders, but Dr. Meffert will relate something about that in his paper.

Dr. Blacher: We have time for one more question.

A colleague from New York: I have a question for Dr. Willner. In one of your papers you mentioned that when a CLAT was associated with poor postoperative outcome another test for organicity was not associated. Could you explain why the CLAT was able to pick up organicity that is important in outcome whereas the other tests failed to do so?

Dr. Willner: I would be happy to explain this. The one test in particular was the WAIS Vocabulary Test. That is a test which is known to be extremely insensitive to organicity and was included so we could have a contrast between a test which was sensitive to brain dysfunction and one that was not. So we thought that the WAIS Vocabulary would not be an effective predictor and it wasn't. One thing we did do that I had not mentioned here is that we had a group of patients that was tested before surgery, 10 days postoperatively, 1 1/2 years later, and 5 years later. These were patients that were tested at all four time intervals. For the WAIS Vocabulary there was no change in test scores over that period. On the other hand, for the CLAT, for the valvular surgery patients there was a slight and nonsignificant decrease from preoperative to postoperatively, followed by a highly significant improvement from postoperative testing to 1 1/2 years later, which was then maintained over 5 years. For the coronary bypass patients there was a slight and nonsignificant increase postoperatively, and then a highly significant increase at 18 months which was then again maintained over the 5-year period. My way of explaining these results would be that the WAIS Vocabulary is not sensitive enough to pick up the impairment that the patient suffered in the first place, and therefore it was not able to register the improvement when it occurred. On the other hand, the CLAT was sensitive enough to pick up the impairment and therefore did show the improvement. The only other test that we used was the WAIS Digit Symbol Test, which is considerably more sensitive to brain dysfunction than the WAIS Vocabulary, and considerably less sensitive than the CLAT. We started using that about halfway through the study, so we got no significant findings for the WAIS Digit Symbol Test. That could very well be because the number of subjects for which it was used was only about half of the sample. Aside from those three tests we did not use any other tests in the study.

Dr. Blacher: Thank you very much. I'd like to thank Dr. Willner and Dr. Götze and Dr. Huse-Kleinstoll and their respective groups for most interesting and stimulating papers. Thank you very much.

III

Organic Findings in Patients with Postoperative Neuropsychiatric Complications

III

Organic Findings in Patients with Postoperative Neuropsychiatric Complications

The Relative Importance of Psychic and Somatic Risk Factors for Postoperative Dysfunctions After Open-Heart Surgery – Preliminary Results*

H.-J. Meffert, B. Flemming, P. Götze, G. Huse-Kleinstoll, Ch. Reimer, H. Speidel

Introduction

It is self-evident for our Hamburg research team that psychopathological dysfunctions after open-heart surgery are mainly a psychosomatic problem [1–3].

We collected a lot of detailed information about the preoperative somatic status and psychological inner and outer conditions of 250 patients. We documented in detail the postoperative psychopathological findings of 168 patients and we are now able to distinguish exactly between different postoperative psychopathological courses [4–10]. We found a large number of meaningful significant correlations between postoperative events and, on the one hand, psychological [10–15] on the other hand somatic predictors [7, 16–21; Huse-Kleinstoll et al., this volume; Spehr et al., this volume].

Concerning the relationship between the patients' pre- and postoperative situation, this distinction between somatic and psychological factors is still common after a number of years research work [22].

Looking into the literature it is difficult to find a combined medicopsychological statistical approach to this problem [23].

We think that only a realistic view of the real relative importance of the preoperative somatic and psychological findings can help to lead to a true understanding of the patients' postoperative psychopathological dysfunctions and to successful therapeutic interventions [15]. A realistic view includes of course the possibility that a somatic finding can mean an irreversible substantial factor or can be a functional, reversible one, for example, because of a psychological disposition. To make a decision it is obviously necessary to look at the patients' psychological structure and situation as well.

The aim in this part of our investigation of a total of 149 valve disease and coronary artery disease patients was to name – in terms of easily understandable and reproducible descriptions – *combinations* of somatic and psychological variables which correlate with different postoperative disorders.

As a statistical approach we used a series of hierarchical multiple regression analyses [24]. With the help of this method it is possible to analyze the relationship between a number of predictor variables and a single criterion variable.

---

* With the aid of the Deutsche Forschungsgemeinschaft, Sonderforschungsbereich 115, Teilprojekt A3

Psychopathological and Neurological Dysfunctions
Following Open-Heart Surgery Ed by Becker et al

The result of such an analysis consists of an equation to predict a criterion value by means of the weights of the predictor variables, and the multiple correlation coefficient, which is the correlation between the predicted criterion value and the real value.

As criterion variables we took the factor values from the varimax-rotated Factor analysis of the AMDP rating scale values of the first 4 postoperative days [8]. (The AMDP system [25] is a standardized psychiatric rating instrument. It was slightly modified for the purpose of our research [7]. The patient's psychic status is documented in the scales: Vigilance, Orientation, Attention/Memory, Formal thinking, Hypochondriac moods/Phobia, Paranoia, Perception, Derealization/Depersonalization, Mood, Psychomotility, Social behavior.)

The three factor solution describes:

1. A *psycho-organic symptomatic,* consisting of the scales vigilance, orientation, attention and memory, formal thinking, and psychomotility,
2. A *paranoid-hallucinatory symptomatic,* consisting of the scales orientation, paranoia, perception, and derealization/depersonalization,
   and
3. *Emotional disorders,* consisting of the scales hypochondriac moods and phobia, mood, psychomotility, and social behavior. This factor mainly describes depressive mood disorders.

As predictor variables we took all those preoperative variables – which had proved to have significant correlations with AMDP data – from the psychologist's and the physician's data sets. That means items from the personality inventories and mood list [10, 11, 13], questionnaire and interview [12, 14, 15], the somatic anamnesis, and actual status inclusive of catheter [16–19] and EEG findings [21; Spehr et al., this volume].

This data set was reduced by correlating the items with the three AMDP factor values. Only the data that showed a significant relationship to AMDP factors were accepted for the multiple regression analysis.

In a first attempt to identify the most important items predicting the criterion variables two findings proved important.

1. There obviously exists not one single valid common data set for all patients (regardless of the diagnosis groups) per criterion variable.
2. It did not prove important to differentiate between patients with aortic and those with mitral valve replacement.

For the remaining two main diagnosis groups – coronary artery disease and valve disease – and the three AMDP criterion variables, six regression equations were computed. The coronary artery disease group consisted of 60 patients, and the valve disease group of 89 patients. The number of variables in the equations ranged from 7 to 14. The resulting multiple correlation coefficients were between 0.61 and 0.80, which is fairly high; all proved to be significant at the 1% level.

Predictors for a Psycho-Organic Symptomatic

Within the group of *valve disease* patients an EEG finding had the greatest influence on the development of a psycho-organic symptomatic: the α frequency at the first decile, that means the slow α component in the posterior temporal region. This finding is highly correlated with an advanced age but seems to be a better predictor of a psycho-organic symptomatic. Hardly less important, and still of significant influence, are an additional diabetes, a higher systolic pressure in the right ventricle and brain emboli. The psychological component has nearly the same influence: little activity and a psychic isolation through a disturbed partner relationship. These patients do not trust their partners and have the feeling of having nobody to talk to about their problems, which are mainly occupational difficulties or – in other words – they cannot open their hearts to anyone.

Within the group of *coronary* patients a disintegrated personality has the most influence on psycho-organic dysfunctions. These patients appear quiet and peaceful but easily irritable, they find it hard to keep to the doctors' orders, they sleep badly, they suffer from financial problems, and they are very doubtful about their future. Somatic parameters are generally less important and characterize the hemodynamically good patient, but neurological findings point to cerebral lesions.

Predictors for a Paranoid Hallucinatory Symptomatic

Within the group of *valve disease* patients a bad hemodynamic status and a higher urea nitrogen level have the greatest influence. These variables do not necessarily describe a purely organic condition, but perhaps point even more to a reversible functional impairment, which is supported by an increased use of sedative and antidepressive drugs. Psychic stressing experiences have an equally important influence: The experience of heart disease leading to death in the environment and war-time experiences.

These experiences can hardly be regarded as essential risk factors because most of our patients have experienced the second world war, and there is no doubt that most heart patients have experienced a cardiac death in their environment. What makes these experience risk factors is probably more a paranoid personality structure, which, with the help of a projective mechanism, distorts these experiences into a menace in their life.

Two more important findings might help to identify these patients: They pretend not to have any problems with their partners or families, and they have difficulties keeping to the doctors' orders.

Within the group of *coronary artery disease* patients an increased systolic aortic blood pressure, which means high amplitudes during catheterization, has the greatest influence on paranoid-hallucinatory symptoms. In combination with the only additional somatic variable which indicates that these patients do not show any lesion signs in the electroencephalogram, a possible explanation might be that the increased blood pressure under catheter stress is more an expression of psychic arousal or emotional tension than a sign of a sclerotic coronary artery system.

The real psychological variables stress this interpretation. They describe as statistically meaningful as the somatic ones, an aggressive character who has got problems with his superiors, who, in view of his illness, does not worry about possible consequences where his family is concerned, and who is not at all happy about his chances regarding the outcome of an operation and therefore took a long time to decide to have it.

Predictors for Emotional Disorders

In both groups, the *valve disease* patients and the *coronary artery disease* group, a psychological disposition turns out to be most important.

The patients within the *valve disease* group are especially prone to becoming depressive, have a pessimistic view of the future, concerning job and family, and suffer from postponements of the operation and the nervewracking time waiting for it. The – in general bad – hemodynamic disposition has only a smaller influence, but patients with double valve disease are more in danger of emotional disorders.

Within the *coronary heart disease* group, the so-called deniers in particular develop emotional disorders. This method of coping reveals itself in the way in which these patients speak about their death as a possible consequence of their illness and the operation without any affection. Another factor is a secondary gain from the illness of rest and time. Of further importance are: psychiatric treatment in the case history, war-time experiences, and actual conflicts concerning job and family. No organic risk factor could be identified in this group.

So far we have described the relative importance of psychic and somatic risk factors for postoperative dysfunctions. With a few final remarks we would like to comment on this study and stress its relevance.

As far as we know this is one of the first attempts to quantify the relative psychological and somatic parts influencing the psychopathology that follows open-heart surgery. We still think about other criterion variables and different methodical proceedings concerning the statistics, and for an even more precise prediction we are planning to differentiate between patients with aortic and those with mitral valve replacement. Therefore, our work might not be perfect and one should look at our results as an approximation of reality.

Our results have thrown light on some interesting relationships between psychic and somatic factors and were helpful for a better understanding of some findings. They have thrown light on the relative influence of these factors on definite psychopathological disorders within different diagnosis groups.

It was shown that altogether *different* somatic and psychic conditions are connected with *similar* psychopathological dysfunctions, depending upon the diagnosis group. Furthermore, our results suggest that only very limited information about and from the patient is sufficient for a prediction of the postoperative situation.

This knowledge might help to identify a risk patient at an early date before the operation, and it should be used for an early therapeutical approach.

Since our results have not yet been validated we have a suggestion to make to the reader: Take a few minutes and think back to a patient you have seen lately. Remember his diagnosis and somatic status and what you know about his personality, his problems, and psychosocial situation. Remember his postoperative psychopathology and think about our results. Do they fit the patient you have in mind?

Acknowledgments. The authors are endebted to Professor Dr. Bernhard Dahme for valuable discussion concerning methodical-statistical questions and to Mr. Mathias Wessel for doing the computerized data processing. Translation was by Kathleen Behnke and Richard A. Bird.

References

1. Speidel H, Dahme B, Flemming B, Götze P, Huse-Kleinstoll G, Meffert H.-J., Rodewald G, Spehr W (1978) Psychosomatische Probleme in der Herzchirurgie. Therapiewoche 28:8191–8210
2. Speidel H, Dahme B, Flemming B, Götze P, Huse-Kleinstoll G, Meffert H-J, Rodewald G, Spehr W (1980) Open-heart surgery unit. Adv Psychosom Med 10:30–56
3. Speidel H, Achilles I, Dahme B, Flemming B, Götze P, Haag A, Huse-Kleinstoll G, Meffert H-J, Polonius M-J, Rodewald G, Spehr W, Strindberg K (1978) Probleme der interdisziplinären Zusammenarbeit in der psychosomatischen Forschung am Beispiel eines Projektes mit Herzoperierten. Gruppenpsychother Gruppendynamik 13:253–261
4. Dahme B, Achilles I, Götze P, Huse-Kleinstoll G, Meffert H-J, Polonius M-J, Rodewald G, Speidel H (1977) Klassifikation psychopathologischer Auffälligkeiten nach Herzoperationen. Thoraxchirurgie 25:245–249
5. Speidel H, Dahme B, Flemming B, Götze P, Huse-Kleinstoll G, Meffert H-J, Rodewald G (1979) Psychische Störungen nach offenen Herzoperationen. Nervenarzt 50:85–91
6. Speidel H, Dahme B, Flemming B, Götze P, Huse-Kleinstoll G, Meffert H-J, Rodewald G (1979) Probleme der Klassifizierung psychopathologischer Auffälligkeiten nach Herzoperationen mit extrakorporaler Zirkulation. Psychiatr Clin (Basel) 12:57–79
7. Götze P (1979) Psychopathologie der Herzoperierten. Psychische und neurologische Störunggen vor und nach Herzoperationen. Enke, Stuttgart
8. Dahme B, Götze P (1980) Objective classification of psychopathological symptoms after open-heart surgery. In: Speidel H, Rodewald G (eds) Psychic and neurological dysfunctions after open-heart surgery. Thieme, Stuttgart, pp 41–48
9. Götze P, Dahme B (1980) Psychopathological syndromes and neurological disturbances after open-heart surgery. In: Speidel H, Rodewald G (eds) Psychic and neurological dysfunctions after open-heart surgery. Thieme, Stuttgart, pp 48–67
10. Flemming B, Meffert H-J (1980) The role of personality traits for psychic disturbances after open-heart surgery. In: Speidel H, Rodewald G (eds) Psychic and neurological dysfunctions after open-heart surgery. Thieme, Stuttgart, pp 169–181
11. Flemming B, Dahme B, Götze P, Huse-Kleinstoll G, Kalmar P, Meffert H-J, Speidel H (1978) Einige psychologische Prädiktoren für psychopathologische Auffälligkeiten nach Herzoperationen. Thoraxchirurgie 26:458–462
12. Meffert H-J, Dahme B, Flemming B, Götze P, Huse-Kleinstoll G, Rodewald G, Speidel H (1978) Psychologische Aspekte der Psychopathologie Herzoperierter. Verh Dtsch Ges Inn Med 84:1560–1562
13. Flemming B, Dahme B, Götze P, Huse-Kleinstoll G, Meffert H-J, Speidel H (1978) Die Beziehung von Persönlichkeitsvariablen von Herzpatienten zu ihrem postoperativen psychopathologischen Status. Med Psychol 3:214–216
14. Meffert H-J, Flemming B (1980) Psychic and psychosocial stress before open-heart operations and their relationship with postoperative psychic disturbances. In: Speidel H, Rodewald G (eds) Psychic and neurological dysfunctions after open-heart surgery. Thieme, Stuttgart, pp 181–188
15. Meffert H-J, Dahme B, Flemming B, Götze P, Huse-Kleinstoll G, Rodewald G, Speidel H (1979) Open-heart surgery from the psychological point of view and resulting therapeutic considerations. Psychother Psychosom 32:148–156

16. Huse-Kleinstoll G, Dahme B, Flemming B, Haag A, Meffert H-J, Polonius M-J, Rodewald G, Speidel H (1976) Einige somatische und psychologische Prädiktoren für psychopathologische Auffälligkeiten nach Herzoperationen. Thoraxchirurgie 24:388–399
17. Huse-Kleinstoll G, Dahme B, Flemming B, Götze P, Meffert H-J, Rodewald G, Speidel H (1978) Die Beziehung zwischen psychischen Störungen nach Herzoperationen und dem prä-, intra- und postoperativen Krankheitsverlauf. Verh Dtsch Ges Inn Med 84:1555–1560
18. Huse-Kleinstoll G, Dahme B, Flemming B, Götze P, Meffert H-J, Rodewald G, Speidel H (1979) Open-heart surgery: Somatic predictors of postoperative psychopathology. Thorac Cardiovasc Surg 27:271–274
19. Huse-Kleinstoll G (1980) Pre-operative somatic factors predisposing to psychic dysfunction following open-heart surgery. In: Speidel H, Rodewald G (eds) Psychic and neurological dysfunctions after open-heart surgery. Thieme, Stuttgart, pp 117–130
20. Pokar H, Huse-Kleinstoll G (1980) Possible intra-operative influences by anesthesia and ECC on post-operative psychic dysfunctions. In: Speidel H, Rodewald G (eds) Psychic and neurological dysfunctions after open-heart surgery. Thieme, Stuttgart, pp 67–74
21. Spehr W, Götze P (1980) Computerized encephalogram before and after open-heart surgery (preliminary results). In: Speidel H, Rodewald G (eds) Psychic and neurological dysfunctions after open-heart surgery. Thieme, Stuttgart, pp 67–74
22. Götze P, Huse-Kleinstoll G, Speidel H (1980) Psychic and neurological dysfunctions following open-heart surgery: A review of the present state of research. In: Speidel H, Rodewald G (eds) Psychic and neurological dysfunctions after open-heart surgery. Thieme, Stuttgart, pp 6–14
23. Kornfeld DS, Heller SS, Frank KA, Moskowitz R (1974) Personality and psychological factors in postcardiotomy delirium. Arch Gen Psychiatry 31:249–253
24. Bortz J (1977) Lehrbuch der Statistik für Sozialwissenschaftler. Springer, Berlin Heidelberg New York
25. Angst J, Battegay R, Benth D, Berner P, Broeren W, Cornu F, Dick P, Engelmeier M-P, Heimann H, Heinrich K, Helmchen H, Hippius H, Pöldinger W, Schmidlin P, Schmitt W, Weis P (1969) Das Dokumentationssystem der Arbeitsgemeinschaft für Methodik und Dokumentation in der Psychiatrie (AMP). Arzneim Forsch 19:399–405

Early Psychic Disturbances After Open-Heart Surgery and Their Relationship to the Postoperative Clinical Course*

G. Huse-Kleinstoll, B. Flemming, P. Götze, H.-J. Meffert, M.-J. Polonius, Ch. Reimer, H. Speidel, G. Wiese

In our study we have tried to throw more light on the relationship between the early postoperative psychic disorders and the early postoperative clinical course.

Morse and Litin [6] have described patients with postoperative psychic dysfunctions, which they classified as delirium, having larger variations of the physiological parameters during the postoperative course in nearly all variables they collected, resulting in alkalosis, anemia, azotemia, hypokalemia, hypochloremia, and hyponatremia etc. Although this was a study of cardiovascular and general surgery patients, the postoperative psychic disorders do not seem to be different in quality compared to our studies involving only patients after cardiovascular operations, with extracorporeal circulation. But it was our aim to be able to view the relationship between the postoperative psychiatric disorders and the postoperative clinical course from a different aspect, namely with regard to the different psychopathological syndromes described by Götze and Dahme [2].

Introduction

In Table 1 the sample for our studies is described. It shows the incidence of the different diagnosis groups. It is a very heterogeneous group with regard to the diagnosis groups. The consequence for the interpretation of our results will be discussed later

Table 1. Main diagnostic groups

Diagnosis group	No. of patients
Congenital defects	12
Heart valve defects	57[a]
Coronary heart disease	26
Combined diagnosis groups	5
Total	100

[a] 1 Patient died intraoperatively

* With the aid of the Deutsche Forschungsgemeinschaft, Sonderforschungsbereich 115, Teilprojekt A3

Psychopathological and Neurological Dysfunctions
Following Open-Heart Surgery. Ed by Becker et al

in connection with the different psychic groups we identified. We investigated the postoperative psychic disturbances by carrying out daily interviews in the ICU from the 1st to 4th postoperative day and assessed them with the help of a 100 item scale, the AMDP scale (as it is called in German-speaking countries) with the following 11 main scales:

Vigilance
Orientation
Attention and memory
Formal thinking
Hypochondriac moods and phobia
Paranoia
Perception
Derealization and depersonalization
Mood
Psychomotility
Social behavior

By statistical analysis we could differentiate between four groups of patients with special psychopathological courses and one group which had subaverage values in all 11 main scales. The latter group we called "unremarkable" and refer to it as group I. The psychopathological groups were classified as follows:

Group II: slight psycho-organic syndrome with affective-emotional and psycho-motor disturbances
Group III: severe psycho-organic syndrome with disturbances of perception and psychomotility
Group IV: paranoid-hallucinatory syndrome with affective-emotional and psychomotor disturbances
Group V: delirious syndrome

According to the psychic disturbances we tried to assess the somatic complications during the early postoperative course. But as Polonius in 1977 [7] had described, the early postoperative course shows divergencies in almost all parameters known since Moore [4] as the postoperative illness, and the question was what is a regular postoperative clinical course. There was a similar difficulty in defining the somatic complications as with the psychiatric. We therefore decided to collect a variety of data, nearly 800 in total, for the day of the operation and the first 4 postoperative days. We assessed them daily, some of them four times a day, for temperature, intracardiac and systemic pressures, etc. and, if it was necessary, the maximum or minimum of a parameter such as arterial pressure or O_2 saturation level etc. At the same time we noted the medication which was given during a particular day by summarizing the doses or noting whether or not a drug was given when a medication was not routinely applied. In addition we collected for each day some more general variables about physical mobilization, pain, sleep, number of blood samples taken, and the number of the nurses' interventions. Thus, we were able to describe the changes in the different variables during the early postoperative period. We were able to demonstrate different courses for different patients' groups such as the five groups with a different postoperative psychic course. In some variables we could compare the preoperative and the postoperative status. For all variables and medications collected we made drawings showing the mean value of a variable as a function of time for the 99 surviving patients (one patient died during the operation because of biventricular heart failure, having mitral stenoses, class IV) and for the different early postoperative psychic groups mentioned above. The groups with the most outstanding psychopathology, group III and group V, contain only four patients each. Therefore the results for these groups must be interpreted as trends.

Results

Table 2 shows the operative procedures and the distribution of age and sex in the unremarkable psychic group. The mean age of the patients in this group was lower than in the psychopathological groups. Forty-nine patients, that is 49.5%, had an "unremarkable" psychic course during the early postoperative period. The clinical course of this group has become the basis for comparison with the other four psychopathological groups. Before the operation the average venous O_2 saturation levels in the pulmonary artery as a measure of the cardiac index were the highest in the "unremarkable" group. In some variables, like the thrombocytes, there was a less deep drop after the operation.

Figure 1 shows the mean value of the hematocrit for the whole sample and for the different psychic groups during the day of the operation and the first 4 postoperative days. The hematocrit had the highest mean values during the first 3 postoperative days in the "unremarkable" psychic group I. Nevertheless it would be erroneous to think that all patients in this group had an uncomplicated physical course. Ten patients stayed longer then 4 days in the ICU which in our unit meant that the discharge to the general unit was delayed by some complication, mostly arrhythmias.

In the following the results for the four psychopathological groups shall be demonstrated.

Table 2. Operation procedure and distribution of age and sex of the "unremarkable" psychic group

Operative procedure	No. of cases	Age mean value	Sex ♂	Sex ♀
Correction of congenital defects	8	34	5	3
Mitral valve replacement	11	48	1	10
Aortic valve replacement	12	41	10	2
Multiple valve replacement	4	46	3	1
Coronary surgery	11	51	9	2
Valve replacement and coronary surgery	3	45	3	–
Total	49	45	31	18

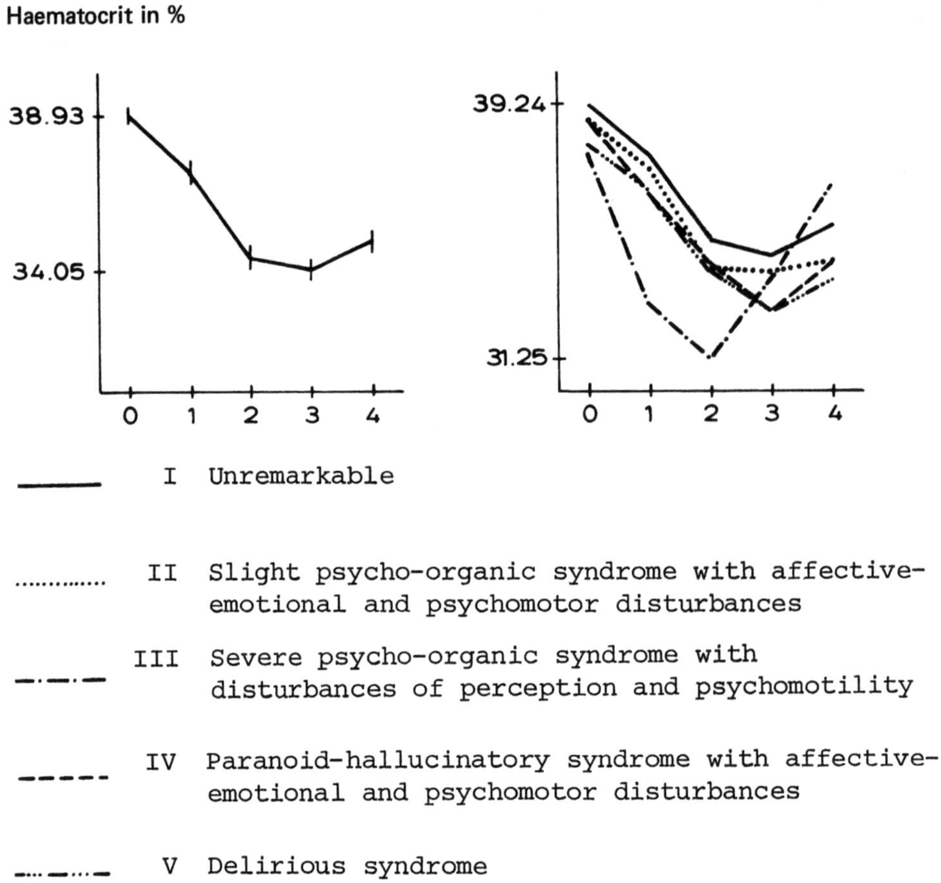

Fig. 1. The early postoperative course for the whole sample and for the five different psychic groups: mean values of the hematocrit

Table 3. Operation procedure and distribution of age and sex of the psychopathological group: "slight psycho-organic syndrome with affective emotional and psychomotor disturbances"

Operative procedure	No. of cases	Age mean value	Sex	
			♂	♀
Correction of congenital defects	3	36	1	2
Mitral valve replacement	4	45	2	2
Aortic valve replacement	9	50	8	1
Multiple valve replacement	6	52	2	4
Coronary surgery	10	52	9	1
Valve replacement and coronary surgery	1	52	–	1
Total	33	49	22	11

Table 3 shows the operative procedures with the mean age and sex of the patients of group II. With one exception all patients with coronary surgery (bypass-surgery and aneurysmectomy) who had psycho-organic symptoms during the early postoperative period were found in this group, where the intensity of these symptoms were only slight. Compared with the preoperative psycho-organic deficits there was no notable increase in these symptoms so that the importance of the influence of the extracorporeal circulation on these patients seem to be rather small compared to the patients with valve replacement. When looking at the relationship between the psychic and somatic conditions, all in all one can say that the postoperative course of this group does not differ very much from the course of the "unremarkable" group. The mean values in nearly all variables were slightly worse compared to group I.

Only in some parameters were there remarkable differences. This was, for example, the average minimal frequency, which in this group was higher than in the normal group and did not drop continually. The arterial oxygen tension was low on the 1st and 2nd postoperative day. The patients in this group had to be paced more often on these first 2 postoperative days.

Figure 2 shows the number of patients in percent who were stimulated by a cardiac pacemaker of the different psychic groups during the early postoperative period and the percent of arrhythmias in these groups. Arrhythmia was relatively seldom in this

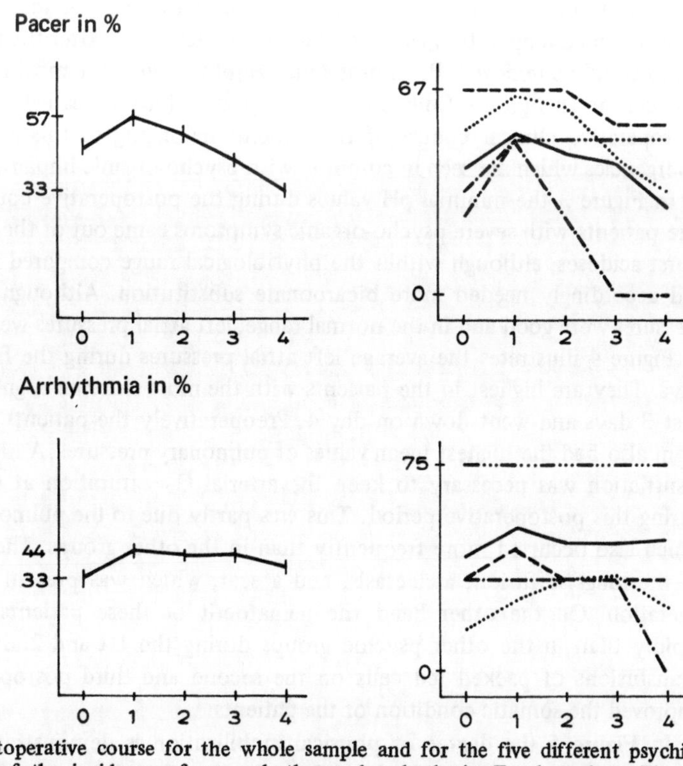

Fig. 2. The early postoperative course for the whole sample and for the five different psychic groups: mean values of the incidence of pacer rhythm and arrhythmia. For legend see Fig. 1

Table 4. Operation procedure and distribution of age and sex of the psychopathological group: "severe psycho-organic syndrome with disturbances of perception and psychomotality"

Operative procedure	No. of cases	Age mean value	Sex	
			♂	♀
Mitral valve replacement	2	56	1	1
Multiple valve replacement	1	51	1	–
Coronary surgery	1	55	1	–
Total	4	54	3	1

group, so that the indication for pacing the patients was rather the necessity to increase the cardiac output.

Now come the results for third group with a severe psycho-organic syndrome with disturbances of perception and psycho-motility (Table 4):

In this group there are only four patients: Two patients with mitral valve replacement, one patient with multiple valve replacement, and one patient with coronary surgery. The patient mentioned last developed left ventricular heart failure ½ hours after extracorporeal circulation because of a thrombosis of the aortocoronary bypass to the left anterior artery. An intra-aortic balloon pump was inserted as a preventive measure and a reoperation was necessary 19 h later, whereafter the intra-aortic balloon pump could be removed. Psycho-organic symptoms were the most outstanding psychic disorders in this group. Compared to the group which we called "unremarkable" the postoperative clinical course of the patients belonging to this group showed many divergencies which are seen in common with psycho-organic impairment.

In Figure 3 the minimal pH values during the postoperative course are to be seen. The patients with severe psycho-organic symptoms came out of the operation with the worst acidoses, although within the physiological range compared to all other groups, and accordingly needed more bicarbonate substitution. Although the arterial blood pressures were good and in the normal range, left atrial pressures were high until day 4.

Figure 4 illustrates the average left atrial pressures during the first 4 postoperative days. They are highest in the patients with the most extreme cognitive deficits on the first 3 days and went down on day 4. Preoperatively the patients with valve replacement also had the highest mean values of pulmonary pressures. A higher rate of oxygen insufflation was necessary to keep the arterial O_2 saturation at an acceptable level during this postoperative period. This was partly due to the pulmonary complications which also occurred more frequently than in the other groups. These were congestion of the lungs, effusion, atelectasis, and a scar, which was present already before the operation. On the other hand the hematocrit of these patients went down more rapidly than in the other psychic groups during the 1st and 2nd postoperative day. Transfusions of packed red cells on the second and third postoperative days visibly improved the somatic condition of the patients.

In Figure 5 the degree of physical mobilization is demonstrated and was rated: 0 immobile, 1 sitting on the bed, 2 getting up, 3 walking around with the physio-

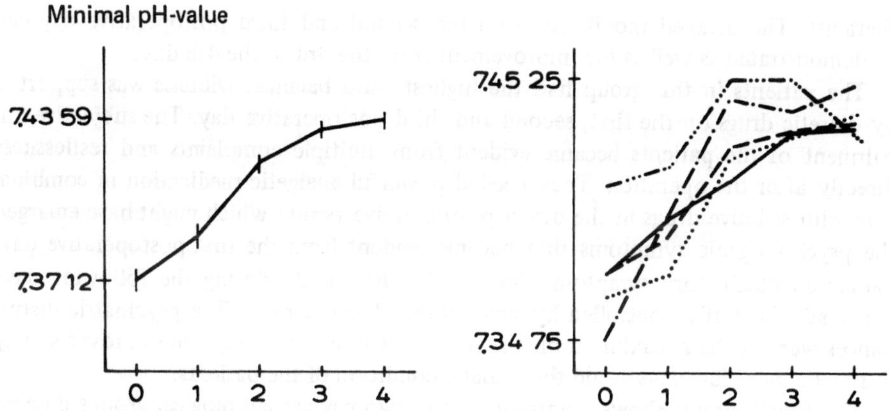

Fig. 3. The early postoperative course for the whole sample and the five different psychic groups: mean values in the minimal pH value. For legend see Fig. 1

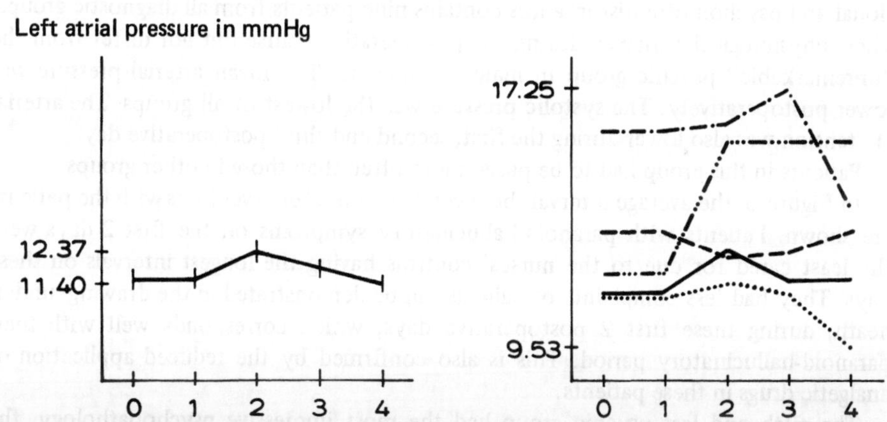

Fig. 4. The early postoperative course for the whole sample and the five different psychic groups: mean values of the left a trial pressure. For legend see Fig. 1

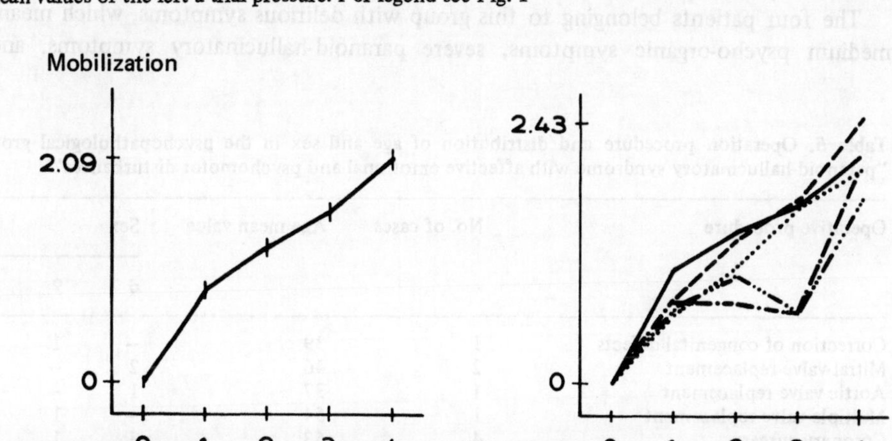

Fig. 5. The early postoperative course for the whole sample and the five different psychic groups: mean values in the rating of mobilization. For legend see Fig. 1

therapist. The delayed mobilization on the second and third postoperative day can be demonstrated as well as the improvement from the 3rd to the 4th day.

The patients in this group had the highest fluid balance. Diuresis was supported by diuretic drugs on the first, second and third postoperative day. The subjective impairment of the patients became evident from multiple complaints and restlessness directly after the operation. They needed powerful analgetic medication in combination with sedative drugs in the direct postoperative period which might have enlarged the psycho-organic symptoms that became evident from the first postoperative day. Paranoid-hallucinatory symptoms developed only slightly during the following days and could be easily controlled by small doses of haloperidol. The psychiatric disturbances were at their maximum on the second postoperative day and improved slowly during the next few days as did the somatic condition of the patients.

The fourth group shows, contrary to the two psychopathological groups demonstrated before, no cognitive deficits (Table 5).

This group of patients with a paranoid-hallucinatory syndrome with affective-emotional and psychomotor disturbances contains nine patients from all diagnostic groups. Their physiological variables during the postoperative course did not differ from the "unremarkable" psychic group in many parameters. The mean arterial pressure was lower postoperatively. The systolic pressure was the lowest of all groups. The arterial O_2 tension was also lower during the first, second and third postoperative day.

Patients in this group had to be paced more often than those in other groups.

In Figure 6, the average intervals between the nurses' interventions with the patients are shown. Patients with paranoid-hallucinatory symptoms on the first 2 days were the least cared for due to the nurses' controls having the longest intervals on these days. They had less complaints of pain, as can be demonstrated in the drawing underneath, during these first 2 postoperative days, which corresponds well with their paranoid-hallucinatory period. This is also confirmed by the reduced application of analgetic drugs in these patients.

The fifth and last psychic group had the most impressive psychopathology, the „delirious syndrome" (Table 6).

The four patients belonging to this group with delirious symptoms, which meant medium psycho-organic symptoms, severe paranoid-hallucinatory symptoms, and

Table 5. Operation procedure and distribution of age and sex in the psychopathological group: "paranoid-hallucinatory syndrome with affective emotional and psychomotor disturbances"

Operative procedure	No. of cases	Age mean value	Sex	
			♂	♀
Correction of congenital defects	1	39	–	1
Mitral valve replacement	2	46	2	–
Aortic valve replacement	1	37	1	–
Multiple valve replacement	1	54	–	1
Coronary surgery	4	53	3	1
Total	9	48	6	3

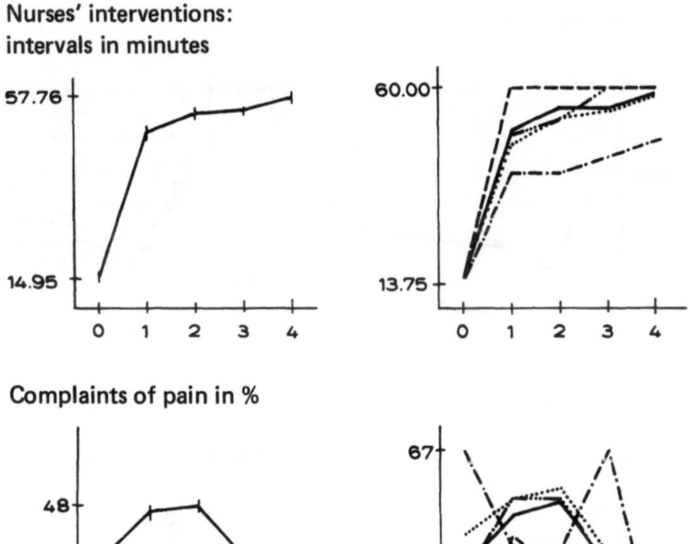

Fig. 6. The early postoperative course for the whole sample and the five different psychic groups: mean values in the intervals between the nurses' interventions and complaints of pain in percent. For legend see Fig. 1

extreme emotional disorders, were all patients with valve replacement. The psychic disorders increased continually from the first to the fourth postoperative day. Compared to the other psychic groups the patients of this group showed special variations which shall be demonstrated here.

Figure 7 shows the average systolic and diastolic pressures after Riva Rocci. The first value is the preoperative value, the second value belongs to the day of the operation after surgery and the following data were noted for the first 4 postoperative days.

Table 6. Operation procedure and distribution of age and sex in the psychopathological group: "delirious syndrome"

Operative procedure	No. of cases	Age mean value	Sex	
			♂	♀
Mitral valve replacement	1	48	–	1
Aortic valve replacement	1	52	–	1
Multiple valve replacement	1	59	1	–
Mitral valve replacement coronary surgery	1	55	1	–
Total	4	54	2	2

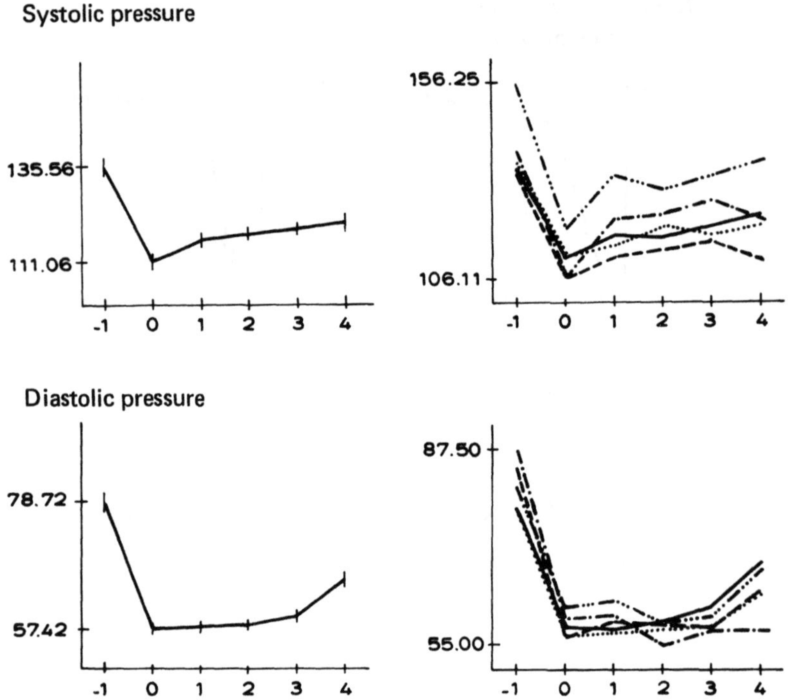

Fig. 7. The early postoperative course for the whole sample and the five early postoperative groups compared to the preoperative status: mean values in systolic and diastolic pressure (Riva-Rocci). For legend see Fig. 1

The average systolic arterial pressures in this group of delirious patients were higher than in the other groups. The systolic pressures were already high before the operation. Three of four patients got NPN directly after the operation and one of them needed antihypertensive drugs during the following days.

Right atrial pressures were high only on the 2nd day, left atrial pressures were in the normal range on the day of the operation and on the first postoperative day, and then went up and stayed high for the following 3 days. There was a positive fluid balance with a rapid rise in the urea-nitrogen level, which shall be demonstrated in Fig. 8.

Figure 8 shows the rise in the average urea-nitrogen level in the delirious patients. There is a gradual rise in the urea-nitrogen levels after surgery in all groups which reflects the diuretic efforts made to remove the water which was retained during the operation with extracorporeal circulation. In some patients this might lead to dehydration, especially if dehydration was already present before the operation. Dehydration seems to make the patients sensible to disturbances of perception, which our working group could demonstrate for preoperative dehydration [3] and other authors like Egerton and Kay [1] and Morse [5] described for postoperative dehydration. The patients in this group had hyponatremia on the first, second and third postoperative day. The arterial O_2 tension went down rapidly from the day of the operation to the third postoperative day. Two patients needed transfusions on the third and fourth postoperative days.

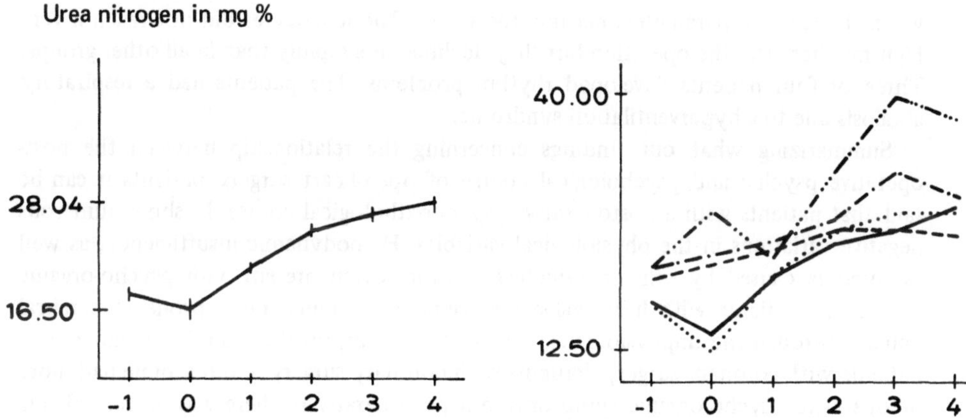

Fig. 8. The early postoperative course for the whole sample and the five different psychic groups compared to the preoperative status: mean values in urea-nitrogen level in serum. For legend see Fig. 1

Figure 9 shows the venous O_2 saturation levels before and after surgery. The most outstanding course of all variables could be found in this parameter for the delirious patients. The average venous O_2 saturation levels were low directly after surgery and stayed low during the following days. This differed extremely from all psychic groups and had a small standard deviation. We presume that the O_2 consumption in these patients was obviously higher than in all other groups, a phenomenon which Polonius et al. [8] had also found in mitral patients with delirious states that he observed in our cardiosurgical intensive care unit. We think that the high O_2 consumption was due to the psychiatric disorders of the patients. With the development of the psychotic symptoms the temperature also rose. The patients' mobilization was retarded on day 3

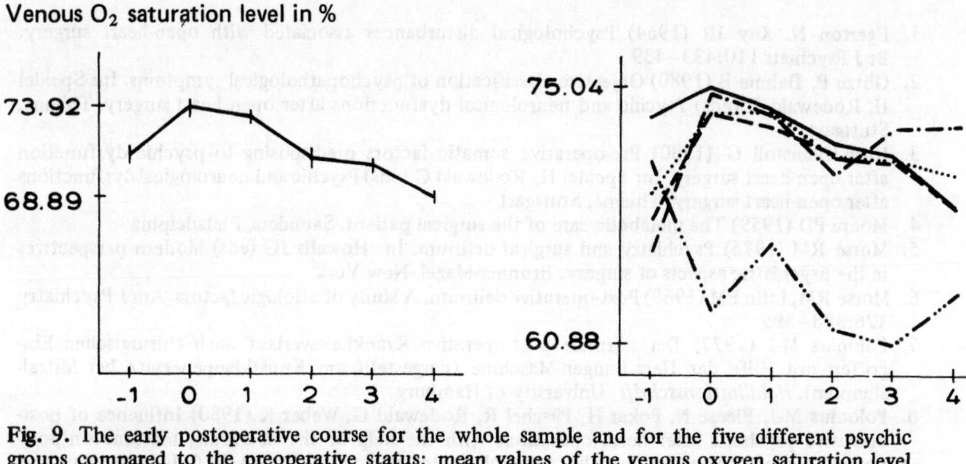

Fig. 9. The early postoperative course for the whole sample and for the five different psychic groups compared to the preoperative status: mean values of the venous oxygen saturation level in percent. For legend see Fig. 1

when the somatic parameters became the worst. The leucocytes did not reach a very high number after the operation but they declined less rapidly than in all other groups. Three of four patients developed rhythm problems. The patients had a respiratory alkalosis due to a hyperventilation syndrome.

Summarizing what our findings concerning the relationship between the post-operative psychic and psychological course of open-heart surgery patients it can be said that patients with a postoperative psychopathological course do show numerous negative variations in the physiological variables. Hemodynamic insufficiency, as well as hypoxia caused by other parameters, is more often present with psycho-organic symptoms. Patients with heart valve replacement are much more prone to cerebral damage through the unphysiological stress of extracorporeal circulation compared to patients with coronary surgery. Patients with coronary surgery in our sample had more preoperative psycho-organic symptoms, but postoperatively there was no remarkable increase in the early postoperative psychopathology, with the exception of one patient who had an intraoperative complication with left ventricular heart failure. The development of early postoperative psycho-organic symptoms is on the onehand correlated to the preoperative clinical state of the patient, and on the other hand it is evident that the improvement of the operative technique and of postoperative care also improves the mental condition of the patients. The development of more complex psychic disorders, such as paranoid-hallucinatory symptoms are favored by psycho-organic deficits and dehydration. Delirious symptoms presumably increase the O_2 consumption of the body and lead to extremely high arteriovenous oxygen content differences ($AVDO_2$) which are easily estimated from the low venous O_2 saturation levels.

Acknowledgments. Processing of the data was performed by M. Wessel. Translation was by Kathleen Behnke und Richard A. Bird.

References

1. Egerton N, Kay JR (1964) Psychological disturbances associated with open-heart surgery. Br J Psychiatr 110:433–439
2. Götze P, Dahme B (1980) Objective classification of psychopathological symptoms. In: Speidel H, Rodewald G (eds) Psychic and neurological dysfunctions after open heart surgery. Thieme, Stuttgart
3. Huse-Kleinstoll G (1980) Pre-operative somatic factors predisposing to psychic dysfunction after open-heart surgery. In: Speidel H, Rodewald G (eds) Psychic and neurological dysfunctions after open-heart surgery. Thieme, Stuttgart
4. Moore PD (1959) The metabolic care of the surgical patient. Saunders, Philadelphia
5. Morse RM (1976) Psychiatry and surgical delirium. In: Howells JG (eds) Modern perspectives in the psychiatric aspects of surgery. Brunner-Mazel, New York
6. Morse RM, Litin EM (1969) Post-operative delirium: A study of etiologic factors. Am J Psychiatry 126:388–395
7. Polonius M-J (1977) Der normale post-operative Krankheitsverlauf nach chirurgischen Eingriffen mit Hilfe der Herz-Lungen-Maschine (dargestellt am Kunstklappenersatz bei Mitralstenosen). *Habilitationsschrift*, University of Hamburg
8. Polonius M-J, Bleese N, Pokar H, Püschel R, Rodewald G, Weber K (1980) Influence of post-operative psychosis after heart operations with the help of the heart-lung machine on post-operative haemodynamics and the metabolism. In: Speidel H, Rodewald G (eds) Psychic and neurological dysfunctions after open-heart surgery. Thieme, Stuttgart

Computerized Electroencephalogram in Open-Heart Surgery: Prediction of Postoperative Psychical Complications*

W. Spehr, P. Götze

Abstaining as much as possible from sophisticated EEG details and speculations, this paper will concentrate on the practical value of computerized EEG in open-heart surgery, i.e., its feasibility and reliability in predicting psychical complications.

Yet some indispensable technical data, though having been presented in previous papers [6, 7], have to be repeated here.

EEG examinations took place around the 5th day before and the 25th day after the operation, using the routine procedure of our laboratory (16-channel Siemens-Elema machine, f = 30, t = 0.15).

In order to test the hypothesis of regional brain dysfunction, precentral, mid-temporal, posterior temporal, and parietal channels of each hemisphere (F3, F4, T3, T4, T5, T6, P3, P4 according to Jasper, reference nasion) were analyzed separately, though simultaneously and on line, using an AEG Telefunken computer (Biosignal-prozessor BIO-16) with special purpose software, applying spectral analysis (by means of FFT) in the frequency domain and Hjorth's parameters "Activity", "Mobility", and "Complexity" [3] in the time domain. Each procedure was based on 160 s of consecutive EEG (frequency resolution: 0.25 Hz, digitizing rate 64 and 128 Hz, respectively).

The whole bulk of "raw data" accumulated per patient thus amounted to 491 520. Some first reduction was already done on line using the special purpose software, applying descriptive statistics (Hjorth: mean and standard deviation; spectral analysis: absolute and relative power, dominant frequency, 1st and 9th decile of frequency distribution for each of the "classical" frequency bands, total power, and theta/alpha ratio [4], – all data for each of eight channels). Data were thus reduced to 416/patient in spectral analysis (0.25% of raw data) and 144/patient in Hjorth's analysis (0.04% of raw data).

These numbers are still too large to cope with without further computer assistance. Therefore, for a "first-glance" information, we use a "Mean Spectrum" [5] computed during the on-line analysis from the above-mentioned eight spectra (channels) and presented in analogue mode only. An example, showing a pre-postoperative shift of dominant frequency (and already familiar to some of you from the first symposium) is presented in Fig. 1.

* With the aid of the Deutsche Forschungsgemeinschaft, Sonderforschungsbereich 115, Teilprojekt A3

Psychopathological and Neurological Dysfunctions
Following Open-Heart Surgery Ed by Becker et al

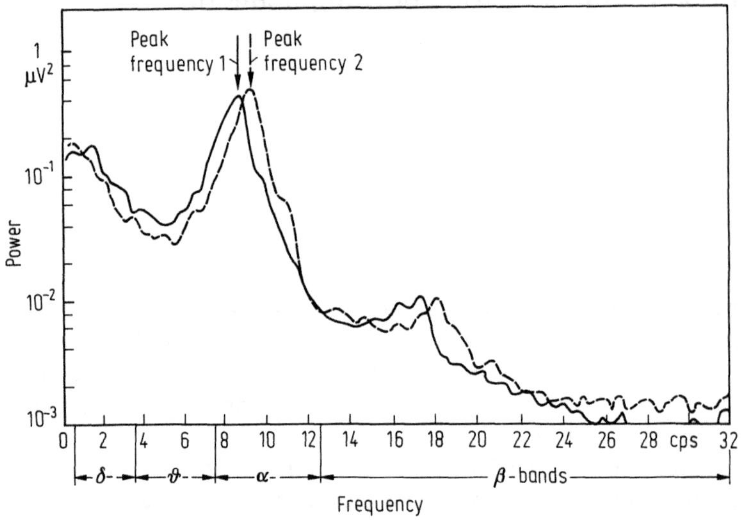

Fig. 1. Intraindividual shift of EEG peak frequency (see text)

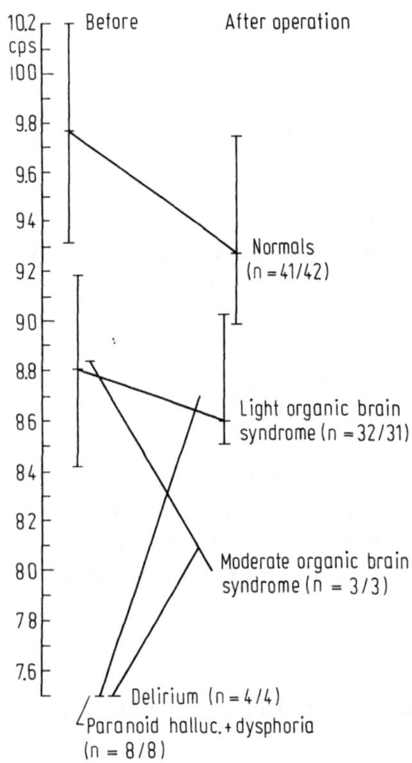

Fig. 2. Estimated peak frequency (mean, 95% C.I.) and postoperative psychical syndrome

As will also be familiar to some of you, an estimated dominant frequency of the combined theta-, alpha- and beta-bands (3.5–32.0 cps) has led to the most powerful prediction of postoperative psychopathology, the latter having been described as kinds of "syndromes" by Goetze [2], applying cluster analysis of AMP rating scale items [1].

In Fig. 2 dominant theta-beta frequency from the preoperative EEG has been grouped according to these postoperative clusters. Differences are apparently significant, preoperative dominant frequency descending with growing severity of postoperative psychical disturbance (caution, of course, has to be exercised with respect to the small-number clusters). From the EEGer's point of view, the two "organic" brain syndromes have a common preoperative situation, the severe one being characterized by a more marked postoperative slowing. Yet, there is no unequivocal connection between prepostoperative shift of dominant frequency and psychical changes. This range of problems has to be postponed for further consideration.

These results are repeated in numerical arrangement in Table 1: psychical disturbance, taken as a whole, can be predicted with high probability from the theta-beta dominant frequency of the preoperative EEG ($P < 0.001$).

To find out whether the predictive power varied with different topographical origin of the signal and/or its special statistical properties, we continued with performing stepwise discriminant analysis, using the EEG of the two somewhat homogeneous clusters of "normals" and "light organic brain syndrome".

This method somehow resembles visual evaluation, taking into account different EEG properties. Accordingly, discriminant functions with a higher percentage of correct classification tended to contain a sometimes puzzling multitude of EEG and localization data. A compromise therefore had to be found between a maximum of correct classification and a minimum of variables.

As to spectral analysis, averaged values from all eight channels (analogous to the abovementioned "mean spectrum") again rendered the best results, as shown in Table 2.

To put it in plain sentences: patients which show a light organic brain syndrome after operation differ from those that do not by an overall higher beta production, a lower frequency at 10% of total alpha power (i.e., the "slower" alpha component), and a slightly higher theta/alpha ratio. The above-mentioned estimated theta-beta dominant frequency does not show up here, as discriminant analysis was performed only with strictly separated bands. We doubt whether this approach is the most rewarding one.

Because of time limitations and more complex problems, we will omit presentation of results with Hjorth's parameters. One result, however, has to be mentioned: discriminating variables were provided by the left hemisphere, with a certain predominance of the temporal regions. This topographical finding has been confirmed by the last methodological approach to be discussed here: the computation of Pearson correlation coefficients of topography, EEG items, and single ratings from the AMP scale, indicating organic rather than psychological disturbance, i.e., disturbances of consciousness, alertness, and orientation. This correlation was done separately for preoperative, early and late postoperative symptoms, and the pre- and postoperative EEG data, respectively. Detailed analysis of the results has not yet been

Table 1. EEG peak frequency within range from 3.5 to 32.0 cps: mean values, standard deviation, and 95% confidence intervals, before and after open-heart surgery

	Peak frequency (cps)						
Group nr.	Psychical syndrome	Before operation	Confidence interval	After operation	Confidence interval	Difference before – after	n before – after
1	Normals	9.76 (1.42)	9.31–10.21	9.37 (1.21)	8.99–9.75	0.39 (0.21)	41/42
2–5	Psych. Disturbed	8.46[c] (1.53)	8.01–8.91	8.66[b] (0.8)	8.42–8.9	−0.2 (0.73)	46/46
2	Light organic brain syndrome	8.8[b] (1.04)	8.42–9.18	8.64[a] (1.03)	8.51–9.03	0.16 (0.01)	32/31
3	Moderate o.b.s. + hallucinations	8.83 (0.76)		8.0 (0.5)		0.83 (0.26)	3/3
4	Paranoid-hallucin. syndr. + dysphoria	7.5 (2.48)		8.69 (1.07)		−1.19 (1.41)	8/8
5	Delirium	7.5 (2.04)		8.1 (0.91)		−0.5 (1.13)	

t-test (difference to normals): [a] t 0.05, [b] t 0.01, [c] t 0.001

Table 2. Spectral analysis variables (mean) from preoperative EEG, discriminating patients with light organic brain syndrome (n = 29) from psychically undisturbed (n = 28) ("normals"), after operation

Spectral variable	Discriminant function coeff.	Postoperative psychical state		
		Light organic brain s.	Normal	t-test
Percentage of beta activity	0.61770	19.29	15.42%	0.047
Alpha frequency at first decile	−0.92397	8.11	8.29 cps	0.027
Theta/alpha ratio	−0.50590	0.48	0.46	
	centroid	−0.41185	0.39730	
Significance: 0.017				
Correct classification in 70.18%				

completed. Nevertheless, we can give a survey of results consistent enough to be more than preliminary.

1. Correlations of psychical and EEG items scarcely exceeded 0.4, – even with significance levels below 0.001.
2. With regard to topography, posttemporal EEG signals appeared to have the most significant predictive value, in that the right side (T6) predicted not only early postoperative psychical disturbances but also those occurring 3–4 weeks after the operation. The left post-temporal region (T5) gave a somewhat specified prediction of disturbed orientation during the early and late postoperative period.
3. As to the predictive value of the EEG frequency content, the most significant correlations of preoperative EEG and postoperative psychopathology were located around the theta-alpha-border (7.5 cps). Frequency distribution within the power of these bands (1st and 9th decile) appeared to be of importance, in that the abundance of slow alpha predicted as well as the abundance of fast theta waves.

Marked enhancement of total EEG power, comprising the delta, theta, and even the alpha band, at T5, appears to be a special predictor of disturbed orientation (note consistency with discriminant analysis of Hjorth's parameters!).

In conclusion, the present state of our EEG research can be summarized as follows:

1. In open-heart surgery, the preoperative EEG, especially when subjected to spectral analysis (FFT) is an efficient method of predicting postoperative psychical complications, especially of a slight to moderate psycho-organic type.
2. Signal analysis from the posttemporal sites (T5, T6) seems most rewarding, when signal averaging from a larger number of channels is not feasible.
3. Alpha-slowing below 9 cps is well correlated with slight psycho-organic symptoms, in prediction as well as in description.
Focal slowing (delta, theta) at the left posttemporal area (T5) appeared to be connected with disturbed orientation.
4. The determination of the predictive EEG features by other clinical factors should be the principal object of future research.

References

1. Angst J, Battegay R, Bente D, Berner P, Broeren W, Cornu F, Dick P, Engelmeier M-P, Heimann H, Heinrich K, Helmchen H, Hippius H, Pöldinger W, Schmidlin P, Schmitt W, Weis P (1969) Das Dokumentations-System der Arbeitsgemeinschaft für Methodik und Dokumentation in der Psychiatrie (AMP). Arzneim Forsch 19:399–405
2. Götze P (1980) Psychopathologie der Herzoperierten. Enke, Stuttgart
3. Hjorth B (1973) The physical significance of time domain descriptors in EEG analysis. Electroencephalogr Clin Neurophysiol 34:321–325
4. Matousek M (1968) Frequency analysis in routine electroencephalography. Electroencephalogr Clin Neurophysiol 24:365–373
5. Spehr W (1976) EEG spectral analysis in laboratory routine work: The biosignalprozessor BIO 16-1. In: Matejcek M, Schenk GK (eds) Quantitative analysis of the EEG. Proceeding of the 2nd symposium of the Study Group for EEG Methodology, Konstanz pp 497–508
6. Spehr W, Götze P (1980) Computerized electroencephalogram before and after open heart surgery (preliminary results). In: Speidel H, Rodewald G (eds) Psychic and neurological dysfunctions after open heart surgery. Thieme, Stuttgart
7. Spehr W, Götze P (1980) Computerized EEG and prediction of psychopathology after open heart surgery. In: Lechner H, Arabinar H (eds) EEG and clinical neurophysiology. Proc. 2nd European Congress of EEG and Clinical Neurophysiology, Salzburg, Excerpta Medica, Amsterdam, p 603

Discussion of Session III

Nwaefuna commented on the preoperative EEG findings in patients with coronary heart disease:

Dr. Spehr said that in coronary heart disease there is no change when the EEG is done. Well, that may be, but the EEG is one of the ways of finding out emotional changes in the individual which may be a contraindication to cardiac surgery. If a patient has an emotional disturbance and he is very worried, under tension, and in fear of the operation, you have to find out any of the causes by asking the relatives or even using hypnosis. If you then mention the cause while they are connected to the EEG you are going to get marked desynchronization, assuring you that the patient is disturbed. This usually means that if you do the operation the patient is going to get a postpsychotic sequela.

Huse-Kleinstoll replied to a question of Scanahan concerning this statistical significance in the four categories of her paper especially related ot the graph of venous oxygen saturation:

We have analyzed it with analysis of variance between the different groups and found that there is a high statistical significance between the groups.

I will give the numbers to you again. Group one with 49 patients; group two with 33; group three with four; group four with nine, and group five with four patients. Regarding your questions concerning the central venous oxygen saturation or the arterial venous oxygen content difference ($AVDO_2$), which is much more correct, clinically you can use the central venous oxygen saturation as you know; over the last years. I did a study on seven patients who belonged to these groups. All these patients had an $AVDO_2$ higher than 5.6, values reaching 7.45. When they were treated by any medication like haloperidol, or something like that, values fell to the normal level, which means that they just cannot compensate the higher oxygen consumption by a higher hemodynamic effort.

IV

Clinical Approaches to the Psychological Care of the Patient Undergoing Cardiac Surgery

Psychological Effects of Preoperative Doctor-Patient Communications*

H. Träger, B. Flemming, J. Nordmeyer, H.-J. Meffert, N. Bleese, H.-J. Krebber

Introduction

The data presented are part of an investigation of psychological aspects of preoperative information carried out on patients of the Department of Cardiovascular Surgery at the University Hospital Hamburg-Eppendorf. The objective of this study was to evaluate the emotional and communicative influences on behavior and experience of patients and physicians during the preoperative information visits in cardiovascular surgery. We want to confine ourselves to the special aspect of preoperative anxiety and the methods used to cope with it.

Hospitalization and surgery are stressful and anxiety-producing experiences. The patient's anxiety in the preoperative situation has some influence on the postoperative period according to the reports of many authors [2, 12]. More important than the amount of preoperative anxiety is the method of coping with the anxiety. The more recent cognitive theories of anxiety [4, 11] emphasizing this point within the concept of cognitive appraisal describe two general coping mechanisms: The tendency to approach or to avoid a threatening stimulus. Coping style as a personality measurement is systematized especially by Byrne [1] within the repression-sensitization construct. Regarding surgery subjects named repressors are patients avoiding or denying the threatening aspects of an impending operation. Patients called sensitizers show anxiety approach behavior as intellectualizing or ruminating and want to know as much possible about their operation. Within our paper we would like to report the influence of those coping styles on the preoperative information process.

Method

Subjects

Fortysix cardiovascular patients (26 male, 20 female, age 20–64 years) who attended the Department of Cardiovascular Surgery at the University Hospital Hamburg-Eppendorf between January 1977 and February 1978 were studied. This sample was re-

* With the aid of the Deutsche Forschungsgemeinschaft, Sonderforschungsbereich 115, Teilprojekt A3

Psychopathological and Neurological Dysfunctions
Following Open-Heart Surgery Ed by Becker et al

presentative of the distribution of three groups of diagnoses including a large proportion of cardiovascular patientship: Surgical treatment for valve disease, coronary artery disease, and patients undergoing varicotomy. Moreover six physicians (three surgeons and three anesthetists) of three different professional levels were included in the study, a surgeon and an anesthetist of equal level at a time.

Assessment Procedures

Preoperative information was given during three periods: Distribution of a consent form to the patient by a nurse in the morning of the day before surgery, and a talk with the surgeon and the anesthetist in the afternoon.

We saw the patients at five points in time (Table 1): In the morning of the day before surgery each patient completed an anamnestic questionnaire and a German version of the Taylor Manifest Anxiety Scale [13]. Before the first talk with one of the two physicians (surgeon or anesthetist) the patient completed a short multidimensional mood scale based on the German scale MSF [7]. After the last talk with the physician (anesthetist or surgeon) each patient completed the mood scale again. Some patients completed the mood scale between both talks too. About 5–10 days after surgery the patient, who was then convalescing, was interviewed using a structured interview about aspects of the preoperative situation, of the experience of surgery, and of information transmission. The patient answered open and structured questions, and self and interviewer assessments were carried out. Besides these procedures further assessments of behavioral and experiental aspects of our patients and physicians were the discussion of made, which is beyond the framework of this paper.

Results

The Patients' Mood Before and After Preoperative Information

The dimensions of the multidimensional mood scale used can be divided into two syndromes (Table 2): First, a general syndrome of anxiety containing the scale state "Anxiety", "Nervousness" within the meaning of anxiety-induced arousal, "Depression" as a reaction to an imagined experience of personal loss which has not yet occurred in reality, and "Aggression" as a sign of frustration. Second, with "Relaxation" as a pleasant mood, and "Activation" as a positive aspect of motivation, we find an activation/relaxation syndrome.

Comparing the moods of our patients before and after the preoperative information procedure we see that remarkable changes have occurred (Table 3). In particular state anxiety – followed by the other dimensions of the anxiety syndrome – was much smaller after preoperative information ($P \leqslant .001$). "Nervousness" and "Depression" also had significantly lower means after the talks with the physicians. But there is no significant change in the means of the two variables of the activation/relaxation syndrome.

Table 1. Data collection schedule

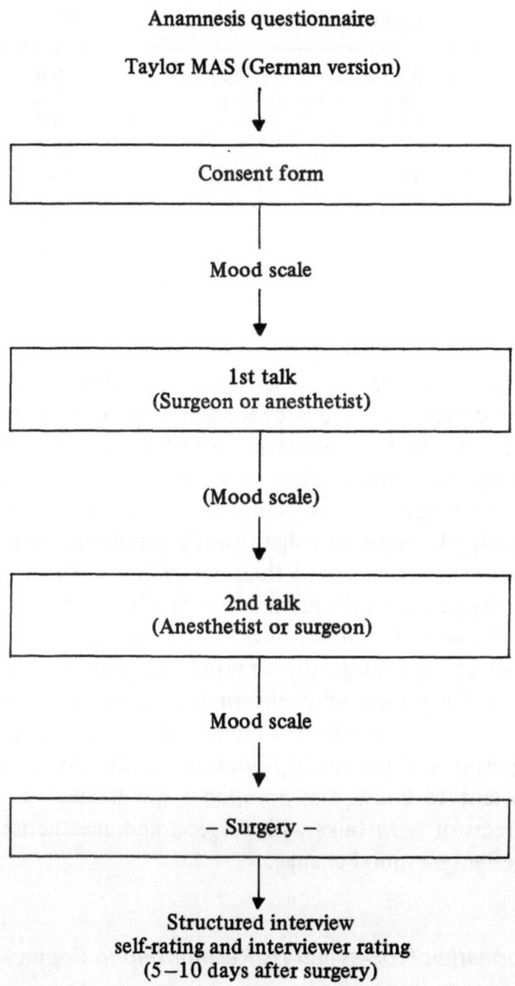

Table 2. Correlation matrix of mood dimensions

		1	2	3	4	5	6
Nervousness	1	1.00					
Depression	2	*0.43*	1.00				
Anyiety	3	*0.64*	*0.73*	1.00			
Aggression	4	*0.47*	*0.41*	*0.43*	1.00		
Activation	5	0.08	0.10	0.17	0.11	1.00	
Relaxation	6	*0.46*	0.29	0.33	0.14	0.61	1.00

Table 3. The patients' mood before and after preoperative information (mean scores)

n = 46	Before		After	*t*-Test
Nervousness	10.5	>	8.6	$P \leq 0.01$
Depression	8.6	>	7.5	$P \leq 0.05$
Anxiety	10.6	>	8.4	$P \leq 0.001$
Activation	15.9		16.5	
Relaxation	16.2	⩽	17.8	($P \leq 0.10$)
Minimum/maximum	5/30		5/30	

In comparison with other groups of subjects (the physicians during the information procedure, clients before and after a psychotherapeutic initial interview) the specific mood changes among our patients were not found among those of other groups. There were no significant changes in the physicians' mood dimensions. This was expected because providing preoperative information is a routine task for surgeons and anesthetists with no intense emotional involvement. Clients before and after an initial interview in psychotherapy [3] showed a significantly greater increase in "Relaxation", but remained in a generally worse mood than our patients. This might be explained by different aims in preoperative information and psychotherapy talks: In the initial interview personal problems and conflicts ought to be elaborated for better perception of one's own. This might be emotionally unsatisfying. The aim of preoperative information is to provide the patient with information about the impending operation and to stabilize his emotional condition. This emotional stabilization was primarily achieved by reducing aspects of the anxiety syndrome under subsistence of relaxation. However, it is important to know that emotional stabilization is only attained by summation of the effects of *both* talks with surgeon and anesthetist, each talk alone having no significant effect on mood change.

The Preoperative Information Process and Its Relationship to Coping with Anxiety

We have just seen that on average the patients' mood is changed positively by the preoperative information talks. Of special importance was the reduction of the anxiety syndrome. We would now like to discuss how our patients cope with anxiety, and which were the mechanisms which reduced anxiety.

The Taylor Manifest Anxiety, Scale and its German version are highly correlated with Byrne's Repression-Sensitization Scale, many authors concluding, therefore, that both scales measure the same and are interchangeable [5, 6, 9]. We therefore used that scale for measuring the style of coping with anxiety.

In our sample we found a clear relation of the two coping styles "repression" and "sensitization" to other variables measured (Table 4). Patients having a tendency for sensitization were more anxious, more depressive, and more nervous before preoperative information than the others. Their anxiety has been strongly reduced by the talks with the physicians. But intellectual understanding of special topics of surgery and

Table 4. Coping style in relation to patient variables (n = 46)

	Sensitization	Repression
Anxiety	+	–
Depression	+	–
Nervousness	+	–
Anxiety reduction	+	–
Intellectual comprehension	–	
Duration of complaints	+	–
Valvular lesions	+	
Coronary heart disease		+

intensive care is reduced. At the first glance this result is discordant, but it may be understood in the frame of information process research [10]: Sensitizers are searching much more for information on problem solving than others; information is reducing anxiety during psychic strain, however, their intellectual processing capability is diminished, i.e., their intellectual understanding is reduced.

With regard to diagnosis there was an unequivocal association of the tendency for sensitization among patients with valvular lesions and of the tendency for repression among patients with coronary heart diseases (Fig. 1). To what extent aspects of chronification and progress of disease play a part besides basic personality characteristics is not yet clearly answered but possible [8]. When including the preoperative risk rated by the physicians we observe an interesting constellation: With increasing preoperative risk – i.e., with greater threat to the patient – the tendency to form a specific coping style (repression or sensitization) becomes greater. Patients with little risk (varicotomy) are not clearly identifiable with regard to coping style. The greater the individual threat – measured indirectly by risk assessment – the greater is the tendency for repression or sensitization behavior.

If patients with different diagnoses have different coping behavior, then preoperative information must be related to the individual coping style. A uniform information

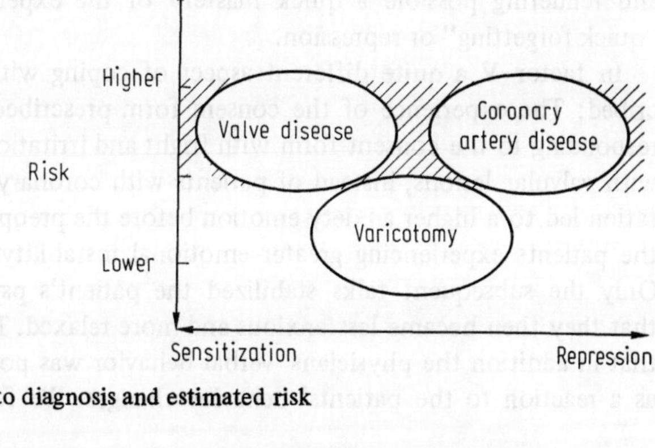

Fig. 1. Relationship of coping style to diagnosis and estimated risk

Table 5. Postoperative evaluation of preoperative information (factor analysis)

I	Effective informedness	(12.8)
II	Postoperative repression	(10.5)
III	Psychic destabilization	(9.7)
IV	Intense need for contact	(9.4)
V	Preoperative sensitization	(8.9)
Amount of total variance		(51.3)

procedure would not have optimal results. But how can such an ideal kind of preparation be realized?

The Retrospective Experience of Preoperative Information with Regard to Coping Behavior

A factor analysis of variables of the postoperative interview yields a factorial structure of five dimensions distinguishing three general features (Table 5): Cognition (factor I), emotion (factors III and IV), and coping (factors II and V). The cognitive aspect includes only characters of information and knowledge. Within the emotional dimension, difficulties in doctor-patient interaction are described which are first induced by the physician's behavior on experiencing the patient as a problem patient (factor III), and which otherwise are induced by the patient distressing the doctor by clinging anxiously to him (factor IV).

Of special interest are the factors II and V related to coping behavior: Factor II represents the behavior of persons who postoperatively pretended to have not been anxious before surgery, and to have gained nothing from the information of the preoperative talks. But these subjects were substantially emotionally strained before surgery – as measured by the mood scale – being very anxious before and after the talks. The consent form was experienced as very stressing and anxiety provoking. It is remarkable that persons represented on factor II have a long anamnesis and great hospital experience, but there is no specific difference between diagnoses. Here we find, first of all, general aspects of coping behavior relating to survival of the operation and rendering possible a quick mastery of the experience of surgery – a kind of "quick forgetting" or repression.

In factor V a quite different aspect of coping with preoperative anxiety is described: The experience of the consent form prescribed by legal regulations. Patients responding to the consent form with fright and irritation are in the first place patients with valvular lesions, instead of patients with coronary heart disease. Fright and irritation led to a higher anxiety emotion before the preoperative information procedure, the patients experiencing greater emotional instability, and less positive motivation. Only the subsequent talks stabilized the patient's psychic condition to the extent that they then became less anxious and more relaxed. This positive effect was so great that in addition the physicians' verbal behavior was positively changed above average as a reaction to the patients' behavior changes. We found no effect of that kind in patients with coronary heart disease. This is plausible with respect to sensitizing coping behavior because searching for information is necessary to reduce anxiety. But if information includes new threats unknown before hand anxiety is increased instead of being reduced by the consent form. Finally, in the personal contact with the physicians, a correlation of negative emotions with explanations of those facts and risks unknown before hand is possible and then has an anxiety reducing effect. This indicates the danger of a global consent form passed on to the patients without further instruction.

Discussion

The results presented indicate that anxiety is a central aspect of the patients' preoperative condition, and that distinct coping styles have different effects on the experience of receiving preoperative information. Especially remarkable is the interrelationship between coping style and diagnosis.

When looking at these results under the aspect of psychological preparation for surgery, there is not only the necessity for a different view of coping behavior but for considering the interrelationship between diagnosis and coping behavior. Patients do not only show different emotional reactions because of different coping styles, but their specific coping style may be – at least partially – influenced by their basic disease. Thus, a different individually adapted preoperative information procedure is of great consequence for a good emotional adaptation to surgery.

We have seen the effect of the consent form as a negative example having bad consequences in persons with sensitizing behavior. On the other hand, comprehensive preoperative information is not useful for each patient – for instance it is not absolutely necessary for patients with a repressive coping style, i.e., we ought not to try to deliver a maximum of information to each patient – which means that we should even renounce giving any information if the preoperative information process bears any danger of emotional breakdown for a patient. The adaptation of preoperative information to the patient's personal needs should be the maxim of preparing the patient for surgery, but because of the cost and time incurred with an individually adapted information procedures which are realistically practicable at any hospital.

Acknowledgment. We gratefully acknowledge the very helpful cooperation of Prof. G. Rodewald (Department of Cardiovascular Surgery, University of Hamburg).

References

1. Byrne D (1961) The repression-sensitization scale: Rationale, reliabilitiy and validity. J Pers 29:334–349
2. Davies-Osterkamp S (1977) Angst und Angstbewältigung bei chirurgischen Patienten. Med Psychol 3:169–184
3. Eckensberger D (1976) Die affektive Reaktion auf das psychotherapeutische Erstinterview als Interaktionseffekt. Med Psychol 2:145–164

4. Epstein S (1967) Towards a unified theory of anxiety. In: Maher BA (ed) Progress in experimental personality research. Academic Press, New York
5. Flemming B (1977) Angst und Angstabwehr bei starker psychischer Belastung vor Herzoperationen. Doctoral dissertation, University of Hamburg
6. Golin S, Herron W, Lakota R, Reineck L (1967) Factor analytic study of the manifest anxiety, extraversion, and repression-sensitization scales. J Consult Psychol 31:564–569
7. Hecheltjen K, Mertesdorf F (1973) Entwicklung eines mehrdimensionalen Stimmungsfragebogens (MSF). Gruppendynamik 4:110–122
8. Kimball CP (1969) Psychological responses to the experience of open-heart surgery I. Am J Psychiatry 125:348–359
9. Krohne HW (1974) Untersuchungen mit einer deutschen Form der Repression-Sensitization-Skala. Z Klin Psychol Psychother 3:238–260
10. Krohne HW, Schroder HM (1972) Anxiety defense and complex information processing. Arch Psychol 124:50–61
11. Lazarus RS, Averill JR, Opton EM Jr (1972) Emotion and cognition with special reference to anxiety. In: Spiegelberger CD (ed) Anxiety. Current trends in theory and research, Academic Press, New York
12. Melamed BG (1977) Psychological preparation for hospitalization. In: Rachman S (ed) Contribution to medical psychology, vol I, Pergamon Press, Oxford
13. Spreen O (1961) Konstruktion einer Skala zur Messung der manifesten Angst in experimentellen Untersuchungen. Psychol Forsch 26:205–223

Reactions to Illness: The Acute Phase*

The Interplay of Environmental Factors
The Intensive Care Unit

Ch.P. Kimball

Introduction

The acute phase of illness, following initial evaluation in a physician's office, patient's home, or an Emergency room is spent in intensive care units of one kind or another. These are specialized units with trained staff and special equipment addressed to the needs of the patient. Our attention has become focused on these *environments of illness* as their number and their special approaches have multiplied. Our interest has been directed to specific problems that arise in these arenas and we have come to think about the effect that environments and what takes place within them have upon the behavior of staff and patients.

The Intensive Care Unit

Thus, the special units and hospitals that have developed as the result of medical specialization and technology have served as laboratories for the study of the behavior of patients and staff during a critical phase of illness. More immediately, our attention was directed to these units because of the frequently disruptive behavior and experiences of patients and staff (Table 1). Indeed, in the early coronary care and the postoperative cardiac units, such behavior was so common as to earn the designation, the intensive care unit syndrome, which Nahum suggested was a disease of medical progress [1]. The behavior of patients described by Blachly as postcardiotomy delirium included a disturbance in perception, cognition, conation, and effect [2]. It sometimes included hallucinations and delusions with increased agitation. Abram and Kornfeld identified staff responses as anxiety, frustrations, sadness, anger, and fatique [3, 4] (Table 2). At first, the bases for these altered states were not always readily apparent. As we began to attend the patients as consultant psychiatrists and internists, our attention was first directed toward the process we observed in the patient, and only later to the interactions between staff and patient, and staff and staff.

---

* Modified after "Reactions to Illness: The Acute Phase – The Interplay of Environmental Factors in Intensive Care Units" in *Symposium on Liaison Psychiatry*. Psychiat. Clinic. No. Amer. 2:307–319, #2, 1979

Psychopathological and Neurological Dysfunctions
Following Open-Heart Surgery. Ed. by Becker et al.

Table 1. The intensive care unit environment

1.	An alien environment
2.	Overstimulation in terms of sounds, number of individuals attending patient, other senses assaulted
3.	Sensory monotony in terms of repetitiousness of sounds, sights, other sensations
4.	Processes that interfere with communication
5.	Absence of familiar individuals
6.	Absence of usual day-night sequence
7.	Physical discomfort of disease
8.	Drugs interfering with cognitive processes
9.	Crowding of beds, resulting in lack of privacy
10.	Illnesses and death of other patients

Table 2. Demands of ICU on staff. After [4]

	Reaction
1. Constant attention of seriously ill patient	Anxiety
2. Constant threat of death in every patient	Fatigue/anxiety
3. Need to work with less experienced house officers	Ambivalence
4. In emergency may have to initiate procedures usually carried out by physicians	Role diffusion

As we listened to our patients, we began to hear first their impressions and secondly their interpretation of these environments. Their descriptions included: "it was like something I could never have imagined existing": "it was like being on a different planet where everything was unfamiliar"; "I didn't know where I was, nothing looked like anything I had ever seen before"; "... even the smells and sounds were unfamiliar"; "everyone was in some kind of uniform or mask"; "there was no way of telling day from night, the lights were always on and there were no windows"; "things were constantly happening, people coming and going, patients dying ... sometimes you didn't know if it was you or someone else". It seemed that oftentimes these experiences lent themselves at first to illusions and subsequently to delusions and hallucinations as part of an altered state of consciousness. When the latter appeared, these were identified by some as psychotic states, either of organic or functional origin. It was our observation that the very designation of craziness served to put greater distance between the patient and his environment, as more anxiety was aroused in the intensive care unit staff and the patient's relatives. This behavior by staff and family further isolated and alienated the patient, lessening communication and even the frequency of medical contacts.

As we spent more time in these environments we began to take stock of our own discomforts, relating these first to the staff and subsequently to the patient who was too often viewed as the source of our discomfort. As time and our research progressed, it became more and more apparent that the discomfort in the patient was not so much the disease as a response to the experience of illness, the environment, and those within it.

The field theory of Grinker, an early extrapolation of a general systems approach to behavior, became a useful model for understanding this phenomenon in general [5]. Not only what is going on the field in which a disease develops, its signs and symptoms precipitated, but also what is going on in the field in which disease and illness is treated became a part of our exploration.

The Phenomenological Approach

With this orientation derived from our explorations with patients and staff living in these environments and from our self-examination and observations made within these environments, we proceeded in our investigations using a phenomenological descriptive approach without too readily or easily applying theoretical formulations which too quickly prejudice our observations. Thus far, our major formulation based on these reports and observations was the idea of an environment as bearing a major relationship to the behavior of the individuals within. While not strikingly novel, this formulation gave impetus to more particulate identification and examination of the behavior within. As we progressed with these studies, attempting to extrapolate concepts formulated within the context of one environment to others, we became aware of the marked differences in appearances, feelings, and activities characterizing the different environments within which illness is treated. Not only are there different tasks imposed on patients and their attendants at different phases of illness, but these are different in different environments at the same relative phase of illness. In order to emphasize this, extrapolations will be made from the studies of coronary care and postoperative cardiac surgical units.

Anxiety and Sadness

Cassem and Hackett [6] have identified a pattern of emotional response which is fairly characteristic of patients surviving an acute myocardial infarction in an intensive care unit (Fig. 1). From the onset of the infarct as measured in the hospital, anxiety mounts, peaking by the 2nd day. It is directly correlated with the intensity and extensity of the symptoms, notably pain. Anxiety is partially defended against by denial which may address the fact of illness, its severity, its treatment and especially feeling. The behavioral counterpart of anxiety and denial is frequently impulsivity. Anxiety gives way to what the authors call depression, which I prefer to identify as sadness, rising to a peak by the 4th day, thereafter dropping off. Some of us experience that this drop-off tapers slowly and remains relatively high throughout the subsequent convalescent period. Depression is defended against by the characterological defenses of the patient. Thus, the individual with obsessive-compulsive traits demonstrates an intensity of these; the patient with impulsive characteristics becomes more impulsive; the patient with depressive orientations more dependent and passive.

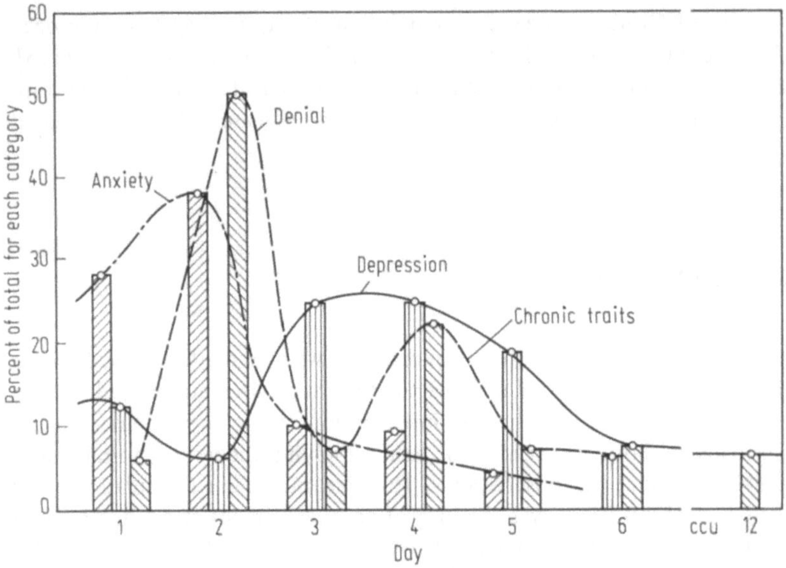

Fig. 1. Psychological responses in a coronary care unit [6]

Altered States of Consciousness (Delirium)

Initially, anxiety was identified as an affective state contributing to an altered state of consciousness, delirium, or an acute organic brain syndrome. The basis of anxiety was viewed as stemming from the patient's self-perception of his illness and its treatment in the environments identified above. Anxiety in these environments may be viewed as a contagious phenomenon, having as its victims staff as well as patients and relatives. It spreads through a unit undermining whatever immunological defenses may be present. When the defenses against anxiety get out of hand, turmoil and unfortuitous circumstances prevail. It is still not uncommon to find a patient in an Intensive Care Unit (arms and legs tied, further pinned down by aides at the shoulder, while a nurse attempts to inject yet another drug, record an electrocardiogram, and remove blood) screaming that he is "being held a prisoner and that they are killing me" – this all before spectator patients in other beds and the roar of several consultants and bystanders offering differing advice. Whatever benefit accrues from such a scene is derived from its review, first allowing for the necessary defensiveness followed by the ventilations of the individuals concerned. When such sessions are held on a regular basis, with physicians as well as nursing staff, these scenes are less often replayed. The staff, by ventilating frustration, are more likely to hear and even give permission for their patient's ventilation with the realization that these processes dissipate rather than increase anxiety. During the convalescent stage, the same therapeutic processes need to be used for sadness and anger. The latter lend themselves to a brief psychotherapy based upon Lindemann's grieving model, which is more formally addressed in the chapters on convalescence [7] (Table 3).

Table 3. Stages and tasks of mourning

(Intensive Care Unit)	1. Overcoming denial
(Intensive Care Unit) (convalescence)	2. Awareness and ventilation of emotion
(Intensive Care Unit) (convalescence)	3. Sorting out of effective *vs* ineffective defenses
(Convalescence) (rehabilitation)	4. Addressing appropriate defenses to conate processes of coping/adaptation

Whereas delirium, as first described by observers working in intensive care units, erupted suddenly 3–5 days following a coronary event and having a course of 5–7 days before its resolution, further studies suggest that delirium is best conceptualized as a process with several stages, that can be identified early in its course, therefore allowing for appropriate intervention (Fig. 2). Not uncommonly, the first symptoms of delirium are those of a hypervigilant state in which patients describe lights as brighter, and sounds as sharper than usual. The individual has heightened perceptivity of the particulate, e.g., a dropped stitch in a sweater or a crack in the ceiling. This stage is associated with irritability, crankiness, and rapid reporting of observations and feelings. The hypervigilant stage is relatively brief and gives way to a mild state of confusion in which orientation, attention and memory, especially recent, may suffer some impairment. There may be some yawning and sighing. A later stage shows more confusion, disorientation and memory impairment with some compromise of judgmental functions and abstraction. A fourth stage might be termed *delirium proper* inasmuch as it is what is usually meant by the term. It is usually the only stage that is identified. In this stage the patient is again more active, frequently agitated, and in addition to confusion, disorientation, memory impairment and abstractive

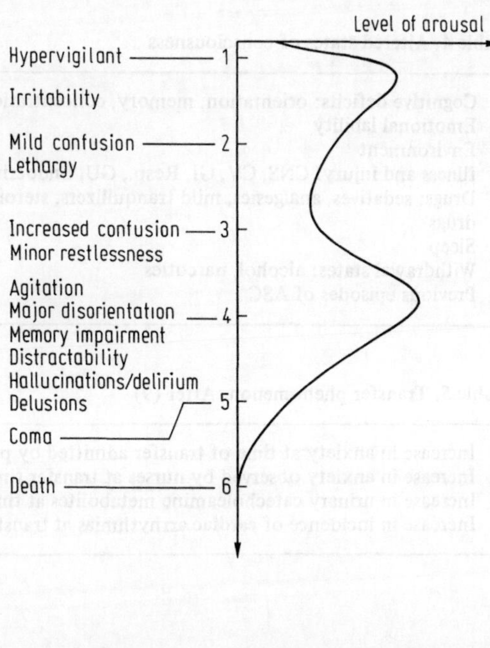

Fig. 2. Stages of delirium

dysfunction, manifests auditory and/or visual hallucinations, as well as delusions. This stage is still frequently designated by terms of acute paranoid state or paranoid schizophrenic reaction. There is little place and no value for this terminology for this condition. Left unattended, this stage either resolves or progresses to a less agitated, more somnolent state and subsequently to coma.

Our extensive examinations of delirium in coronary units identify correlations in the order of the following frequency: hypnotic sedatives, analgesics (esp. pentazocine), withdrawal states, steroids, metabolic and physiologic factors relating to the illness, the environment, communication difficulties (stemming from tracheostomies to human relationships) (Table 4). Other factors have specificity for specific environments, e.g., hypothermia in cardiac surgery units, patched eyes in post-operative ophthalmology units (Black Patch Delirium) [8], isolation in some chemotherapy units. Thus for each environment, studies need to be conducted in order to identify factors specific and unique to each and the association of these with behavioral states. At times, extrapolations from one unit to another are in order.

Transfer Phenomenon

At this point, we talk of transition points, the transfer from one unit to another. One does not transcend these easily. Klein has identified the concurrence of anxiety at the time of transfer with patient verbalization, nurses' observations, biochemical variables and cardiac arrhythmias [9] (Table 5). Patients' verbalization of this period include: "It's like a bird being pushed out of the nest ... you either fly ... or ..." and "when they unhooked my monitor, I had to keep beeping or my heart would stop ...". For others, the progress is even rougher. The questions of readiness are on hand. Again, there is uncertainty. "Will I make it?" "What will it be like out

Table 4. Altered states of consciousness

1. Cognitive deficits: orientation, memory, concentration, abstraction (concreteness)
2. Emotional lability
3. Environment
4. Illness and injury: CNS, CV, GI, Resp., GU, Endocrine, Hematologic, Metastatic
5. Drugs: sedatives, analgesics, mild tranquilizers, steroids, anticholinergics, specific drugs
6. Sleep
7. Withdrawal states: alcohol, narcotics
8. Previous episodes of ASC

Table 5. Transfer phenomenon. After (9)

1. Increase in anxiety at time of transfer admitted by patient
2. Increase in anxiety observed by nurses at transfer time
3. Increase in urinary catecholeamine metabolites at time of transfer
4. Increase in incidence of cardiac arrhythmias at transfer

Table 6. Tasks of illness

	Staff	Patient	
1st Phase Acute	1. Permission to be ill	Accepts partial dependent position based upon acceptance of illness	
	2. Permission to ventilate	Talks about fears, sadness, anger	Grieves
	3. Accepts ventilation	Tries various defenses	
	4. Accepts and helps shape appropriate defenses	Accepts therapist's suggestions and encouragement	
2nd Phase Convalescent	5. Accepts patient's convalescence	Conservation withdrawal	
	6. Allows patient to grieve	Uses increasingly sophisticated mechanisms of defense	
	7. Eshorts patient to self-care	Accepts self-care	
3rd Rehabilitative	8. Supports positive coping and adaptive strategies	Prepares self for the event of home-coming	

there?" "Will there be enough care?" For most, these questions go unsaid, perhaps unfelt. The next environment is strange too. It has different customs. The pace is different. There are new customs to learn and new tasks to accomplish. Not the least of these is to find one's sea-legs again after a virtual week of confinement to bed during which there may have occurred a tremendous loss of muscular strength and altered emotional control. Resolution is a major task of recovery from illness, of the process of going from patienthood to nonpatient status. Before resolution, there is the task of acceptance of illness which may be viewed as a process of mourning (Table 6). Denial must be overcome; the emotions of anxiety, anger and sadness expressed; the thoughts of mortality, uncertainty verbalized; and the trial and error process of testing out which available defenses will or will not prove adaptive. This requires time and needs to be replayed several times over. Resolution occurs much later after emotional processes have taken place. For effective coping and adaptation, resolution appears essential. Of coping and adaptation, we have much to learn. Since these processes more likely take place outside of the acute hospital situation, comparatively little work has been done in this area.

Therapeutic Process

In working with the staff and patient in situations of delirium, anxiety, and depression, the first approach is usually that of re-establishing communication (Table 7). This is easier than it may appear, providing that there are few interruptions and there is relative quiet. Communicative processes need not be elaborate. In fact, most is accomplished when they are matter of fact and simple. *Re-orienting* statements, identification of staff and patient, a clarification of what has happened, supportive statements regarding present and future, and allowing a patient to ventilate his feelings and concerns constitute the bedside therapeutic approach. Occasionally, structuring statements

Table 7. Treatment of altered states of consciousness

1. Do not leave patient alone!
2. Nurse's aide
3. Direct simple repeated orienting reassuring remarks
4. Review medications, chemistries
5. Identify other possible causes
6. Reduce environmental confusion; change
7. Butyrophenone, haloperidol
8. Assess for further therapy

involving limit-setting or confirming the patient's own positive reflections are useful. Most of all, these bedside chats require both brevity and frequency. Cassem and Hackett [6] have demonstrated that full-blown delirium can be readily attended by the above approach, sometimes with the assistance of a butyrophenone (haloperidol). Usually the process is best approached by identifying and removing incriminated factors. Sometimes these are relatives. In these communications we are not surprised to find that patients bring with them a preoccupation with other environments, those of home and business. Preoccupation with the affairs of these, for whatever reason, takes priority over the preoccupation with the present. Difficulty with compliance may result less from anxiety or conflicts with authority than from concern over specific events occurring in the illness-onset situation. When viewed from the vantage-point of life phase, expectable events may be identified. For the middle-aging individual, these concerns will be with marriage, children and job generally and more specifically with separation, departing children, promotions or sense of stagnation. As the interviewer hones down with the patient and the family, important particulates invariably emerge. But looking backward, there is a horizon beyond what was happening in the illness-onset situation, which once reached and explored may contribute to both the patient's and the therapist's understanding. Fair game is soliciting information regarding responses to other illnesses and through these to the vital statistics of growth and development in the areas of physical, social, educational, and psychological development. These will give data contributing to an understanding of the patient's personality and the life from other environments he brings with him and which is now on the line. With this information personality emerges as a variable subject to the environment's relation to it. Further back, a distant mirror may be reflected identifying biological and psychological markers genetically and familially transmitted. Into the present, crowd the environments of the past, awaiting accommodation with the forebodings of an uncertain future.

References

1. Nahum LH (1966) Madness in the recovery room from open heart surgery or "They Kept Waking Me Up". Conn Med 29:771–772
2. Blachly PH, Starr A (1964) Post-cardiotomy delirium. Am J Psychiatry 121:317–375

3. Abram H, Gill BF (1961) Predictions of postoperative psychiatric complications. N Engl J Med 265:1123–1128
4. Kornfeld DS, Zimberg S, Malm JR (1965) Psychiatric complications of open-heart surgery. N Engl J Med 273:287–292
5. Grinker R (1960) Open system psychiatry. Am J Psychoanal 26:115–126
6. Cassem NH, Hackett TP (1971) Psychiatric consultation in a coronary care unit. Ann Intern Med 75:9–14
7. Lindemann E (1944) Symptomatology and management of acute grief. Am J Psychiatry 101:141–148
8. Weisman AD, Hackett TP (1958) Psychosis after eye surgery: Establishment of a specific doctor-patient relation in the prevention and treatment of "black-patch delirium". N Engl J Med 258:1284–1289
9. Klein R, Kliner VA, Zipes DP (1968) Transfer from a coronary care unit. Arch Intern Med 122:104–108

The Control of Anxiety by Hypnosis and Anxiolytics in Open-Heart Surgery

A. Nwaefuna

Introduction

It is accepted that about 50% of patients who undergo open-heart surgery develop neuropsychiatric sequelae. The type and severity of the complications depend on the prepsychiatric morbidity, sex, age, and environmental variables of each individual case.

The heart is under the control of the autonomous nervous system which is controlled by the limbic system, which also controls human emotional reactions. Hypnosis regulates the activities of the caudal and rostral ends of the reticular formation and therefore controls the emotional discharges of the limbic system to the heart.

The anxiolytic drugs chlorozapate dipotassium (Tranxene) and lorazepam (Ativan) have a direct action on the higher centers and amygdala (center for anxiety and aggression) of the limbic system. The latter drug, being pharmacologically a dependency drug, is not advisable for prolonged drug therapy.

Neuropsychiatric Sequelae of Open-Heart Surgery

Postcardiotomy Syndrome. This consists of generalized chest pain like a dull ache. This has its psychopathology in stress and anxiety.

Postoperative Hallucinosis. This consists of visual hallucinations of fearful animals besides the patients' bed. Patient may hear auditory hallucinatory voices of persecution after recovery from the operation.

Toxic Psychoses. This may occur due to extracorporeal circulation; micro-embolism may irritate basal ganglia causing temporarily psychotic episodes.

Acute Situational Psychosis. This may be self-limiting and could be caused by fear and doubts about surviving the operation.

Indefinite Period of Unconsciousness. This is invariably due to the death of rostral cells of the Reticular Activating System due to anoxia. This condition is usually irreversible. These patients remain mute for days on end.

Psychopathological and Neurological Dysfunctions
Following Open-Heart Surgery Ed by Becker et al

Postoperative Delusion of Grandeur. Some patients awake and imagine themselves as prophets and saviours of the world. Others imagine themselves to have been endowed with supernatural powers and could do almost anything – could make either side in a football match score a goal.

Psychopathology

The sensory imput ascending through the median lemniscus and trigemenal lemniscus enter the reticular formation. The rostral cells of the Reticular Activating System relay these impulses to the cerebral cortex including the superior cingulate gyrus which is the higher center for the limbic system. Some of the impulses are relayed from the thalamus, which is a part of the limbic system, to the sensory cortex (area 3.1.2) (scc Fig. 1).

There is a two way relay system between the nuclei of the limbic system (see Fig. 2). These impulses reaching the limbic system are then relayed to the amygdala mass of nuclei (see Fig. 3) of the limbic system, which is the center for anxiety and aggression. The limbic system also controls memory and emotion.

The impulses originating from the limbic system are discharged through the hypothalamus (see Fig. 4) which itself is a part of the limbic system. The hypothalamus in turn discharges through the autonomic nervous system. The parasympathetic originate from the anterior aspect while the sympathetic originate from the posterior. These two groups of fibers unite to form the dorsal longitudinal bundle which sends autonomic nerve fibers including vagus nerves to the heart and sympathetic fibers to the heart from the cervical ganglia. From this dorsal longitudinal bundle autonomic fibres are sent to all organs of the body endowed with autonomic innervation and these organs in turn are susceptible to psychosomatic disorders. Through this route, all emotional changes in the limbic system, including fear and anxiety, affect the heart.

The thalamus is a part of the limbic system as already stated, and is also a part of the basal ganglia involved in the Inhibitory Circuit. With an increase in emotional discharge from the limbic system the basal ganglia increases its discharge of dopamine, most abundant in the substantia nigra and bringing about hallucinations, delusions, and paranoid ideas.

Psychic Scan and Hypnotherapy

In the past some people held esoteric views about the nature of hypnosis [1, 2], though nowadays most workers have generally recognized [3–5] the fact that the hypnotic state involves a temporary alteration in the subject's awareness of his external and internal environments or, in other words, in his span of attention.

The altered state of perceptual awareness is due to changes in the neurological mechanisms that underly the process whereby one is aware of one's environment in a global sense, and in a specific sense.

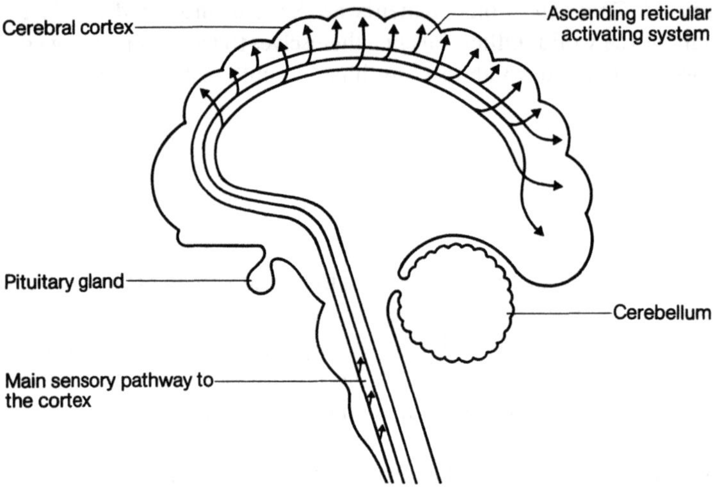

Fig. 1. The cortex. Sensory stimuli entering the brain travel either directly or via the reticular system to the cortex. There the stimuli are evaluated and the decision about the necessary response is made. The decisions are then returned to the body. either through the reticular system or directly from the motor centers. The cortex is mainly responsible for deciding the direction the individual's response to stimuli should take.

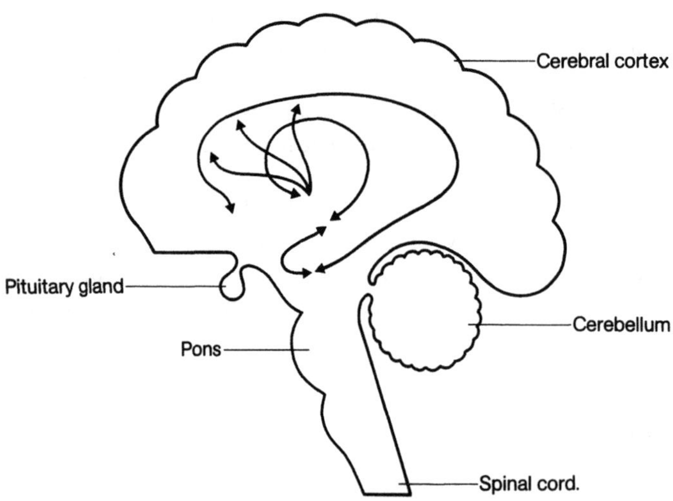

Fig. 2. The limbic system. The limbic system consists of a group of structures: the cingulate gyrus, amygdala, anterior thalamic nuclei, reticular formation, hippocampus, hypothalamus. Stimuli which enter the brain also reverberate through the structures of the limbic system. These structures are associated with the emotions such as fear, rage or anxiety, which color and intensify the response decided upon in the cortex. The limbic system provides the emotional component and determines the intensity of the individual's response to a stimulus. The thalamus relays the stimuli to the basal ganglia and the inhibitory circuit. The *arrows* indicate main pathways of nerve impulses through the limbic system

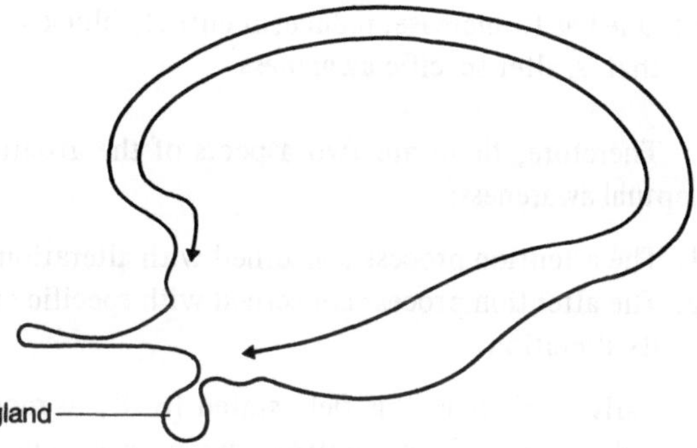

Fig. 3. The amygdala. In controlling the intensity of the individual's response to a stimulus the various components of the limbic system have different functions. As far as anxiety is concerned the amygdala seems to be the most important. Stimulation of the amygdala produces anxiety and aggression. The *arrows* show a push-pull relationship

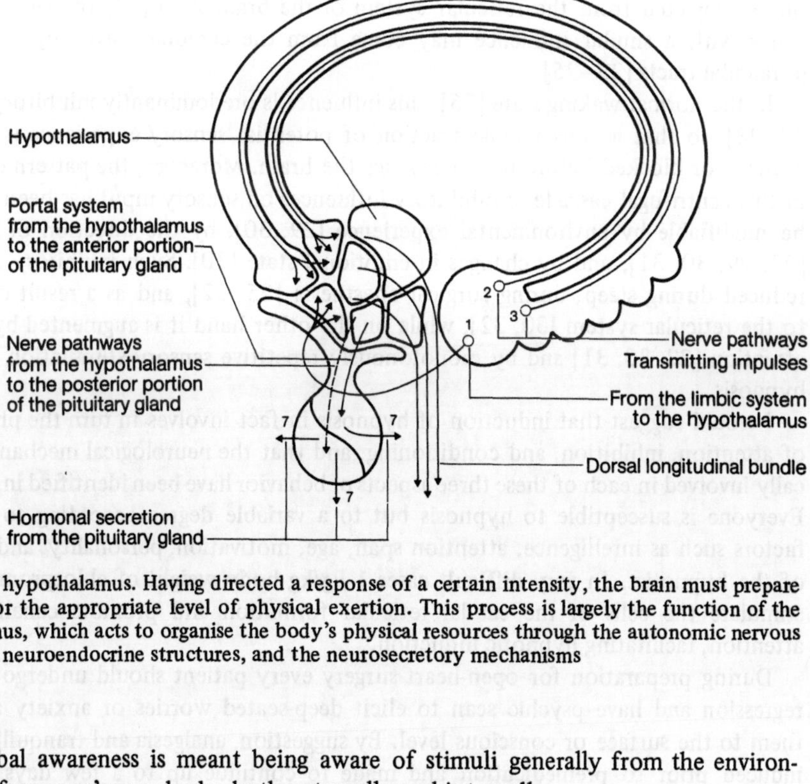

Fig. 4. The hypothalamus. Having directed a response of a certain intensity, the brain must prepare the body for the appropriate level of physical exertion. This process is largely the function of the hypothalamus, which acts to organise the body's physical resources through the autonomic nervous system, the neuroendocrine structures, and the neurosecretory mechanisms

By global awareness is meant being aware of stimuli generally from the environment and from one's own body, both externally and internally.

By specific awareness is meant being aware of a particular stimulus from the environment or from one's body externally or internally. In order to alter perceptual awareness:

a) One has to increase, reduce, or totally eliminate the awareness of sensory input at the cortical level, that is, alter global awareness, and/or

b) One has to increase, reduce, or entirely block specific sensory inputs into the C.N.S., that is, alter specific awareness.

Therefore, there are two aspects of the attention process affected in altering perceptual awareness:

1. The attention process concerned with alterations of global awareness.
2. The attention process concerned with specific awareness or perceptual selection and its alteration.

Early workers in this field stated [6–8], as most of you are aware, that the electroencephalogram of a hypnotized subject was in no way different from that of the same subject in the normal waking state. The brain waves are influenced by hypnotic suggestion [6, 9–12] and this is the basis of hypnotherapy and hypno-aversion therapy. The work of the last few years [13–18] has clearly established that incoming impulses from sensory receptors can be selectively facilitated or inhibited [30] at their point of entry into the neuraxis, by activity delivered through centrifugally directed nerve fibers projected from the reticular system of the brain stem [13, 18, 19–22]. Some fibres with a similar influence may come from the cerebral cortex by way of the pyramidal tracts [23–25].

In the normal waking state [26], this influence is predominantly inhibitory [16, 18, 27, 28], so that a considerable fraction of potential sensory experience is normally reduced or blocked before it ever reaches the brain. Moreover, the pattern of activity in this centrifugal cascade of inhibitory influences on sensory input has been shown to be modifiable by environmental experience [29, 30], by the direction of attention [22, 29, 30, 31], and by changes in emotional state [30]. Such inhibitory activity is reduced during sleep, during surgical anesthesia [25, 32], and as a result of damage to the reticular system [30, 32], while on the other hand it is augmented by directed attention [22, 30, 31] and by monotonously repetitive sensory stimulation [22] as in hypnosis.

I would suggest that induction of hypnosis in fact involves in turn the phenomena of attention, inhibition, and conditioning, and that the neurological mechanisms basically involved in each of these three aspects of behavior have been identified in hypnosis. Everyone is susceptible to hypnosis but to a variable degree according to different factors such as intelligence, attention span, age, motivation, personality, and expertee of the hypnotist. In very difficult cases 1 μg/kg body weight of chlorpromazine can stimulate the cells of the caudal reticular formation and promote canalization of attention, facilitating hypnotic induction.

During preparation for open-heart surgery every patient should undergo hypnotic regression and have psychic scan to elicit deep-seated worries or anxiety and bring them to the surface or conscious level. By suggestion, analgesia and tranquility can be induced prior to premedication and made to continue up to a few days after the operation. This facilitates the work of the anesthetic team and the surgical team but most important prevents the postoperative psychiatric sequelae. The hypnotherapy can be repeated a few times postoperatively. The anesthetic or surgical procedure could not give rise to psychiatric disorders observed postoperatively if the patients' preoperative psychic problems were first dealt with and rectified prior to the operation. This is supported by the fact that the advent of hypothermic cardiac arrest and systemic or cardioplegic cardiac arrest have not prevented the psychiatric sequelae experienced when ischemic cardiac arrest was the main procedure in open-heart surgery. Psychiatry has been ignored by many surgeons throughout the world for centuries and until the surgeons learn to withhold their scalpels until the psychiatrist in the team gives the green light, the psychiatric sequelae following open-heart surgery will not be checked.

Anxiolytics

Chlorozapate dipotassium (Tranxene) is the best anxiolytic we have found so far to produce inner tranquility without sedation, does not produce dependence, and does not increase REM sleep or rebound phenomena. The dosage can be varied according to the individual patient's requirement – 5 mg bd, 10 mg bd, or thrice daily, or it can be given once daily preferably at night.

Lorazepam (Ativan) is another fairly good anxiolytic but it is a dependency drug and causes sedation. The dose is 1 mg or 2 mg bd or thrice daily to be started before the operation and continued postoperatively. Any of these drugs can be used in open-heart surgery in the absence of a hypnotist in the operating team, in conjunction with psychotherapy. This will help to allay some of the anxiety that could precipitate psychiatric sequelae postoperatively.

Discussion

It has been shown that while suggestions are being made to the subject to induce hypnosis, the cerebral electrical activity that he displays when awake and relaxed is desynchronized [8, 33] in the same manner as when his attention is directed in any specific direction. As the subject enters a light trance, a well-synchronized alpha rhythm returns [8, 33, 34], and it remains unchanged unless hypnosis be deepened as shown in EEG frequency [8, 33] or unless further specific suggestions be made to him, when it desynchronizes briefly after each suggestion [8, 33], or unless specific suggestions of sleep be made – in which case his electroencephalogram develops the patterns characteristic of natural sleep [8, 33]. Suggestions of increased or decreased emotional tension have also been shown [34] to produce desynchronization and synchronization of brain waves; while desynchronization was found [34] to occur with hypnotically induced age regression to earlier periods of life associated with marked anxiety.

It is imperative that prior to open-heart surgery every patient should be seen by a psychiatrist, preferably a psychiatrist hypnotist, to check emotional disorders, and an electroencephalogram should be considered obligatory to identify serious desynchronization of brain waves. This should be considered an important contra-indication to surgery if one wants to avoid postoperative psychiatric sequelae. Finally, the patient for open-heart surgery should be under hypnosis throughout the operation as a hypnotised subject reacts to only one stimulus in his environment and that is the hypnotist.

Summary

In this study, the pre- and postoperative psychological sequelae following open-heart surgery have been discussed.

The control of these sequelae using deep hypnotherapy and anxiolytic drugs – chlorozapate dipotassium (Tranxene) and lorazepam (Ativan) – has also been discussed, bearing in mind that the heart is under the control of the autonomic nervous system which originates from the hypothalamus, a component of the limbic system which also controls anxiety, emotion, memory etc.

The control of the rostral end of the Reticular Formation which feeds information into the limbic system and the subsequent control of the limbic system must be regarded as conditio sine qua non in open-heart surgery.

Acknowledgments. My gratitude goes to my friend Dr. Barry Wyke, Director of Neurological Laboratories, Queen's Square, London, and also to Dr. Yankah, Consultant Cardiothoracic Surgeon, J.F. Kennedy Medical Center, Monrovia, Liberia, and finally to Mrs. Elizabeth Ademisoye for her relentless secretarial services.

References

1. Ambrose G, Newbold G (1956) A handbook of medical hypnosis. Bailliere, Tindall & Cox, London
2. Meares AA (1957) A working hypothesis as to the nature of hypnosis. Arch Neurol Psychiatry 77:549–555
3. Editorial (1958) Medical use of hypnosis (A.M.A. Mental Health Council Report). JAMA 168:186–188
4. Barahal HS, Spiegel H, Werner WEF, Wood PM (1959) Symposium: hypnosis and its use in the medical arts. NY State J Med 59:1552–1568
5. Mathieu M (1959) L'hypnotisme dans ses lignes générales. Union Med Can 88:64–69
6. Loomis AL, Harvey EN, Hobart G (1936) Brain potentials hypnosis. Science 83:239
7. Dynes JB (1947) Objective method for distinguishing sleep from the hypnotic trance. Arch Neurol Psychiatry 57:84–93
8. Barker W, Burgwin S (1949) Brain wave patterns during hypnosis, hypnotic sleep and normal sleep. Arch Neurol Psychiatry 62:412–420
9. Blake H, Gerard RW (1937) Brain potentials during sleep. Am J Psychol 119:692–703
10. Marinesco G, Sager O, Kreindler A (1937) Etudes electroencephalographiques: le sommeil naturel et le sommeil hypnotique. Bull Acad Natl Med (Paris) 117:273–276
11. Lundholm H, Lowenbach H (1942) Hypnosis and the alpha activity of the electroencephalogram. Character Personality 11:145–149
12. An electroencephalographic study of the hypnotic dream. J Psychol 20:109–113
13. Jasper HH, Proctor LD, Knighton RS, Noshay WC, Costello RT (eds)
14. Bruner JS (1958) Neural mechanisms in perception. Res Publ Assoc Res Nerv Ment Dis 36:118–143
15. Dawson GD (1958) The central control of sensory inflow. Proc R Soc Med 51:531–535
16. Magoun HW (1958) The waking brain. Thomas, Springfield
17. Hernandez-Peon R (1959) Sensory perception and centrifugal control of sensory input to the brain. Electroencephalogr Clin Neurophysiol 11:373–374

18. Livingston RB (1959) Central control of receptors and sensory transmission systems. In: Field J, Magoun HW, Hall VE (eds) Handbook of physiology. vol 1, sect 1. American Physiological Society, Washington, pp 741–760
19. Brouwer B (1933) Centrifugal influences on centripetal systems in the brain. J Nerv Dis 77:621–627
20. Harlow HF, Woolsey CN (eds) (1957) Biological and biochemical basis of behaviour. University of Wisconsin Press, Madison
21. Hernandez-Peon R (1955) Central mechanisms controlling conduction along central sensory pathways. Acta Neurol Latinoam 1:256–264
22. Jouvet M, Hernandez-Peon R (1957) Mecanismes neurophysiologiques concernant l'habituation, l'attention et le conditionnement. Electroencephalogr Clin Neurophysiol [Suppl] 6:39–49
23. Chambers WW, Liu C-N (1957) Cortico-spinal tract of the cat. An attempt to correlate the pattern of degeneration with deficits in reflex activity following neocortical lesions. J Comp Neurol 108:23–55
24. Lindblom UF, Ottosson JO (1957) Influence of pyramidal stimulation upon the relay of coarse cutaneous afferents in the dorsal horn. Acta Physiol Scand 38:309–318
25. Hagbarth K-E, Fex J (1959) Hippocampal electrical activity in centrifugal influences on single unit activity in spinal sensory paths. J Neurophysiol 22:321–338
26. Lindblom UF, Ottosson JO (1953) Effects of spinal sections on the spinal cord potentials elicited by stimulation of low threshold cutaneous fibres. Acta Physiol Scand [Suppl 106] 29:191–208
27. Hagbarth K-E, Kerr DI (1954) Central influences on spinal afferent conduction. J Neurophysiol 17:295–307
28. Wolff HG, Goodell H (1943) The relation of attitude and suggestion to the perception of and reaction to paid. Res Publ Assoc Res Nerv Ment Dis 23:434–448
29. Dechaume J, Jouvet M, Courjon J, Schott B, Allegre G, Vautrin C (1957) Etude neurophysiologique de l'attention chez l'homme. Ses mécanismes sous-corticaux. Lyon Med 45:473–480
30. Hagbarth K-E, Hojeberg S (1957) Evidence for subcortical regulation of the afferent discharge to the somatic sensory cortex in man. Nature 179:526–527
31. Barker W, Burgwin S (1948) Brain wave patterns accompanying changes in sleep and wakefulness during hypnosis. Psychosomat Med 10:317–326
32. Ford WL, Yeager CL (1948) Changes in the electroencephalogram in subjects under hypnosis. Dis Nerv Syst 9:190–192
33. True RM, Stephenson CW (1951) Controlled experiments correlating electroencephalogram, pulse and plantar reflexes with hypnotic age regression and induced emotional states. J Pers 1:252–259
34. Kline NS (1958) Pharmacotherapy retrospective and prospective. Annual Proceedings of American Pharmaceutical Manufacturers Association

Consultation-Liaison in Intensive Care Units

H. Freyberger

Introduction

With regard to our *consultation liaison* in *intensive care unit* patients, I intend to present the following *two* relevant *supportive-psychotherapeutic* strategies:

1. The psychotherapeutic dealing with the two *defense mechanisms* "Secondary hypochondria" and "Denial" for the purpose of *stimulating* the patient's *insight capacity.*
2. The clinicopsychological steps in patients who are treated by *artificial respiration.*

Our experience is based on the long-term consultation liaison in general medical and surgical intensive care units as well as in the intensive care room of a renal transplant unit [1–3].

The Psychotherapeutic Dealing with the Two Defense Mechanisms "Secondary Hypochondria" and "Denial"

Firstly, let me give some comments concerning the two defence mechanisms "Secondary hypochondria" and "Denial".

The Two Defense Mechanisms

Secondary hypochondria is the organically ill patient's modality to make the impaired organ, the resulting failing bodily functions, and the connected therapeutic processes the main concern of his self interest.

This hypochondriasis, as an overlay of the organic disease, concerns a complainer whose chronic complaints seem relatively fixed. The secondary hypochondria can occur in *two* ways:

Either in the sense of a *transitory* state which will decrease after the disease has been cured or in the sense of a *permanent* state which applies to patients whose disease tends toward a chronic development [6]. The secondary hypochondria defense quality is made clear by the following *two* facts: The patient's imaginary idea that he is able to partially psychically "control" and "master" the disturbed somatic functions as well as the patient's strong need to bring, at least partially, his painful secondary hypochrondriac emotions to conscious catharsis with a resulting psychic relief.

As the direct consequence of this secondary hypochrondria, we observe a *limited insight capacity* in the patient for certain differentiated psychic functions – e.g., the

Psychopathological and Neurological Dysfunctions
Following Open-Heart Surgery Ed by Becker et al

self-reflective ability – are restricted due to the prevalance of the secondary hypochrondriac self-interest.

We observe in the intensive care unit patient similarly impairing effects concerning the insight capacity as the consequence of *denial* because of the fact that a partial suppression of that self-reflective ability is performed which concerns all the psychic thoughts and feelings which are outside the immediately present medical problems by which the patient is overwhelmed. In the patient's view, these central medical problems are: "The emotional acceptance of the disease situation" and "The understanding of the therapeutic measures". If the denial leaves a certain amount of the patient's intrapsychic capacity intact so that the patient is able to perceive and sufficiently control his own psychic situation concerning his needs and emotions, then a *realistically adapted* denial occurs. In contrast to this, the *highly intensive* denial concerns a nearly total repudiation or suppression of the illness and the inherent feelings as well as of the understanding concerning the therapeutic necessity. A further pathological denial quality, the *insufficient* denial, includes the patient's tendency to overestimate the seriousness of the illness and perceive too strongly the inherent feelings with the consequence of relapsing states of death anxieties and/or hopelessness.

The Psychotherapeutic Dealing

Concerning our supportive-psychotherapeutic dealing with these two defence mechanisms, we start from the statement that a possibly optimal insight capacity is very relevant in intensive care unit patients for, then, the somatotherapeutic cooperation ability and the motivation concerning the psychotherapy are promoted on the one hand. On the other hand, it is our clinicopsychological hypothesis that the realistically adapted denial favors more the intensive care unit patient's survival than in the case of the highly intensive deniers and the insufficient deniers.

Concerning this hypothesis we refer to the well-known findings of Hackett et al. [4] that no one major denier died in the case of their 50 myocardial infarction patients. In our view, Hackett's term "major denial" corresponds to our term "realistically adapted denial".

Concerning the psychotherapeutic dealing with secondary hypochondria, the therapist in a sense gives permission to the patient for the *ventilation* of his *secondary hypochondriac displeasures.* In the patient, these verbalization and the connected cathartic-off reactions provide both a considerable psychic relief and a mitigation of his limited insight capacity.

In the case of highly intensive or insufficient denial, the attempt concerning the (re-)stabilization of the patient's nonrealistically adapted denial can be realized on the basis of the satisfying of his strong *oral-narcissistic* needs. The main way with regard to the realization of satisfying these needs is the building-up of a stable object relationship which will be created through regular visits of the psychosomaticist.

These visits include short interviews for the duration of 20 min which concentrate exclusively on the patient's emotional needs. The satisfying of the oral-narcissistic needs, particularly the building of object relationships, positive transference, answering questions and offering good advice, only brings positive results when the patient is made fully aware of the psychosomaticist's continuous potential availability.

Following these two psychotherapeutic procedures with regard to secondary hypochondria and denial, the intensive care unit patient should be regularly addressed to such personal problems which are evident at present. The resulting *mutual reflecting* over these problems by both patient and therapist is furthermore suitable for *increasing* the patient's *insight capacity.*

This psychotherapeutic dealing with the intensive care unit patient's defense mechanisms "Secondary hypochondria" and "Denial" occurs in the following *consulation liaison setting:*

1. There exist agreements between the doctors'-nurses' group and the psychosomaticist that the doctors and nurses may be initially engaged in the solving of the patient's problems following the secondary hypochondriac and the denial function which lead to the patient's particular limited insight capacity. However, the psychosomaticist is available if the doctors and nurses are not able to cope with the patient.
2. The psychosomaticist is not, however, working on the consultation basis alone. Independent of the doctors' and nurses' calls for consultation, the psychosomaticist makes short *informal impatients' visits* to each patient at least three times weekly. The particular aim of these visits is to find out which patients show too strongly marked secondary hypochondria or traits of highly intensive or insufficient denial which are not sufficiently recognized by the doctors and nurses.

Following his short informal inpatients' visits and his resulting psychotherapeutic treatment, it is very useful for both consultation and teaching that the psychosomaticist *regularly* meets the doctors and nurses to *discuss* the patient's individual psychological situation. In our experience, it is very advantageous to connect repeatedly mutual discussions with such *conferences* in which the emotional troubles and the interactional problems of the doctors'-nurses' group are discussed.

The Clinicopsychological Steps in Patients who Are Treated by Artificial Respiration

I would now like to make some comments about *artificial respiration.* The second *supportive-psychotherapeutic* strategy in intensive care units, which I intend to present, concerns artificial respiration which represents both a very important therapy procedure and an extremely stressful experience in most intensive care units.

The Patient's Secondary Psychic Reactions

Our clinicopsychological program stems from the following three *secondary psychic* reactions which can regularly be found in these patients:

1. Excessive feelings of *total dependency* on the doctors and nurses, together with the patient's hypersensitivity vis-à-vis the geographical distance from these, including

traits of *helplessness, depression,* and *separation anxiety* with the particular culmination of this psychopathology in the case of total paralysis due to a curare-like drug.
2. The marked *reduction* of the patient's *verbal ability;* particularly concerning his communicative utterances (e.g., speaking) and his cathartic affective reactions (e.g., displeasure, anger).
3. The patient's *heightened emotional sensitivity* vis-à-vis the doctors and nurses because of his highly anxiety-provoking state "acute dyspnea" and his strong dependency on the doctors' and nurses' "positive" or "negative" quality with regard to their intensive care therapeutical activities; namely: patient's feelings of "being well cared for" (with resulting supporting effects) resp. patient's feelings of "not being well cared for" (with resulting marked anxieties and hopelessness).

The Six Clinicopsychological Steps

Starting from these three secondary psychic reactions, the strict consideration of the following *six* clinicopsychological rules is very desirably in patients who are treated by artificial respiration:

1. *The Preceding Information*
Under ideal circumstances, we are able to carefully prepare the patient for his traumatizing experience, e.g., in situations where the doctors and nurses feel there is a possibility that the patient may require a period of artificial respiration following surgery. In this way, later on, the patient's motivation with regard to cooperation is facilitated.
2. *The Verbal Company of Each Single Therapeutic Step*
During the artificial respiration procedure, each single therapeutic step should be explained. Because the patient may not be able to ask detailed questions, the doctors and nurses should make an effort to anticipate his concerns and provide as many reassuring answers as is realistically possible [5]. This regular verbal company is experienced by the patient in the sense of a relevant conscious illustration of the therapy program. Therefore, the feelings of being well cared for are increased and a circumscribed emotional delivering from the respirator is mediated. These relaxing effects are strengthened if the *same* nurses (in the particular day- or night-shift) are present.
3. *The Doctors' and Nurses' Offers with Regard to Information Given by the Patient in a Verbal, Written, or Gesture Way*
On the basis of the patient's information given in a verbal, written, or gesture way the doctors and nurses are able to realize the patient's cathartic-off reactions and to concentrate on his strong needs. This procedure particularly concerns the staff's "reading" and interpreting of the patient's head and eyelid movements as well as his capability to lip-read; other patients may have to use an alphabet or word board (Kornfeld 1980).
4. *The Clarification of the Reasons for the Patient's Changes Concerning his Psychic State*
If any changes in the patient's psychic state are manifest then the doctors and nurses should try to clarify the basic causes as soon as possible. The patient's emotional security feeling is strengthened by this procedure.

5. *The Avoidance of Talks in the Presence of the Patient*
Any talks within the doctors'-nurses' group, which do not directly concern the patient's medical or psychological problems, should be strictly avoided in the presence of the patient. The staff's defective discipline still exists to discuss vis-à-vis the patient's medical problems and/or private matters which have nothing to do with the present strong needs of the patient.
6. *Possible Low Dosage concerning the Psychotropic Drugs*
The dosage of psychotropic drugs should be low if possible so that an open communication level from the patient to the staff and vice versa can be maintained.

If these *six* rules are be systematically realized, then a stable object relationship between patient and doctors'-nurses' group occurs. This relationship includes the following *three* psychologically relieving effects:

1. The patient's *feelings* of dependency and helplessness as well as the separation anxiety and depression are *reduced.*
2. Therefore, the patient's *motivation* concerning his cooperation ability and his stamina *increases.*
3. As a consequence of this weaning patients from the respiratory is easier to realize in a patient who has not been sedated before hand in contrast to the originally severely sedated patient who is completely nonprepared concerning weaning.

Final Consultation Liaison Aspects

According to our experience, *student auxiliary therapists* represent a further relevant possibility with regard to consultation liaison activities in intensive care units. The students, who belong to a larger pool of auxiliary therapists, work in the departments of Medicine and Surgery of the Hannover Medical School. These students are supervised in so-called *Balint groups* at weekly intervals. On the one hand, the students are acting both as psychotherapists dealing with the two defense mechanisms as well as at the occąsion of the informal inpatients' visits and the following contacts with the doctors and nurses concerning the patient's findings, while on the other hand, the student auxiliary therapists are also active in close connexion with the clinicopsychological steps during artificial respiration. In particular they do not only act as consultants and teachers but also as psychotherapists if the respirated patient's clinicopsychological situation is too complicated.

This special consultation liaison, performed by the students and the supervisor, is greatly suitable for filling a relevant vacuum in the field of psychotherapy with regard to the primary organically ill patients. Furthermore, it is the accepted opinion of the students and the supervisor that there exists no better teaching method with regard to students than his combination consisting of treatment of a patient and supervision in Balint groups.

References

1. Freyberger H (1976) Psychosomatic aspects of an intensive care unit. In: Howells (ed) Modern perspectives in the psychiatric aspects of surgery. Brunner-Mazel, New York
2. Freyberger H (1980) Consultation liaison in a renal transplant unit. In: Levy (ed) Psychological factors in hemodialysis and renal transplantation. Plenum, New York
3. Freyberger H (1980) Psychotherapeutic interventions in intensive care units. In: Speidel H, Rodewald G (eds) Proceedings of the International Symposium on psychopathological and neurological dysfunctions following open heart surgery. Thieme, Stuttgart
4. Hackett TP, Cassem NH, Wishnie HA (1968) The coronary care unit. An appraisal on its psychological hazards. N Engl J Med 279:1365–1370
5. Kornfeld DS (1980) The intensive care unit in adults: Coronary care and general medical/surgical. Adv Psychosom Med 10:1
6. Nemiah J, Freyberger H, Sifneos PE (1976) Alexithymia, a view of the psychosomatic process. In: Hill (ed) Recent advances in psychosomatic medicine. Butterworth, London

Rehabilitation Following Open-Heart Surgery – From a Surgeon's Point of View

G. Rodewald, P. Kalmar, H.-J. Krebber

Introduction

The risk of open-heart surgery has decreased considerably during the past decade. Somatic and physical results have improved continuously due to better techniques, devices, and equipment. Thus, psychological results influencing the long-term result have be come the center of attention [2].

Overall hospital mortality today is approximately 2.8% at our institutions and similar at other centers. The differences between various procedures are still present due to the influence of duration of the disease and secondary organ damage induced by the defect.

Isolated mitral valve replacement procedures represent a risk of 3.1%, aortic valve replacement of 1.6% and coronary vein graft procedures of 1.2% [1, 3, 4].

Late results are encouraging too, as far as mortality is concerned. Overall annual mortality is calculated for our patients following open-heart procedures as being 3.1%,

Table 1. Annual death following valve replacement (actuarial method of Anderson)

Year postop.	Aorta	Mitral	Double	Total
1.	4% 9/223	4.3% 10/235	7.4% 5/68	4.6% 24/526
2.	1.9% 3/158	3.5% 7/200	7.0% 3/43	3.1% 13/420
3.	3.5% 4/144	0.7% 1/136	7.4% 2/27	2.5% 7/277
4.	2.2% 2/93	1.6% 2/122	10.6% 2/19	2.7% 6/222
5.	4.5% 3/66	0 0/83	7.7% 1/13	2.5% 4/162
6.	4.9% 2/41	1.9% 1/54	20.0% 1/5	4.0% 4/99
7.	4.2% 1/24	0 0/26	0 0/1	2.0% 1/51
Per year	25.2:7 = 3.6%	12:7 = 1.7%	60.1:7 = 8.6%	21.4:7 = 3.1%

Psychopathological and Neurological Dysfunctions
Following Open-Heart Surgery Ed by Becker et al

varing between 1.7% for mitral patients, 3.6% for aortic patients, and 8.6% for those who underwent double valve replacement (Table 1).

With in-time surgical treatment of patients with acquired valvular heart disease or coronary artery disease, it will be possible to achieve a normal or near normal physical performance in more than 90% of the cases. However, the aim of surgical procedures is not only to preserve and to prolong life but to improve the quality of life by reconstituting the physcial performance and the ability to lead a normal life.

The grade and rate of reintegration into working life of patients in the working age group (16–65 years for male and 16–60 years for female patients) could probably be a more subtle indicator of the quality of the surgical results than mortality statistics alone.

We therefore evaluated patients who had valve replacement and coronary artery surgery in a follow-up study and established some objective criteria for physical performance as well as the grade and rate of reintegration into their preoperative employment.

Patients and Methods

The composition of the group studied is listed according to diagnosis, sex, and age (Table 2). One hundred and twenty eight patients underwent aortic valve replacement (AVR), 137 had mitral valve replacement (MVR), and 100 patients underwent coronary bypass procedures (ACB). As expected, there was a predominance of male patients in the aortic group while in the mitral group the ratio of male to female was 1:2. Among the patients who had coronary artery surgery there was a reversal of the distribution with a ratio of 4:1 males:females. The AVR group had a mean age of 47 years, the MVR group a mean age of 46 years, and the ACB group a mean age of 58 years.

All patients were analysed using objective (clinical data) and subjective (interviews and patient questionaires) criteria, comparing their symptomatology pre- and postoperatively. Some of the results of this analysis for the AVR group can be seen in Table 3. Preoperatively 50 patients were diagnosed as having Class II symptoms, 66 patients as having Class III symptoms, and 12 patients as having Class IV symptoms. Postoperatively, out of the 12 patients originally with Class IV symptoms, only two remained in this class with only little relief. In the Class III group, out of 66 patients

Table 2. Patients studied

Diagnosis	n	Sex distribution in %		Mean age in years
		♂	♀	
Aortic valve disease	128	75	25	47
Mitral valve disease	137	31	69	46
Coronary artery disease	100	81	19	58

Table 3. Pre- and postoperative class according to NYHA in 128 patients with aortic valve replacement (48 months postop.; min.-max. 12–72 months)

	Preop.		Postop.	
NYHA	n	%	n	%
I	0	0	39	30
II	50	39	76	59
III	66	52	11	9
IV	12	9	2	2
Total	128	100	128	100

11 remained unchanged. The largest symptomatic class following surgery was Class II with 76 patients. Finally, postoperatively there were 39 patients in Class I. These shifts in NHYA classification seem to suggest a postoperative trend to Class I and II symptomatology after 12–72 months following surgery.

Results

Table 4 shows the hemodynamic changes in the mitral group preoperatively and 6 months postoperatively. The markedly increased pulmonary artery pressures seen before surgery, with a mean of 68 mmHg at rest and 103 mmHg after exercise, were found to be considerably lower postoperatively; however, with a mean of 40 mmHg, normal values at rest were still not achieved. A more obvious postoperative improve-

Table 4. Hemodynamic findings before and 4–6 months after mitral valve replacement

	Systolic pulmonary artery pressure (mmHg)		
	Normal	Preop.	Postop.
At rest	20 (± 8)	68 (± 42)	40 (± 23)
After 5′ 50 Watt	30 (± 7)	103 (± 55)	56 (± 20)
	Oxygen saturation of venous mixed blood (% HbO_2)		
	Normal	Preop.	Postop.
At rest	78 (± 6)	68 (± 10)	75 (± 5)
After 5′ 50 Watt	62 (± 9)	34 (± 11)	55 (± 8)
n	30	55	33

Abbreviations: n, number of studied patients; (±), standard deviation

Table 5. Comparison of self assesment of physical capability with the rate of employment of 43 male and 94 female patients with mitral valve replacement

	43 ♂		94 ♀	
Physical performance		employed		employed
None	6	1	10	5
Poor	13	7	38	21
Active in sports, gardening etc.	24	6	46	22
Total	43	14	94	48

ment was seen after 5 min of treadmill exercise at 50 W with an increase to 56 mmHg only in contrast to 103 mmHg preoperatively. Another important parameter of cardiac performance is oxygen saturation in central venous mixed blood.

The preoperative value at rest was slightly below normal with 68% of oxygen saturation, and returned to normal postoperatively with 75% of oxygen saturation. The postoperative improvement was even more evident after 5′ of exercise for there was an increase from 34% preoperatively to 55% postoperatively. The subjective statements of the patients, taken from interviews and questionaires, correlated very well with the objective or clinical findings obtained pre- and postoperatively.

Table 5 shows the statements of the aortic and mitral patients concerning their postoperative physical condition in comparison to how they felt before surgery. 120 of 128 AVR patients and 121 of 137 MVR patients judged their physical capability to be better or much improved after surgery.

The correlation of objective findings and self-assessment in terms of symptomatology can be carried over for the aortic patients with regard to their record of pre- and postoperative employment: Out of 128 aortic patients 102 returned to work postoperatively. The behavior of mitral patients was in strong contrast to that of the aortic patients, where only 62 out of 137 returned to their jobs postoperatively (Table 6).

When analyzing the MVR patients in terms of their sex and their working habits we found that only 14 out of 43 *male* patients went back to work after surgery. In contrast to that the number of *female* patients involved in home-centered work

Table 6. Postoperative employment of patients with valve replacement

	Patients with aortic valve replacement n = 128	Patients with mitral valve replacement n = 137
	Postop.	Postop.
Employed	102	62
Unemployed	26	75

Table 7. Postoperative employment of 137 patients with mitral valve replacement

	Postoperative	
	♂	♀
Employed	14	48[a]
Unemployed	29	46
Total	43	94

[a]14 in business, 34 "full-time" housewives

Table 8. Subjective statement on physical capability of patients with valve replacement in comparison to preoperative

Feeling	Patients with aortic valve replaced n = 128		Patients with mitral valve replaced n = 137	
Much better	54	94%	51	88%
Better	66		70	
Unchanged	6		8	
Worse	1	6%	7	12%
Much worse	1		1	

on a fulltime basis was 48 out of 94 (Table 7). There is no real correlation between the physical load the patient feels capables of and the postoperative employment rate as demonstrated in Table 8. It became evident that out of 24 *male* patients who were active in sports or busy with gardening or similar exercise only six were back to their previous jobs, while out of 46 *female* patients at least 22 were working again.

Table 9 shows the clinical results of 100 patients 2–6 years following ACB surgery. Seventy three of these patients had marked relief from their preoperative symptoms and 17 patients had slight improvement. Only ten patients experienced no change in their preoperative condition and three of these patients felt even worse following surgery. Angina in varying degrees was present in 27 patients.

When analyzing the postoperative complaints of these 100 patients, and relating these findings to the number of patients returning to work, we found that out of 73 patients with no, or much less, symptoms 46 (= 68%) were back at work, while out of 17 patients with less symptoms ten (= 58%) were working again, but even out of the ten patients who were unchanged or worse five were working. Thus it became evident that there is no correlation between the severity of complaints postoperatively and the patient's return to work (Table 10).

When comparing the mean age for the group who returned to work and those individuals who remain unemployed and unwilling to work, we found the working group to be 11 years younger.

Table 9. Clinical results in 100 patients (n) 2–6 years following ACB procedures

Postoperative symptoms	n	With angina (pectoris)	With signs of congestive heart failure
None	32	–	–
Much less	41	9[a]	6
Less	17	11[b]	4
Unchanged	7	4[c]	2
More	3	3	3

[a]At severe exercise, no medical treatment
[b]At exercise, occasional medical treatment
[c]As preoperative or worse, continuous medical treatment

Preoperative: no myocardial infarction, 28; 1 myocardial infarction, 42; 2 and more myocardial infarction, 30. 95 angina (pectoris) and continuous medical treatment

Table 10. Severity of subjective symptoms and rate of employment in 100 patients 2–6 years following ACB procedures

Postoperative symptoms	n	Employed	Unemployed
None	32	25	7
Much Less	41	21	20
Unchanged	17	10	7
More	3	1	2
Total	100	61	39
Mean age	58	51	62

Discussion

This study revealed that the rate at which patients returned to an active business life, following open-heart surgery, was not a good indicator of the quality of surgical results for all patients, as a correlation was only given for AVR patients where almost 80% returned to work. On the other hand, among patients who underwent mitral valve replacement the rate was approximately 45% and 60% for the ACB patients. This 80% rate of return to employment in AVR patients corresponds with the increased objective and subjective physical ability in these patients. In the patients who underwent mitral valve replacement the portion of improved patients was considerably higher (88%) than the number of patients in that group who returned to work (45%). Similar, but not as marked, were the differences in the ACB group.

The difference between objective findings and subjective statements on one side and the number of patients returning to work on the other side still remains to be explained.

It is interesting to note that those patients who continued to work until shortly before surgery were more likely to return to work than those who have had a prolonged period of inactivity before surgery. A factor influencing the length of inactivity before surgery. A factor influencing the length of inactivity is the limited capacity for open-heart procedures in Germany.

Further more, younger patients were found to return to work more often than older ones. Patients in private enterprise, however, tended to return to work earlier and sometimes even when close to or beyond retirement age. These controversies might be explained by socio-economic, psychological, and medical factors.

One of the *socio-economic factors* is given by the social security system in West Germany. Patients who are treated medically for a long period of time and/or have to wait a long time for their surgery are no longer supported by compulsory medical insurance (so-called Krankenkasse) but receive their income from retirement funds. These patients therefore live under the same conditions as retired people, that is they became used to a somewhat restricted but still sufficient financial situation. The higher unemployment rate, especially among older people, contributes to the fact that the employers quite often refuse to put individuals back into their previous position following open-heart surgery.

Psychological factors are explained in detail by Meffert et al. and Speidel et al. (this volume). Further more, interrelationships between patients and between the patient and his family are of considerable importance [2, 5].

A *medical factor* is the treatment of patients by certain family physicians who tend to be overprotective. The physician might fear complications beyond his control for which he could be responsible, this behavior being partially based on uncertainty and partially on ignorance. This is true of physicians asked for their opinion concerning the definite retirement of the patients as well.

Concerning occupational accidents there has already existed, for many years in Germany, a well-established and worldwide recognized system of judging specialists (orthopedic surgeons), who give their opinion on the degree of the impairment. For patients following open-heart surgery such a system is still to be developed, although there are already existing objective measurements to assess the physical capability of heart patients.

Conclusion

The limiting factors for open-heart procedures are no longer the immediate risks but rather those factors which impair the long-term results. In order to achieve better results we have to schedule surgery as early as is needed rather than as late as possible when lasting impairment is already present. This implicates reduced time of preoperative inactivity which allows the patient to lead an active life until shortly before surgery.

Psychotherapy started prior to surgery and continued in combination with physical training beyond the recovery period is greatly needed. The continuous education and postgraduate training of family physicians and judging physicians has to be improved in this respect. Those goals can only be achieved by cooperation of all who are working in this field, that is surgeons, cardiologists, and psychologists to mention only a few.

References

1. Bleese N, Darup J, Pokar H, Rödiger W, Rodewald G (1980) Causes of death in complicated open heart procedures (Abstr). Thorac Cardiovasc Surg 28:35
2. Götze PA (1980) Psychopathologie der Herzoperierten. Enke, Stuttgart
3. Rodewald G, Polonius M-J (1980) Cardiac surgery in the Federal Republic of Germany during 1978. Thorac Cardiovasc Surg 28
4. Rodewald G, Guntau J, Bantea C, Krebber H-J, Rödiger W, Tilsner V (1980) The risk of reoperation in aquired valvular heart disease. Thorac Cardiovasc Surg 28:77–88
5. Speidel H, Dahme B, Flemming B, Götze P, Huse-Kleinstoll G, Meffert H-J, Rodewald G (1979) Psychische Störungen nach offenen Herzoperationen. Nervenarzt 50:85–91

Characteristics of Postoperative Patient Education Programs for Open-Heart Surgery Patients in the United States

R.A. Frantz

Introduction

To the patient suffering the debilitating effects of cardiovascular disease the prospect of cardiac surgery offers the potential to reverse restrictive lifestyle patterns and become more active and independent. For many patients this reversal requires modification of deep-rooted work habits and living patterns. Patient teaching programs have been developed based on the belief that people can and must be educated to desire, preserve, and restore health. Compliance with the medical regimen specified in the teaching programs has generally been inadequate. Rates of noncompliance have been shown by Davis [1] and Ley and Spelmann (1965) to be increased when the regimen requires a change in life patterns or patient judgments. Riley [5] and Sapolsky [6] noted that when the significance of the regimen is not clearly conveyed to the patient there is a reciprocal failure of the patient to comply. Johannsen et al. [4] identifies psychological readiness as a critical factor in patient compliance.

Statement of the Problem

At the present time little is known about the effect of program timing and specific teaching strategies on patient compliance following open-heart surgery. As a basis for investigating the effect of these variables on compliance, it was necessary to collect detailed information regarding teaching methods used to deliver existing educational programs to open-heart surgery patients.

Methodology

This study surveyed, via questionnaire, the 512 hospitals in the United States and its territories which the American Hospital Association's Joint Commission on Accreditation listed as ones which perform open-heart surgery. This includes surgery carried out for single or multiple valve repair, repair of congenital anomalies of the heart, and/or the coronary artery by-pass graft procedure. The 37 item questionnaire used in this study asked about: 1) the type of health personnel who conduct their postoperative patient teaching program for open-heart surgery patients, 2) the major

Psychopathological and Neurological Dysfunctions
Following Open-Heart Surgery Ed by Becker et al

areas of content included in this program, 3) the type of teaching methods and/or tools used, 4) how patient readiness for the program is determined, 5) if postdischarge follow-up visits are a part of the program, 6) if a patient learning or compliance evaluation is done, and 7) the factors seen as supportive or as impeding the delivery of the postoperative patient teaching program for open-heart surgery patients. The "postoperative teaching program" was defined as one designed to assist patients in learning the information and procedures necessary for them to follow the medical regimen prescribed for them upon discharge from the hospital.

Subject Population

The questionnaires were sent to Directors of Nursing Service in each of the 512 hospitals asking that a nurse familiar with their institution's ongoing education program for open-heart surgery patients be asked to complete the questionnaire. Of the 402 questionnaires returned, 358 indicated that open-heart surgery was still performed at the hospital. Of the nurses responding, 54% were in direct patient contact positions, 39% were in administrative position, and 7% had an educational type position.

Data Analysis

Hospital Profile

Only 237 (66%) of the 358 hospitals performing open-heart surgery indicated that they provide a program to facilitate patients' acquisition of the knowledge needed to follow their medical regimen after discharge. Although over 50% of the hospitals had been performing open-heart surgery for more than 7 years, only 18% had a postoperative teaching program operating for more than 7 years. While older surgical programs tended to be initiated without a corresponding teaching program, since 1972

Table 1. Areas of learning included in postoperative teaching programs (3, p. 138)

Frequency of inclusion	Areas: Diet	Drugs	Activity levels	Potential complications	Support services
Always	167	192	195	119	114
Almost always	53	34	32	74	48
Occasionally	13	4	4	24	49
Seldom	1	4	0	14	16
Never	0	0	3	4	4
No response	3	3	3	2	6

educational programs were begun more consistently with the introduction of the surgical procedures.

Methods and Materials Utilized in Postoperative Teaching Programs

The extent to which specific content areas are included in postoperative teaching programs are identified in Table 1. The most frequently included content area is activity level, followed by drugs, diet, and potential complications. The least often included content area is support services, which were defined as those resources available after discharge which provide assistance should problems arise. In only 45% of the hospitals with teaching programs is the content delivered according to a planned instructional sequence.

The most frequent primary teacher varied with the content being taught. The nurse is most often the principal teacher of activity, drugs, and support services. The dietitian most frequently provides diet instructions with potential complications most often being taught by the physician. The nurse is the second most frequent provider of instruction in diet and potential complications. However, in over 50% of the programs each of the major content areas are not taught consistently by the same person.

In over 40% of the teaching programs patient readiness to begin learning is not evaluated or is assessed using nonpatient-oriented criteria. When readiness was determined, the factor most frequently sited was the patient's physical condition. This factor, combined with patient anxiety level and patient requests for information provided the major criteria utilized in judging readiness.

The types of teaching methods and tools used in the postoperative teaching programs are noted in Table 2. As can be seen, the predominant teaching is done using individual contact with the teaching supports of pamphlets, pictures, and diagrams.

Table 2. Types of teaching methods and tools used in the postoperative teaching programs (3, p. 139)

	No. of hospitals which use method or tool	No. where it is used as primary method or tool
Method:		
Individual contact	233	233
Group discussion	47	14
Lecture	27	6
Tool:		
Pamphlets	145	10
Pictures-diagrams	135	85
Books	45	14
Films-filmstrips	30	18
Instruction sheets or tapes	26	26
Models	15	0
Patient-mended heart Society	5	0

Table 3. Content areas reviewed for compliance (3, p. 140)

Content area	No. of programs
Diet	103
Drugs	115
Activity level	114
Potential complications	98
Support services	75

Characteristics of Follow-up Visits After Discharge

Follow-up visits after discharge were not a part of 40% of the teaching programs. In the 60% who include follow-up visits, 38% schedule at least two visits with half having over five follow-up visits. The data noted in Table 3 raise some questions regarding the extent to which patient compliance with the medical regimen is evaluated. Less than half of the programs use follow-up visits to review the patients' compliance in any one of the five content areas of their teaching program. Only two programs of the 157 with follow-up visits include additional areas of instruction beyond those related to diet, drug therapy, activity level, potential complications, or support services. However, a number of programs provided additional instruction in these five areas. The two programs where new content areas were added during follow-up visits included instruction in the effects of smoking and methods of coping with the psychological adjustment to new lifestyle patterns.

Factors Which Support or Impede Delivery of the Postoperative Teaching Programs

The factor most frequently sited as supportive of delivering a postoperative teaching program was a knowledgeable staff who perceived their teaching activities to be of

Table 4. Factors which support the delivery of a postoperative teaching program (3, p. 140)

Support factors	No. of programs
Knowledgeable staff	80
Motivation of nurses	51
Physicians see teaching as a priority	41
Teaching is assigned to a specific person	40
Support from nursing administration and/or physicians	38
Continuity of care with patients	25
Availability of teaching tools	22
Support from auxiliary departments	21
Good physician-nurse rapport	17
Positive feedback from patients	13
Available resources for assistance	8
Part of staff training	8
Stability of nursing staff	4
Stability of medical staff	3
No response	31

Table 5. Factors which impede the delivery of a postoperative teaching program (3, p. 140)

Impeding factors	Number of programs
Inadequate time	87
Inadequate staff	43
Physicians do not want nurses to teach	41
Lack of knowledge of how to teach	32
Heavy patient load	25
Lack of formal, structured program	18
Unstable nursing staff	18
Frequent patient transfers	15
Lack of follow-up program	13
Lack of patient acceptance	13
Lack of teaching resources	8
Difficulty in getting discharge orders	8
Unstable medical staff	7
Lack of money for teaching	6
No response	32

importance (Table 4). The most frequently indicated impediments to an effective teaching program were inadequate time and lack of adequate numbers of staff (Table 5). As with the supportive factors, the factor ranked third relates to physician support of the teaching role of the nurse. It is noteworthy that while motivation of the nurse ranked second in supporting factors, it is perceived as having much less impact as an impediment. The fourth most frequently sited impediment was lack of knowledge of how to teach. It appears that the staff must be knowledgeable not only of content, but also of how to teach if an effective postoperative teaching program is to be delivered. The probability of having a successful postoperative teaching program seems to be improved by the presence of an adequate number of knowledgeable, motivated staff, who have physician and nursing administration support and reasonable continuity of contact with patients.

Discussion

The survey results suggest that a number of problem areas exist in postoperative education programs currently delivered to open-heart surgery patients. The content areas included in the teaching programs appear to be directed primarily at physiological and basic safety and security need areas. Only one program indicated that it included in its teaching plan a learning experience aimed at the development of belonging and assistance in adjusting to new lifestyle patterns. The importance of these content areas is noted by Frank et al. [2] who reported that psychological adjustment and return of emotional well-being progressed very slowly following cardiac surgery.

Articulation of the teaching effort appears to be another problem area in these teaching programs. Only 45% of the programs have a planned instructional sequence and more than 50% do not provide continuity in their teaching personnel. Such a lack of emphasis on the importance of the medical regimen has been noted by Johannsen et al. [4] to increase the risk of noncompliance.

The interaction of factors noted to be supportive of the teaching program with those identified as impediments suggests deficiencies in the instructional methods and materials. Individual contact, the most time consuming of teaching methods, is used in 94% of the programs. However, lack of adequate time and available staff are the most frequently sited impediments to an effective teaching program. It is conceivable that the lack of those factors perceived as supportive to the teaching program is contributing to this situation. Specifically, the lack of knowledgeable staff with teaching skills, who perceive their teaching role as one of importance, may promote extensive use of the less formalized individual interaction to deliver instructional content. It may be necessary to delegate the responsibilities of a teaching program to a few specially prepared individuals. This should promote optimum use of time and personnel and increase accountability for teaching.

Assessment of learner readiness is another problem area in postoperative teaching programs. Regardless of the quality of the teaching program, learning may not occur because the patient is physically or emotionally incapable of processing the instruction. With over 40% of the programs either not judging readiness or using nonpatient-oriented criteria, a significant number of teaching programs may not be designed to meet individual needs.

The lack of follow-up evaluation of the teaching program's effectiveness was a commonly occurring deficit. Systematic review of previous learning or evaluation of patient compliance was not done on a consistent basis. Studies by Riley [5] and Sapolsky [6] indicate that the degree of patient compliance corresponds with the clarity of teaching. It would appear that evaluation of program effectiveness is essential to insure maximum benefit to the patient. Furthermore, the ongoing process of psychological adjustment after open-heart surgery may continue for several months after discharge. If a teaching program is to facilitate the patient achieving optimum well-being, it would appear that additional teaching in the area of adapting to changing lifestyle patterns might well be incorporated into the educational program.

Conclusions

The results of this study suggest a number of areas for further investigation. Future studies are needed to determine the patient variables most significant in determining readiness for learning. In addition, systematic investigation is needed of the factors which enhance patient compliance with the prescribed regimen following discharge. Studies should also be conducted to determine specifically what additional areas of learning are necessary to promote optimum adjustment to altered lifestyle patterns. Having defined more clearly these characteristics of the learner and the learning task, efforts can be directed at identifying specific teaching methods which will efficiently and effectively deliver the required instruction to patients.

References

1. Davis MS (1967) Predicting noncompliant behavior. J Health Soc Beh 8:265–271
2. Frank KA, Heller SS, Kornfeld DS (1972) A survey of adjustment to cardiac surgery. Arch Intern Med 130:735–738
3. Hart LK, Frantz RA (1977) Characteristics of postoperative patient education programs for open heart surgery patients in the United States. Heart Lung 6:137–142
4. Johannsen WJ, Hellmuth GA, Sorauf T (1966) On accepting medical recommendations. Arch Environ Health 12:63–69
5. Riley CS (1966) Patients' understanding of doctors' instructions. Med Care 4:34–37
6. Sapolsky A (1965) Relationship between patient-doctor compatibility, mutual perception and outcome of treatment. J Abnorm Psychol 70:70–76

Model of an Integrated Psychotherapeutic Approach to the Heart Surgery Patient*

H. Speidel, B. Flemming, P. Götze, G. Huse-Kleinstoll, H.-J. Meffert, Ch. Reimer

During the first few years of work of our Hamburg group, we were under the impression that we ought in future to carry out a controlled therapeutic study, with which we should be able to prove to ourselves and the heart surgeons that psychological aids for heart surgery patients in the ICU are useful. We had hoped to be able to prove one day that under the influence of psychotherapeutic treatment, postoperative psychic disturbances would occur less frequently, in a milder form, and be of shorter duration. In other words, we wanted to be able to substantiate with hard facts Kimball's [8] supposition when he said: "We attributed our low finding of classical delirium to several factors: [1] the careful and lengthy preparation of our patients and [2] the role of the clinical investigators throughout the pre- and postoperative stages".

We have abandoned this plan in the meantime for three reasons and have started to become interested in a different manner of dealing with psychotherapeutic aids for the patients of the heart surgery unit:

1. The research of the last 15 years [13] has produced evidence enough that psychic factors do play a role in the development of postoperative psychic disturbances and thus that psychological aids are fundamentally significant. Caston [1] and Speidel et al. [12], by way of theoretical models, have provided the reasons why even such, or precisely such, postoperative disturbances which are to be classified as psycho-organic, need psychotherapeutic attention.

The exact statistical "evidence" that the observations made hitherto are correct appeared to us, to an increasing extent, to be more the problem of a questionable scientific understanding, not so much the task for the application of meaningful psychotherapeutic aids accompanied by science in practical heart surgery.

2. The findings of the various working teams, including those of our own [13] show that that section which was the main object of psychological-psychiatric studies not only of our own working team, but also that of most of the other groups, namely, the early postoperative phase, is too narrow. There are numerous indications that psychic problems which become manifest under the conditions of the postoperative situation, in the form of dramatic symptoms in some cases, have precursors. They can, in some instances, be traced back to early childhood [7] and in fact they form

* With the aid of the Deutsche Forschungsgemeinschaft, Sonderforschungsbereich 115, Teilprojekt A3

Psychopathological and Neurological Dysfunctions Following Open-Heart Surgery Ed by Becker et al

the personality structure. Other origins are to be found in current job and family conflicts. These conflicts, on the other hand, are not independent of experiences and behavioral patterns specific to the personality. Other relevant factors are the problems surrounding the illness, the organization of the surgical treatment, the relationship to doctors and nursing staff as well as how the explanatory talks by the heart surgeons and anesthetists have been conducted (Träger et al., this volume).

All these factors have shown themselves to be causally significant for the occurrence of postoperative psychic disturbances [13]. For the first time, Meffert et al. this volume) try to determine the relative weight of these psychological factors for postoperative psychic disturbances in relationship to the somatic factors. Here it is shown that for coronary heart disease and valve patients differing and differently significant psychological factors do play a role in the development of the postoperative psychic disturbances, but that overall they are important though not predominant. From these investigations the necessity for psychic aids emerges as the inevitable consequence.

However, these findings, too, apply to only a fraction of the overall problem. Various authors [5, 7, 9; Reimer et al., this volume] have shown that in the course of convalescence and rehabilitation, psychic problems arise which remain mute to some extent because in the meantime the patients have moved out of the reach of the heart surgeons and because they are no longer part of the observation system of an institution. For this reason it has hitherto escaped the attention of the medical and other social authorities that heart surgery patients were suffering under the weight of psychic problems which, inter alia, are of great social significance [Rodewald et al., this volume]. Heart surgery patients have no institution of their own which systematically takes care of their psychic situation, as is the case, for example, with chronic hemodialysis patients, who are under the constant care of doctors, some of whom are very interested in and knowledgeable about psychosocial matters [10].

In the case of heart surgery patients, this applies only to a limited extent, namely in rehabilitation clinics where these patients and those who have suffered infarction receive follow-up treatment. In these centers and in the self-help sports clubs for infarction patients as outpatients, although the heart surgery patients are treated in close proximity to infarction patients, the former's actual participation in sports groups in each case depends on the initiative of each one; there is no institution set up for them.

If we observe the activities in these rehabilitation clinics, as they exist in the Federal Republic of Germany, we can see that they are built up on an ideology in which the psychic factors play almost no part or no part at all [A. Boll, U. Röttger, personal communication]. On the contrary, in their physical training programme, they embody precisely the ideal which the coronary patients set themselves from the beginning and which perhaps is one of the very risk factors which led to the cardiac infarction. The impression is created that the ideology of this form of rehabilitation, which is part of the social security system in the Federal Republic of Germany, is not really sufficiently well thought out. It is thus not certain whether the lack of such social security, as in the USA, really constitutes a disadvantage.

3. If we doctors, as psychotherapists and psychologists, consider this important aspect in our observations, then we can no longer be satisfied with such restricted therapeutic concepts as the care of postoperative patients in the ICU.

All these reasons have been instrumental in our trying to find a comprehensive therapeutic approach which will cover all relevant aspects which have been acknowledged.

In the study we are planning, we want to describe the various fields of psychological-psychotherapeutical-psychiatrical influence, to examine the effects and the problems, and to draw conclusions concerning a practically applicable model.

The type and range of therapy possible are best classified according to the stages at which they are applied.

1. The time between the first clinical cardiological or cardiosurgical examination and admission to the clinic:

   a) When the patient is put on the waiting list for the heart operation, an extensive programme of diagnosis ought to be carried out to make it possible to assess the following sectors:
   the primary socialization conditions (among others, infantile neurosis) and their influence on coping with the disease, the mental attitude to the illness and the operation, the question of the secondary illness gain, the current domestic and vocational problems in connection with psychogenetic aspects and social conditions, the personality structure and the correlated defence mechanism and coping styles, and, in turn, their correlation to the impending operation [Möhlen et al., this volume].

   b) If the operation does not immediately succeed the initial diagnosis, the patient should be offered two things:
   Regular somatic and psychic control examinations, which will enable observation not only of the development of the patients' physical condition but also of the psychic state and, if the need arises, make it possible to derive therapy from this observation.
   In principle, a series of talks, either individual or in groups, should be offered. The problems surrounding the impending operation and waiting for it, the vocational and domestic situations, can then be dealt with.
   During this phase, organizational problems (how the cardiosurgical centre deals with waiting lists) can be observed and, if necessary, be corrected in the interdisciplinary discussion.

2. The time between admission to the clinic and the operation:

   a) Individual talks ought to make it possible for the patients to come to terms with their fears and to find a realistic way of coping with the impending event.

   b) Systematic inclusion of the family, or a central reference figure, is intended to mobilize their supportive potential, inter alia, by reducing anxiety and coping with problems of uncertainty about the imminent operation and the ensuing attitude to the patient. This is also meant to prepare the way for their therapeutic involvement in the early postoperative phase.

   c) The crucial significance of the talks the heart surgeons and anesthetists have with the patient is to be duly taken into account by offering to supervise these preparatory talks; the object is to achieve a helpful conversational technique and to reconcile the expectations on each side (the doctors expect factual information and the patients expect psychic support, cf. [Träger et al., this volume].

3. The time spent in the ICU:
   a) Care of the patients by a constant person of reference is significant precisely in respect of cognitive deficits and their compensation ("psycho-organic disturbances").
   b) These functions could possibly be fulfilled by a central person of reference (the partner, for example), providing he or she has been prepared for this function (see above). In this phase, the partners should be offered supportive advice.
   c) In the interests of improving psychological competence and relief from anxiety in dealing with the patients' problems, the training of all staff by means of sustained group work on the lines of the Balint groups, appears to be of vital importance in reducing, inter alia, postoperative psychic complications. That is to say, group work should be carried out in every ward, with all nursing and medical staff participating.
4. In-patient treatment from the date of transfer from the ICU to the rehabilitation clinic:
   The psychic processes which play a part at this stage, (withdrawal, grieving process) have been described by Kimball [7]. The offer of individual talks, advice to relatives, and staff training (see above) all appear equally important at this stage.
5. The period spent in the rehabilitation clinic:
   At this stage, the most important thing is to mobilize the doctors' awareness that the physical training program represents at the most, only a part of the work to be done, and that in addition, questions of the revised life plans, i.e., psychohygienic problems, dealing with the partner, and vocational problems, must play an essential part. If the prerequisites can be created for this, then group discussions with the patients and supervisory groups for doctors and nursing staff ought to be offered.
6. The period after discharge from the rehabilitation clinic:
   This phase is characterized by a wealth of very serious problems – concerning work, the family, and the partner [7]. The discrepancy between the relatively good physical and the frequently poor psychosocial state is remarkable. The latter endangers the success of the operation [3, 4, 6, 9].
   a) Awareness of the correlated problems is of vital importance to the overall success of the surgery. In this phase patients should be offered individual and group discussions.
   b) The investigations undertaken by G. Dahme et al. [2] showed that the important persons of reference are decisive in coping with this phase. For this reason, it appears to be a matter of urgency that relatives be actively involved.
   c) In addition, the doctors and medical officers of health who will be responsible for treatment and assessment should be sought out. With them, it is often the case that they do not know enough about the opportunities heart surgery patients have [Rodewald et al., this volume]. For this reason, they often promote the patients' regressive inclinations rather than their (vocational) autonomy. An attempt should be made to set up a working team of the doctors who will continue dealing with the patients, a group in which specific further training will be made.

An overriding objective ought to be to improve the currently inadequate cooperation between the doctors and institutions involved.

We do not have an equivalent of the self-help organization, "Mended Hearts" [7] in the Federal Republic of Germany, but we want to try to encourage patients to take up such activities.

The scientific accompaniment of this therapeutic program is, in the first place, to be in the shape of carefully recording the observations. A seminar, in which the therapeutic experiences can be dealt with practically and theoretically, and from which fundamental conceptual conclusions are to be developed, will be the focal point.

Comparative examinations of patients from our own and other heart surgery centers during their stay in the rehabilitation clinic, and parallel investigations in other centers, will provide clues as to the effects of such an extensive program of psychological care. We hope to obtain more information from the investigation of patients of the Hamburg cardiosurgical unit which was carried out prior to this project. The knowledge thus gained will help us to decide exactly which of the activities carried out in the program of investigation can be practicably transferred to a care-orientated rather than a research-orientated cardiosurgical unit.

Our deliberations hitherto have naturally been orientated to the local conditions in Hamburg and the Federal Republic of Germany. To date, we do not yet know how many and what parts of our plan will be realised. The object of our investigation, however, is to check the possibilities. Transferability to other countries with different social and medical systems will not be immediately possible but it is precisely from the exchange of experience, as is possible at symposiums like this and from the international study planned, that we hope to have the opportunity to learn from each other about improving therapeutic care.

We hope to be able to report about our experiences with our project at the next or one of the next symposiums.

Acknowledgment. Translation was by Kathleen Behnke and Richard A. Bird.

References

1. Caston JC (1980) Inside the heart of darkness: A journey through cardiotomy. In: Speidel H, Rodewald G (eds) Psychic and neurological dysfunctions after open-heart surgery. Thieme, Stuttgart, pp 19–37
2. Dahme G, Dahme B, Kornemann J, Vollers A, Huse-Kleinstoll G (1980) Fulfilment of patient's expectations concerning outcome of open-heart surgery. In: Speidel H, Rodewald G (eds) Psychic and neurological dysfunctions after open-heart surgery. Thieme, Stuttgart, pp 228–236
3. Frank KA, Heller SS, Kornfeld DS, Malm JR (1972) Long-term effects of open-heart surgery on intellectual functioning. J Thorac Cardiovasc Surg 64:811–815
4. Heller SS, Frank KA, Kornfeld DS, Malm JR, Bowman FO Jr (1974) Psychological outcome following open-heart surgery. Arch Intern Med 134:908–914
5. Heller SS, Kornfeld DS, Frank KA, Barsa J (1980) Delirium after coronary artery bypass surgery. In: Speidel H, Rodewald G (eds) Psychic and neurological dysfunctions after open-heart surgery. Thieme, Stuttgart, pp 156–162

6. Henrichs TF, Mackenzie JW, Almond CH (1971) Psychological adjustment and psychiatric complications following open-heart surgery. J Nerv Ment Dis 152:322–345
7. Kimball CP (1976) The experience of cardiac surgery and cardiac transplant. In: Howells JG (ed) Modern perspectives in the psychiatric aspects of surgery. Brunner-Mazel, New York, pp 243–266
8. Kimball CP (1980) The experience of open-heart surgery VI. Research and consultation-liaison psychiatry. In: Speidel H, Rodewald G (eds) Psychic and neurological dysfunctions after open-heart surgery. Thieme, Stuttgart, pp 215–228
9. Lützenkirchen J, Lamprecht K, Walter J, Dietz A (1980) The sociomedical situation and personality after heart surgery. In: Speidel H, Rodewald G (eds) Psychic and neurological dysfunctions after open-heart surgery. Thieme, Stuttgart, pp 188–192
10. Speidel H, von Kerekjarto M, Knauf B, Probst P (1975) Psychische und psychosoziale Probleme bei Prothesenträgern; ein Vergleich zwischen Patienten mit Hüftendoprothesen, künstlichen Herzklappen und unter chronischer klinischer Hämodialyse. Med Psychol 29:127–158
11. Speidel H, Dahme B, Flemming B, Götze P, Huse-Kleinstoll G, Meffert HJ, Rodewald G, Spehr W (1978) Psychosomatische Probleme in der Herzchirurgie. Therapiewoche 28:8191–8210
12. Speidel H, Dahme B, Flemming B, Götze P, Huse-Kleinstoll G, Meffert HJ, Rodewald G (1979) Probleme der Klassifizierung psychopathologischer Auffälligkeiten nach Herzoperationen mit extrakorporaler Zirkulation. Psychiatr Clin (Basel) 12:57–79
13. Speidel H, Dahme B, Flemming B, Götze P, Huse-Kleinstoll G, Meffert HJ, Rodewald G, Spehr W (1980) Open-heart surgery unit. Adv Psychosom Med 10:30–56

Discussion of Session IV

Meffert added to Träger's paper: The time the surgeons spent with each patient varied between 20 min and about an hour. The anesthesiologists and the surgeons were aware of the study because they had to fill in special forms and the talks were taperecorded with their and the patients' permittance. The possible influence of this knowledge was that the physicians certainly tried to give their very best in terms of sensitivity and appropriate amount of information, and that this probably influenced the outcome in a positive way, in terms of less anxiety on the part of the patients. The investigation did not take into account the psychological effects of nursing interventions during the patients' preoperative stay in hospital. It was a first attempt to study in a controlled design the psychological effects of the doctors' explanatory talks on the patients.

Blacher commented on Trägers' paper concerning the patients massive denial from his own experience and in the light of several studies reported, for instance, the Merav and Robinson study. When one asks the patient what the surgeon did during surgery, fewer than half of the patients have any recollection that the heart would be open in open-heart surgery. According to the Merav and Robinson study, in which the investigators each spent about an hour preparing the patients for their operation, including physical examination, the patients' total recollection, more or less, was that the doctor spent a little time with them, listened to their chest, and said that they were going to do a little bit of surgery. They were concerned about this because of certain medical legal problems, which were brought up in the Träger paper, too, in terms of the informed consent. Blacher mentioned the fact that some of the patients in the Träger study got more anxious, and he suggested that this reflects a certain anxiety on the part of the people preparing them. According to Blacher, the patients, if one really queries them, will, when one asks them what the risk of their surgery is, say that they have a 1% or a 5% chance of mortality, according to what the surgeons will tell them in giving them informed consent. But if one pushes the patients further one will find that an almost universal fantasy is that their surgery has a 50 : 50 chance of mortality. This seems to be a universal statistic that cardiac patients have, which reflects not only the view of the danger of the heart surgery, but also the role of the heart as a binary organ – it either works or it doesn't.

Willner pointed to the useful methodological technique in Träger's investigation controlling the assumption that the explanatory talks influenced anxiety by investigating emotional states before and after the doctors' interventions.

Concerning the use of hypnosis in the field of psychoses after open-heart surgery, Nwaefuna stressed that hypnosis is used as a preventive measure for anxiety and many other psychotic episodes, but not as a treatment for psychoses. For treating delusions, hallucinations and paranoid ideas of any form he suggested specific drugs (dopamine-antagonists) to block excessive secretion of dopamine.
Willner suggested that documentation for the usefulness of hypnosis as a preventive measure for psychosis is needed. He pointed to the well-controlled study of Sermon and Hackett in which the authors had found that preoperative preparation using hypnosis did not result in any improved adaptation for surgery, either in the incidence of delirium or in other measures like pain, anxiety, depression. Also they did not find any difference between the group which received hypnosis and the control group which did not. To Willner this does not mean that hypnosis is not effective. He suggested that perhaps there is a particular group of patients who might be able to make more use of hypnosis or perhaps many more sessions need to be done with the patients preoperatively.

Nwaefuna reminded the participants of the varying expertises of the hypnotists, of the varying motivation of the patients and the varying sociability. According to him everybody can be hypnotized except somebody who is mentally subnormal. Referring to his paper, he suggested that if somebody becomes resistant to hypnosis, one of the things one can do is to treat him with chlorpromazine, which actually removes the resistance, and then one can hypnotize anyone straight away. However, Nwaefuna would not hypnotize a patient who is delirious.

Meyendorf commenting on Kimball's paper stated that there is no question that anxiety and specific fears can be ameliorated and should be ameliorated by a specific patient-doctor relationship. But he suggested that one should be careful not to confuse the causes and the treatment of special symptoms arriving in cardiac surgery. He had the impression from Kimball's paper that delirium and psychosis and what might be called typical cardiac delirium might also be caused by the environment of the intensive care unit. From Meyendorfs' point of view the intensive care unit may play a role in giving the psychosis a special aspect, but he suggested that a careful differentiation be made between different types of psychiatric disorders, the not psychotic and the psychotic disorders. He stressed that the typical cardiac psychosis is not caused by the intensive care unit because very many other symptomatic or organic psychoses do exist and are caused outside the intensive care unit.

Kimball stressed the difficulty of segregating the psychotic element from the delirium element or the toxic psychoses, which he thinks is a word that should be abandoned. He suggested the use of the term delirium for the majority of the post-surgical psychological events. Two things were quite important in differentiating delirium from psychotic states:

1. The content of the delirium is most often ego-alien as opposed to egosyntonic with the patient, (the patient says I'm hearing this, I'm seeing this, I'm feeling this, I think this is going on – but I know it isn't so),

2. With relatively modest doses of phenothiazines or haloperidol the state of delirium is reversible within hours if it is treated appropriately. The development of these disordered states of consciousness is slowly progressive and malignant; it interacts with what is going on in the course of treatment of the patient, both physiologic-

ally in terms of specific metabolic abnormalities and probably in sleep-disturbance, and certainly in terms of medication, largely with the abuse and misuse of anxiolytic medication which alters the state of consciousness and the perception of the individual.

Looking at it in this way, Kimball was confident that one could reduce by at least 75% the number of so-called psychotic disturbances postoperatively. He furthermore pointed out that it still cannot be stated whether some things are organic and some things are functional in psychopathology. Both factors contribute to the manifestation of an altered state of consciousness, not the least of which is anxiety, and anxiety is not a psychological state alone. By definition it is a physiological state and it has its physiological measurements.

Answering a question from Rodewald, Kimball described the patients' course of consciousness during the early postoperative period as typical for all open-heart surgery patients, stating that any patient coming out of surgery is in an altered state of anesthesia and other drugs given at the same time as anesthesia. Frequently one sees an obtunded state but the patients come up from that obtunded state with the merging consciousness. Then there is the vigilant stage with more or less hyperactivity and irritability. Then there comes a stage where the patient's senses are sharper, and he identifies louder noises, louder sounds etc. It is the lower senses that are still overshooting in terms of their awareness of the environment. This is a rather transitory stage and in most patients it decreases relatively quickly, usually occurring around the second day. This decrease takes place relatively quickly and is accompanied by more lethargy and turning away. At this stage the patient tends to withdraw and unless one is really familiar with him/her, one has no idea what they are thinking or how they are feeling. He is quiet, acts normally enough, causes no difficulty, and receives little attention. During this period of time some of these patients, particularly when they are under heavy doses of anxiolytic agents, begin to misinterpret the environment – become confused concerning day, night, and who is who, lose track of time and become a little disoriented. An altered state of consciousness is present in every postoperative patient, but the majority of them never reach a level of detection, because it is only when they begin to say things which disturb other people that they get any attention. However, if careful observations were made by the nurses, the mental status tested daily, and five or six questions asked of the patient three times a day, one will find that there is an impairment in every patient.

Only in the smaller group has the incidence of delirium in terms of a major altered state of consciousness in postcardiotomy situations decreased markedly over the last few years. Kimball considers this to be due to the preoperative counseling by physicians and the nursing staff, to decreased use of medications, particularly hypnotic sedatives, to improved operative procedures, reduction in operation time etc., and is another statistic in support of the idea that much of what was observed in these patients is more aptly characterized and diagnosed as delirium rather than as a psychotic or functional psychosis.

V

Neuropsychological Considerations in the Care and Treatment of Children Undergoing Cardiac Surgery

Cardiac Surgery in Infancy Using Profound Hypothermia and Circulatory Arrest: Late Developmental Progress*

P.M. Clarkson, B.A. MacArthur, B.G. Barratt-Boyes, R.M. Whitlock, J.M. Neutze

Introduction

Children with congenital heart disease destined to become important symptomatic are often in serious difficulty prior to 1 year of age. In an attempt to improve the results of primary repair in infancy a number of groups have adopted surgical techniques using profound hypothermia, in order to provide a sufficient period of circulatory arrest in which to perform an accurate repair within a totally relaxed bloodless heart.

This study [2] was undertaken to assess the late developmental progress in children whose congenital heart defects were repaired using profound hypothermia and circulatory arrest.

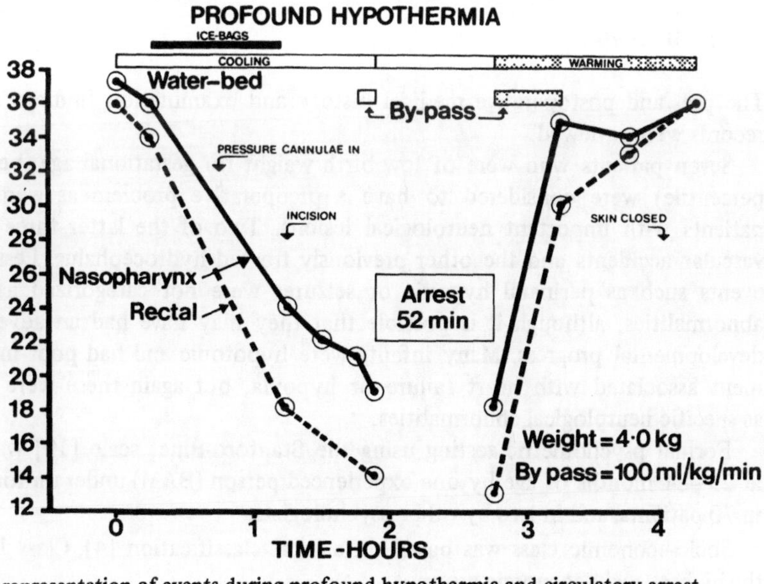

Fig. 1. Graphic representation of events during profound hypothermia and circulatory arrest

---

* This investigation was supported by the Medical Research Council of New Zealand

Surgical Technique

The anesthetised infant lies on a water bed through which cooled water is circulated. Ice bags are placed on the front of the body and around the head. The nasopharyngeal and rectal temperatures fall (Fig. 1). Usually, a short period of cardiopulmonary bypass (CPB) with cooled perfusate is used which results in further cooling prior to arresting the circulation. Repair is performed with the heart arrested. Once the repair is completed CPB is resumed with warm perfusate and warm water circulated through the water bath [1]. In the patients reported here the mean nasopharyngeal temperature was 22 °C, the mean rectal temperature 20.5 °C, and the mean duration of circulatory arrest 48 min.

Material and Methods

Clinical Material

Seventy two of 76 consecutive long-term survivors who had surgical repair of congenital heart lesions at 11 days–26 months of age using profound hypothermia and circulatory arrest, from the beginning of our experience in July 1969 until December 1971 were evaluated late postoperatively.

Testing Methods

The pre- and postoperative medical history and examination findings and operative records were reviewed.

Seven patients who were of low birth weight for gestational age (below the 10th percentile) were considered to have a preoperative problem as were three other patients with important neurological lesions. Two of the latter three had cerebrovascular accidents and the other previously treated hydrocephalus. Less well-defined events such as perinatal hypoxia or seizures were not categorized as neurological abnormalities, although it is possible that they may have had an adverse effect on developmental progress. Many infants were hypotonic and had poor motor development associated with heart failure or hypoxia, but again these were not regarded as specific neurological abnormalities.

Formal psychometric testing using the Stanford-Binet scale [10] was undertaken at 29–84 months of age by one experienced person (BAM) under uniform conditions in 70 patients, and in two by other psychologists.

Socio-economic class was based on a local classification [4], Class 1 representing the highest socio-economic group.

Linear regressions were constructed by the least squares method in an attempt to determine whether a number of variables related to preoperative status and perioperative events were associated with postoperative performance as judged by IQ. Results were considered to show a significant correlation at the 5% level. Comparisons between groups were made using the unpaired Student's t-test, differences being considered significant when $2P < 0.05$.

During the period when this study was undertaken another group of 69 children also had Stanford-Binet tests administered by the same investigator. This group was randomly selected from a larger sequential group of infants born at one hospital, who met certain criteria based on birth and neonatal characteristics with a view to providing an "ideal" group for comparison with other infants who had pre or perinatal problems. It consisted of Caucasian singletons, 38–42 weeks gestation, weighting 3000–4000 g and without evidence of congenital malformation, neonatal illness or other adverse features. They were tested as preschoolers at an average age of 57 months.

Results

Relation to Operative Events

The mean IQ of the 72 patients tested was 92.9 (1SD = 16.5). Stanford-Binet scores bore no relation to the duration of circulatory arrest (Fig. 2) or to other aspects of surgical technique [2]. The mean score of those who had ventilatory or circulatory support in the postoperative period was similar to the score of those who did not require this assistance. There was no demonstrable relationship between intelligence test results and age at operation, age at assessment, race (Caucasian vs Polynesian), or sex.

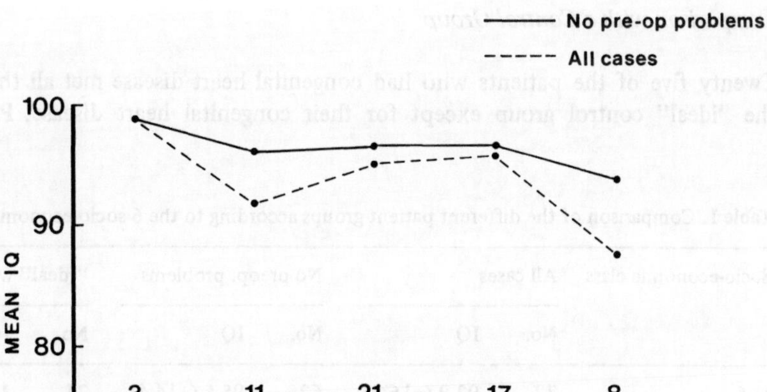

Fig. 2. Mean IQ (Stanford-Binet) at varying durations of circulatory arrest in 69 patients in whom the arrest time was less than 70 min [2]

Effect of Pre- and Postoperative Events

The ten patients who were of low birth weight for gestational age or had important neurological problems preoperatively had a mean IQ of 76.5 (1SD = 20.0) which was significantly lower than the mean obtained by those in whom these problems were absent (95.5, 1SD = 14.4).

Two patients had choreoathetotic movements postoperatively. Both had developmental abnormalities before operation and mild neurological residua at follow up. Test scores were 65 and 82. Another patient who had a total circulatory arrest time of 89 min, interrupted by an additional period of cooling CPB, had a cardiac arrest postoperatively and showed important neurological abnormalities on discharge. These largely resolved and IQ at review was 79. No permanent adverse effects were noted in four patients who had transient seizures after operation.

General

No major differences were found in mean intelligence test scores amongst patients in socio-economic classes 1–4. Patients in socio-economic classes 5–6 (Table 1) had a mean IQ of 85.6 (1SD = 15.3) as compared with 97.6 (1SD = 15.4) in classes 1–4 ($2P < 0.005$). The difference between these groups remained significant when patients with preoperative problems were excluded ($2P < 0.01$).

Patients with ventricular septal defect, tetralogy of Fallot, and transposition of the great arteries made up 75% of the study group. No significant difference in mean IQ was found between patients in these diagnostic categories.

Comparison with a Control Group

Twenty five of the patients who had congenital heart disease met all the eriteria of the "ideal" control group except for their congenital heart disease. Psychometric

Table 1. Comparison of the different patient groups according to the 6 socio-economic class

Socio-economic class	All cases		No preop. problems		"Ideal" with CHD	
	No.	IQ	No.	IQ	No.	IQ
1–6	72	92.9 (±16.5)	62	95.5 (±14.4)	25	101.4 (±13.9)
1–4	43	97.6 (±15.4)	38	99.3 (±14.4)	17	105.9 (±12.6)
5–6	29	85.6 (±15.3)	24	89.2 (±11.7)	8	91.7 (±12.0)
					"Ideal" controls	
1–6					69	106.2 (±11.6)
1–4					53	108.1 (±10.7)
5–6					16	99.7 (±12.5)

Figures in parentheses refer to 1SD

testing was undertaken in this subgroup of patients at an earlier mean age (43 months) but it was not considered that this affected the comparison between them and the "ideal" control group, as all were tested prior to 6 years of age. The "ideal" group of 25 children with congenital heart disease (Table 1) had a mean IQ of 101.4 (1SD = 15.0) while the "ideal" control group of 69 children had a mean IQ of 106.2 (1SD = 11.6). This difference is not statistically significant.

Discussion

Cerebral damage may result from a number of operative events. On this basis of experience with CPB techniques the most common cause would appear to be cerebral air embolism, although particulate emboli can also occur. Despite meticulous attention to surgical technique and careful control of temperature gradients, the completeness of de-airing of the left ventricle remains conjectural and air from this source could be a cause of early or late intellectual impairment [1]. Apart from the risk of air or particulate emboli, these infants were liable to cerebral damage from the circulatory arrest per se, as the safe period of arrest at any given temperature is uncertain. In the early series of infants reported here we based arrest time on that recommended by Hikasa et al. [6] who suggested that for a 60-min arrest period a rectal temperature of 20 °C was appropriate. In fact, we preferred nasopharyngeal temperature to rectal temperature in the belief that it reflects brain temperature more accurately. We were surprised that the mean nasopharyngeal arrest temperature in this group of patients turned out to be 22 °C. This was in part due to the selection of a temperature of 22 °C–24 °C in most patients where the surgeon considered the defect could be repaired within a relatively short arrest time. Mean rectal temperature was lòwer – 20.5 °C. However, a relatively poor correlation between arrest temperature and arrest time was noted [2] indicating that this practice was not wise, and for some time now we have stabilized the prearrest nasopharyngeal temperature at 18 °C. It is probable that 60 min should be regarded as the maximum arrest time for a nasopharyngeal temperature of 20 °C. With a nasopharyngeal temperature of 16 °C–18 °C current results suggest that an arrest time of up to 70 min is safe.

The data show that the mean intelligence score of the study group differs from normal. The difference between patients and controls with similar birth and neonatal characteristics is, however, negligible. The four patients not included in the study would not have affected the comparison with the control group, as none would have been included in the "ideal" subgroup of patients with congenital heart disease.

In particular there was no correlation between the IQ and duration of circulatory arrest. The results obtained here are very similar to those obtained form other studies [3, 5, 7–9].

The data from this study do not provide conclusive information on the incidence or severity of cerebral damage using profound hypothermia circulatory arrest techniques. To obtain this it would be necessary to assess intelligence of individual patients before, as well as after, operation. Assessment before repair was not feasible due to the young age of the subjects and their often critical illness. On the other hand, we have not been able to demonstrate any deleterious effect attributable to the operative technique used with our patients. Rather it would seem that postoperative intelligence test scores reflect characteristics related to the individual patients.

References

1. Barratt-Boyes BG (1976) The technique of intracardiac repair in infancy using deep hypothermia with circulatory arrest and limited cardiopulmonary bypass. In: Ionescu MI, Wooler GH (eds) Current techniques in extracorporeal circulation. Butterworths, London, pp 197–228
2. Clarkson PM, MacArthur BA, Barrat-Boyes BG, Whitlock RM, Neutze JM (to be published) Developmental progress following cardiac surgery in infancy using profound hypothermia and circulatory arrest circulation
3. Dickinson DF, Sambrooks JE (1979) Intellectual performance in children after circulatory arrest with profound hypothermia in infancy. Arch Dis Child 54:1–6
4. Elley WB, Irving JC (1976) Revised socio-economic index for New Zealand. NZJ Educat Stud 11:25–36
5. Haka-Ikse K, Blackwood MJA, Steward DJ (1978) Psychomotor development of infants and children after profound hypothermia during surgery for congenital heart disease. Dev Med Child Neurol 20:62–70
6. Hikasa Y, Shirotani H, Mori C et al. (1967) Open heart surgery in infants with an aid of hypothermic anesthesia. Arch Jap Chir 36:495–508
7. Messmer BJ, Schallberger U, Gattiker R, Senning A (1976) Psychomotor and intellectual development after deep hypothermia and circulatory arrest in early infancy. J Thorac Cardiovasc Surg 72:495–502
8. Stevenson JG, Stone EF, Dillard DH, Morgan BC (1974) Intellectual development of children subjected to prolonged circulatory arrest during hypothermic open heart surgery in infancy. Circulation 49–50:11, 54–59
9. Subramanian S, Vlad P, Fischer L, Cohen MF (1976) Sequelae of profound hypothermia and circulatory arrest in the corrective treatment of congenital heart disease in infants and small children. In: Kidd BSL, Rowe RD (eds) The child with congenital heart disease after surgery. Futura, New York, pp 421–431
10. Terman LR, Merrill MA (1961) Stanford Binet intelligence scale. Manual for the third revision. Harrap, London

Psychiatric Complications in Children After Open-Heart Surgery*

G. Jänsch, K. Bühlmeyer, R. Meyendorf, F. Sebening, E. Tacke, Ch. Tröndle

Introduction

Our studies with children suffering from congenital heart disease were inspired by the observations made with adult patients with cardiac defects. Many authors report consistently that a certain number of adult patients show a psychotic reaction after cardiac surgery in the pattern of the "exogener Reaktionstyp Bonhoeffer" [4, 5, 7, 8]. This postoperative delirium or "cardiac psychosis" presents mainly as a syndrome of disorientation, visual and auditory illusions and hallucinations, and paranoid ideas. In addition Meyendorf [8] enumerates the following characteristics:

1. The delirium normally occurs between the 3rd and 6th day after operation.
2. Its duration normally varies between 3 and 7 days.
3. It occurs significantly more often after open- (26%) than after closed-heart surgery (17.4%).

Two main causes, which may very well interact, are discussed in today's literature on the subject:

1. Organic factors: Meyendorf [8] supposes that the extracorporeal circulation encourages the development of microembolis and thus increases, by way of hypoxic changes in brain metabolism, the probability that a postoperative psychosis might occur.
2. Psychological factors: Kornfeld et al. [6], e.g., hold the psychological strain in the intensive care unit to be responsible for the psychotic reaction.

Systematic observations of children after heart surgery are much rarer than those of adult patients, and the described reactions are much less uniform. Egerton and Kay [4] report postoperative deliriums in children similar to those observed in adults. Furthermore, they found that the children had depressed reactions with refusal to eat. Kornfeld et al. [6] found no abnormal reaction to operation in 20 children. Barnes [1], Bergouignan et al. [2] and Danilowicz and Gabriel [3] describe a syndrome with the following symptoms:

* The reported data were gained in two studies for a final examination in psychology (Diplomarbeiten) at the Ludwig-Maximilians University in Munich in 1978

Psychopathological and Neurological Dysfunctions Following Open-Heart Surgery Ed. by Becker et al.

1. Emotional instability
2. Fearfulness
3. Confusion
4. Reduction of speech, sometimes absolute mutism.

Bergouignan et al. [2] could also observe that these psychological symptoms often coincide with distinct choreiform movements.

These heterogeneous results led to the main questions of our own study.

Questions and Suppositions

Our investigation was based on the main hypothesis that the psychotic reactions which some patients show in response to cardiac surgery are caused by organic factors. This led to the following questions and suppositions:

1. Do children show psychotic forms of reaction following cardiac surgery?
   We expected a small number of children to develop psychotic symptoms after surgery, but not before.
2. How many children show psychological signs of minimal brain dysfunction *before* and *after* surgery?
   We expected to find such signs significantly more in children after than before the operation.
3. What are the intellectual abilities of the children before and after surgery?
   We expected the average IQ to be within the norm before the operation and to remain unchanged or even decrease a bit afterwards.
4. In how many children can behavioral disturbances be observed before and after cardiac surgery?
   We expected that a great number of children would show behavioral disturbances already before the operation and that their number would significantly increase postoperatively.

   Furthermore, we were interested in the following questions:

5. What meaning does the heart have for children?
6. What is the body image like of children suffering from congenital heart disease?
7. How do children experience the intensive care unit?

   The last two questions were only investigated for part of the sample.

Sample

We examined all children between the age of 4 and 13 years suffering from congenital heart disease who were operated on in the "Deutsches Herzzentrum" in Munich during the time between August 1977 and February 1978. Only children with severe mental retardation and those whose native language was not German were excluded.

Thus, we got a sample of 41 children who were divided into two groups:

- The first group consisted of 21 preschool children at the age of 4–7 years.
- The second group consisted of 20 school children at the age of 8–13 years.

There were 25 boys and 16 girls. Thirty children underwent open-heart surgery, ten closed-heart surgery. One school boy died before the operation.

Methods

The same psychological procedures were used before and after surgery (Table 1).

The questionnaire for parents and nurses was submitted to the parents before the operation and to the nurses afterwards.

The children were rated on 33 different variables (12 rating scales and 21 alternative variables) which were based on the questionnaire, the interview, and the behavioral observation. The full psychological examination before surgery took place in the afternoon of the day of arrival in the hospital because most children were operated on the following day. After surgery the examination was divided into two parts:

1. The less tiring tests were carried out on the 3rd or 4th day after the operation.
2. The intelligence tests and the Benton test were performed shortly before their dismissal from the clinic (15th–18th day).

Statistical Analysis

The pre- and postoperative data were analysed with regard to the level of statistical significance. For this analysis three different statistical methods were used according to the three different levels of measurement:

1. For data on an interval scale (for example the IQ): the t test for related samples.
2. For data on an ordinal scale (rating scales): the sign test by Siegel.
3. For data on a nominal scale (check lists): the binomial test variant of the McNemar test.

Results

Psychotic Reactions

None of the children showed the classic picture of an exogenous psychosis after the operation that one observes in adult patients. A reaction similar to psychosis was diagnosed in four *preschool children*. All four of them showed disturbances in social behavior: a marked emotional reserve culminating in a total refusal of contact in one case and accompanied by partial mutism.

Table 1. Psychological procedure

	For the preschool children	For the school children
1.	Draw-a-man-test by Ziler with the instruction to draw themselves	Draw-a-man-test by Ziler with the instruction to draw themselves
2.	Raven Coloured Progressive Matrices	Benton-Test
3.	The performance subtests of the German form of the WPPSI (called HAWIVA)	A short form of the German form of the WISC (called HAWIK) consisting of the four subtests "information", "similarities", "picture order", and "block design" plus the two subtests "digit span" and "figure symbols"
4.	Two pictures of the Children's Apperception Test by Bellak	The "Kinder-Angst-Test" by Thurner and Tewes, a standardized questionnaire for measuring anxiety in children
5.	A self-devised questionnaire for parents and nurses respectively	A self-devised questionnaire for parents and nurses respectively
6.	A partly standardized interview with the child	A partly standardized interview with the child
7.	Behavioral observation	Behavioral observation

Table 2. Number of cases showing a psychotic form of reaction

Group	Before surgery	After surgery	Level of significance
Preschool n = 21	0 (0%)	4 (19%)	–
School n = 20	1[a] (5%)	0 (0%)	–

[a] This was the little boy who died before the operation

Among the *school children* no child showed a psychotic form of reaction to the operation. There was only one child with psychotic symptoms; this was the little boy who died before surgery. He showed illusory misperceptions and a distorted feeling of reality shortly before his death.

There was also a significant increase ($P < 0.05$) in the variable "slight disorientation concerning time" in the school group after the operation.

Thus the first hypothesis, i.e., that children show after-heart-surgery symptoms of a "cardiac psychosis", could not be confirmed.

Minimal Brain Dysfunction

In both groups the psychological signs of minimal brain damage did not increase significantly after the operation. In most of the tests that were used for the diagnosis of brain dysfunction the average performance even improved significantly after surgery. However, this result must be seen in the context of a general postoperative improvement in all intellectual areas. Therefore, an isolated interpretation is not possible.

Table 3. Number of cases suspected of minimal brain damage

Group	Before surgery	After surgery	Level of significance
Preschool n = 21	0 (0%)	4 (19%)	–
School n = 19[a]	10 (53%)	6 (32%)	–

[a] The child who died before surgery was excluded

It should be noted, however, that there was one single test in which there was found to be no postoperative improvement, but even a slight decrease in the average performance. This was the subtest "digit span" in the WISC for the school group. This was the result of a considerable deterioration of short-term memory in some children after surgery, which brought about a statistical compensation for the rest of the group.

Thus the second hypothesis, i.e., that the signs of minimal brain damage increase after surgery, could not be confirmed either.

It should be noted that the four preschool children who showed signs of minimal brain damage postoperatively were the same four children who showed transitory psychotic symptoms after surgery. All four underwent open-heart surgery.

In the school group, however, the results are much less consistent. Of six children who showed signs of minimal brain damage after surgery only two underwent open-heart surgery. They were not identical, either, with the disoriented children or with those whose short-term memory had been impaired.

Intellectual Abilities

As Table 4 shows there was a highly significant increase in the average IQ in both groups after the operation. The draw-a-man-quotient also *increased* in the *preschool group*, though not significantly. The only exception was the draw-a-man-quotient in the *school group*, which showed a highly significant *decrease* after the operation. Since

Table 4. Intellectual abilities

Group	Test	Before surgery	After surgery	Level of significance
Preschool	WPPSI-IQ	94.2	98.1	$P < 0.01$
n = 21	Draw-a-man-quotient	104.1	108.4	–
	Right answers in the Raven-test	14.9	16.2	$P < 0.05$
School	WISC-IQ	108.5	116.3	$P < 0.001$
n = 19[a]	Draw-a-man-quotient	92.3	86.5	$P < 0.001$

[a] The child who died before surgery was excluded

Several reasons may account for the postoperative increase in the average IQ:

1. Getting experienced with the test by repetition.
2. There was no postoperative fear and excitement.
3. Increasing familiarity with the environment.
4. The children knew by now the examiner and the test situation.
6. The time of the examination was more convenient: The children were tested in the morning and not in the afternoon.
7. The operation might have brought about better oxygenation of the brain.

The third hypothesis, i.e., that the IQ would be in the norm and remain unchanged, or even decrease a bit after the operation, could only partially confirmed.

Behavioral Disturbances

The rate of children with neurotic behavior was already very high in both groups prior to the operation. Thus part of the fourth hypothesis could be confirmed. Postoperatively the scores tended to increase but there were no statistically significant differences. The main observed behavioral disturbances were biting of nails and thumb-sucking, hyperactivity, eating problems, different tics, symptoms of autonomic nervous disorder, aggressive behavior, and a strong wish to be at the center of attention.

In both groups the anxiety and tension observed and rated by the examiner decreased significantly after surgery. In the school group the stanine scores of the children's anxiety test showed a significant postoperative decrease too. These results probably reflect the relief of the children that all was over.

Table 5. Number of cases with behavioral disturbances

Group	Before surgery	After surgery	Level of significance
Preschool n = 21	20 (95%)	19 (91%)	–
School n = 19[a]	14 (74%)	16 (84%)	–

[a] The child who died before surgery was excluded

Table 6. Anxiousness

Group	Variable	Before surgery	After surgery	Level of significance
Preschool n = 21	Number of children rated "anxious"	16 (76%)	10 (48%)	$P < 0.05$
School n = 19[a]	Average stanine-score in the KAT	5.1	4.6	$P < 0.05$

[a] The child who died before surgery was excluded

The Meaning of the Heart for the Children

Before the operation we asked all the children if they knew what the heart is for. The meaning of the heart was deduced from their answers.

There were five types of answers:

1. Eleven children (26.8%) gave objectively correct answers, i.e., answers which described correctly one or more functions of the heart. All 11 children came from the school group.
2. Seven children (17.1%) gave objectively wrong answers, e.g., "we need the heart for breathing" or "the heart presses the food into the stomach".
3. Eleven answers (26.8%) referred directly to the vital importance of the heart, e.g., "one can't live without a heart".
4. Three children (7.3%) – all from the preschool group – identified the function of the heart with the impending operation, e.g., "we need the heart for surgery".
5. Fourteen children (34%) gave no answer at all. They too were all preschool children.

These results suggest that most of the younger children were not informed very clearly about the meaning and functioning of the heart, whereas for the older children – as in fact for most adults – the heart represents "life".

Body Image

This question was examined for the school group only. The draw-a-man-quotient averaged 92.3 points before the operation, which is close to the lower limits of the norm (97–99 points for children of this average age) and suggests that the children's relation to their body was already slightly disturbed before surgery. The operation seems to have additionnally impaired the body image, since the average draw-a-man-quotient dropped to 86.5 points postoperatively. This difference is highly significant ($P < 0.001$). The disturbed body image was mainly characterized by the following mistakes in the drawings:

1. incomplete or wrong presentation of parts of the body, especially the hands.
2. wrong or distorted proportions.
3. presentation as a portrait which was interpreted as a reduction of themselves to a head only.

Experience of the Intensive Care Unit

After the operation we asked each child what disturbed them most and what they liked best in the intensive care unit. The answers cannot be discussed in full length here. The most important result was that many children pointed out how relieved they were that their mothers were allowed to be with them during the greater part of the day.

This could even lead to the speculation that perhaps the more severe postoperative disturbances have been avoided by the presence of the mothers.

Discussion

As for the results of our study one wonders first of all why there was no typical psychotic reaction after surgery in a single child. This finding is actually in harmony with the observations of other authors, who found – if at all – less psychotic reactions with children than with adults [4, 6]. One could think of two explanations for this phenomenon:

1. It is possible that the psychological care for children in hospital is better than that for adults. For example in the "Deutsches Herzzentrum" in Munich the mothers are allowed to be with their children in the intensive care unit immediately after the operation.
2. The infantile brain and psychological development is not yet as "matured" as in adults, so that the psychopathological reactions of children to heart surgery may principally be different from those of adults, and on the whole less dramatic. Psychotic reactions do not manifest themselves in paranoid and hallucinatory syndromes as clearly as in adults. Perhaps children are tending more to neurotic than to psychotic reactions. This would also explain the high rate of behavioral disturbances in our study.

However, the rate of behavioral disturbances was surprisingly high before surgery, and this asks for an explanation, too. We think that overprotection by the parents towards the ill child plays an important role here. This is certainly a big problem because the children do not learn to cope adequately with disagreeable situations and therefore react to them with behavioral disturbances. Thus, it is possible that a child may gain complete physical health by the operation and yet will never be able to be really accepted by his peers and thus live from then on a normal life. Therefore, in many cases psychological guidance of the parents seems to be as important as the medical treatment of the child.

References

1. Barnes CM (1975) Levels of consciousness indicated by responses of children to phenomena in the intensive care unit. Matern Child Nurs J 4:215–285
2. Bergouignan M, Fontan F, Trarieux M, Julien J (1961) Syndromes choréiformes de l'enfant au décours d'intervention cardio-chirurgicales sous hypothermie profonde. Rev Neurol 105:48–59
3. Danilowicz DA, Gabriel PH (1971) Postoperative reactions in children: "Normal" and abnormal responses after cardiac surgery. Am J Psychiatry 128/2:185–188
4. Egerton N, Kay JH (1964) Psychological disturbances associated with open heart surgery. Br J Psychiatry 110:433–439
5. Kimball CP (1969) Psychological responses to the experience of open heart surgery I. Am J Psychiatry 126:348–359
6. Kornfeld DS, Zimberg S, Malm JR (1965) Psychiatric complications of open heart surgery. N Engl J Med 273/6:287–292
7. Meyendorf R (1976) Psychische und neurologische Störungen bei Herzoperationen. Prä- und postoperative Untersuchungen. Fortschr Med 94:315–320
8. Meyendorf R (1976) Hirnembolie und Psychose. Unter besonderer Berücksichtigung der Basalganglienapoplexie bei Herzoperationen mit extrakorporaler Zirkulation. J Neurol 213:163–177

Comparison of Personality and Social Development After Heart Surgery Using Profound Hypothermia, Normothermia Perfusion, and Cardioplegia in Children

J. Wada, Y. Takanashi, H. Matsui, M. Iwasa, M. Nakazawa, A. Takao, R. Umezu

Introduction

A neuro-psychiatric problem with heart surgery is not common but can be fatal or significant for the patient's life.

This report is presented to discuss the validity of conventional open-heart surgery by reviewing the incidences and prognosis of convulsive episodes in 134 children operated upon for noncomplicated ventricular septal defect or d-transposition with respect to the type of bypass conditions, degree of hypothermia, and the method of anesthesia. The former was extracted from 361 ventricular septal defect closure operations and the latter was from 34 performed at the Heart Institute of Japan, Tokyo Women's Medical College, between Jan. 1975 and Dec. 1979.

Material and Method

One hundred thirty four patients operated on for ventricular septal defect or d-transposition under 6 years old between January 1975 and December 1979 were assessed.

Closure of ventricular septal defect was carried out in 110 patients. Patients were devided into three groups according to the surgical approach.

In group one (17 patients), the procedure was performed under deep hypothermia and circulatory arrest using GOF anesthesia or ether anesthesia.

In group two (35 patients), the procedure was undertaken under deep hypothermia and low flow perfusion using GOF anesthesia.

In group three (58 patients), the procedure was performed under moderate hypothermia and higher flow perfusion using GOF anesthesia.

Septation for d-transposition was undertaken on 24 patients. They were divided into three groups. These are group four, five, and six.

In group four (ten patients), the surgery was performed under deep hypothermia and circulatory arrest with GOF anesthesia.

In group five (eight patients), the procedure was performed under moderate hypothermia and higher flow perfusion with GOF or morphine anesthesia.

In group six (six patients), patients were operated on under deep hypothermia and circulatory arrest with ether anesthesia.

Psychopathological and Neurological Dysfunctions
Following Open-Heart Surgery. Ed. by Becker et al

In the entire series, deep hypothermia was induced with surface cooling, while moderate hypothermia was established only with cor cooling. GOF or ether was used for anesthesia. In GOF anesthesia, chlorpromazine and in ether anesthesia methyl-prednisolone was given before initiation of extracorporeal circulation or surface-cooling. In the early postoperative period special attention was given to detecting any signs of seizure manifestation and intensive observation was continued for at least 1 week, particularly when neurological complication was suspected. When there was any clinical evidence or indication of neurological complication, particularly seizure, repeated electroencephalography and computerized tomographic scanning obtained.

Result

In group one, 2 of 17 patients died. Cause of death was surgical and was not related to neurological problems (Table 1). Three patients had transient convulsive episodes which were not fatal. Neurological complication was found in two patients, while it was transient in one. One patient had monoparesis with motor weakness of the left arm, and another patient developed evidence of diffuse encephalopathy with severe and diffuse electroencephalographic abnormality associated with persistent convulsive seizures.

In group two, 3 of 35 patients died from nonneurological causes. While two patients developed transient convulsive episodes, another died 3 months postoperatively with a nonneurological condition.

In group three, 1 of 58 patients suffered a surgical death unrelated to neurological causes. Three patients presented postoperative convulsive episodes. Transient seizure with normal computerized tomographic scanning, but persistent paroxysmal electroencephalographic abnormality, was observed in one patient. Another patient had convulsive episodes prior to surgery which had been persistent following a pump operation.

Table 1. Three groups with ventricular septal defect

Group 1	Total	Death	Convulsion episode	%
Deep hypothermia with circulatory arrest	17	2	3	18%
Group II Deep hypothermia with low flow perfusion	35	3	2	6% *
Group III Moderate hypothermia with high flow perfusion	58	1	3	5% **
	110	6	8	7%

* $P > 0.1$
** $P > 0.1$

Table 2. Prognosis after convulsive episodes in ventricular septal defect and d-transposition

	Age	Prognosis
Group I		
Y.O.	4 m	Paresis of right side of face, motor weakness of left arm
N.Y.	3 m	Persistent convulsion, diffuse EEG abnormality
Y.K.	3 m	Transient
Group II		
S.N.	4 m	Transient, died 3 months postoperatively with a nonneurological condition
H.I.	7 m	Transient
Group III		
K.N.	2 y	Persistent convulsion, epilepsy in EEG
T.M.	1 y	Transient, abnormality in EEG with normal findings in CT scan.
Y.K.	1 y, 3 m	Convulsive episodes prior to surgery, abnormal EEG findings with mild atrophy in CT Scan.
Group IV		
M.T.	1 y, 3 m	Transient
K.T.	1 y, 2 m	Hyperextension of lower extremities
K.M.	1 y, 3 m	Transient
Group V		
M.T.	9 m	Transient

In closure of ventricular septal defect, 8 of 110 patients developed convulsive episodes (Table 2). Episodes were only transient in three but persistent in five patients with some evidence of continued neurological dysfunction. Retrospective evaluation indicates that surgical conditions such as temperature, duration of bypass, and circulatory arrest are not related to neurological complications (Table 3).

In group four, four of ten patients died from nonneurological causes (Table 4). Three patients had convulsive episodes which were transient in two patients and persistent in the other with hyperextension of lower extremities.

In group five, one of eight patients died from surgery but had no neurological complications. Only one patient developed transient convulsive episode.

In group six, two out of six patients died after surgery without any evidence of neurological complication.

Summarizing then, with the septation procedure for d-transposition in 24 patients, three patients developed transient convulsive episodes, while the other showed evidence of persistent neurological abnormality (Table 2).

Discussion

In cardiac surgery using deep hypothermia, neurological complications have been recognized as a serious postoperative problem. The earlier reports by Björk and Hult-

Table 3. Operative conditions for ventricular septal defect and d-transposition

	Rectal temperature	Duration	
		Bypass	Arrest
Group I Deep hypothermia with circulatory arrest	17 °C (13°–26 °C)	63 min (36–104 min)	23 min (2–32 min)
Group II Deep hypothermia with low flow perfusion	27 °C (18°–35 °C)	78 min (25–261 min)	–
Group III Moderate hypothermia with high flow perfusion	28 °C (22°–32 °C)	79 min (38–137 min)	–
Group IV Deep hypothermia with circulatory arrest, GOF anesthesia	19 °C (16°–23 °C)	76 min (62–136 min)	44 min (7–63 min)
Group V Moderate hypothermia with higher flow perfusion, GOF or Morphine anesthesia	24 °C (16°–28 °C)	139 min (89–208 min)	–
Group VI Deep hypothermia with circulatory arrest, ether anesthesia	13 °C (11°–14 °C)	64 min (51–93 min)	56 min (46–70 min)

Table 4. Three groups with d-transposition

	Total	Death	Convulsion episode	%
Group IV Deep hypothermia with circulatory arrest and GOF anesthesia	10	4	3	30%
Group V Moderate hypothermia with higher perfusion flow and GOF or morphine anesthesia	8	1	1	13% *
Group VI Deep hypothermia with circulatory arrest and ether anesthesia	6	2	0	0% **
	24	7	4	17%

* $P > 0.4$
** $P > 0.2$

quist [1], and Egerton et al. [2] had stressed the existence of significant neurological and psychological dysfunction after open-heart operations, while Silverstone et al. [3], Stevenson et al. [4], and Brunberg et al. [5] in contrast, reported that the neurological complication is rather infrequent by means of assessing postoperative neurological status and intellectual development through employment of intelligence quotients. The results showed that all the survivors possessed normal intelligence. The final conclusion was that the hypothermic technique did not appear to cause gross neurological or intellectual impairment. Brunberg et al. [5] evaluated 22 infants neurologically before and after the cardiac procedures. They found only six normal clinical examinations prior to the operation. Developmental delay and/or hypotonia persisted in one-half of the patients, although usually to a minor degree. Meanwhile Kilman et al. [6] suggested that a high flow normothermia technique may also carry postoperative neurological risk due to air or fat embolism.

In our series the incidence of convulsion after surgery was higher in the deep hypothermia and circulatory arrest group than in the remaining groups, but it is not significant statistically. In contrast to GOF anesthesia, our current impression is that ether anesthesia seems to carry less postoperative neurological risk. Probably in ether anesthesia hemodynamics were more stable during surface cooling. Several other factors may be responsible for increased incidence of neurological complication after the pump procedures: for example diminished microvascular cerebral perfusion, gas fat, and platelet and microparticulate emboli during cardiopulmonary bypass. Neurological complication may also have been induced by deep hypothermia which may result in uneven cerebral cooling. Rapid cooling and rewarming may produce significant temperature gradient between blood and neural tissue.

Neurological complications previously repeated, had included convulsion, altered consciousness states, hypotonia, paresis, rigidity, choreoathetosis, and personality and intellect changes.

Brunberg et al. [5] reported that the depth of cooling and the period of cardiopulmonary bypass and circulatory arrest were not related to postoperative neurological complication.

In this study convulsive episodes were selected as an important indication of neurological complication. Half of the convulsive episodes in 12 patients were transient, but the other half showed persistent evidence of abnormalities such as monoparesis, convulsive seizures, extrapyramidal dysfunction, and abnormal electroencephalogram.

If transient convulsion due to postoperative change in PH, low serum glucose, or calcium in some infant is excluded, the incidence of postoperative convulsive episode could have been much less than the incidence documented above.

Neurological complications in other patients with cardiac disease undergoing extracorporeal circulation surgery are also under investigation, with the hope of making surgical approach as safe as possible in terms of minimizing postoperative morbidity and mortality.

Summary

Neurological complications among 134 patients undergoing surgery for ventricular septal defect or d-transposition between 1975 and 1979 were studied. Although the deep hypothermia and circulatory arrest group showed higher incidence, other groups also developed the neurological complications.

Our study suggests that not only the long-term postoperative evaluation of higher nervous function, but also detailed preoperative assessment, are needed in order to develop better insight into safe surgical management approach which enables rapid and safe rehabilitation of patients undergoing cardiac surgery.

References

1. Bjork VO, Hultquist G (1962) Contraindications to profound hypothermia in open heart surgery. J Thorac Cardiovasc Surg 44:1
2. Egerton N, Egerton WS, Kay JH (1962) Neurologic changes following profound hypothermia. Ann Surg 157:366
3. Silverstone JT, Tannahill MM, Ireland JA (1970) Psychiatric aspects of profound hypothermia in open-heart surgery. J Thorac Cardiovasc Surg 59:193
4. Stevenson JG, Stone EF, Dillard DH, Morgan BC (1974) Intellectual development of children subjected to prolonged circulatory arrest during hypothermic open heart surgery in infancy. Circulation [Suppl 2] 49–50:II–54
5. Brunberg JA, Reilly EL, Doty DB (1974) Central nervous system consequences in infants of cardiac surgery using deep hypothermia and circulatory arrest. Circulation [Suppl 2] 49–50: II–60
6. Kilman JW, Williams TE Jr, Kakos GS, Craenen J, Hosier DN (1973) Surgical correction of the transposition complex in infancy. J Thorac Cardiovasc Surg 66:387

Chronic "Life-Threatening" Illness in Childhood and Adolescence: Developmental, Cognitive and Psychotherapeutic Considerations in the Care of Children Facing Open-Heart Surgery – Selected Isreaeli Experience*

R.D. Becker

When an infant, child, adolescent, or indeed adult patient comes to a hospital, he or she is not just the incidental carrier of a disease process or lesion that is intended to be treated, possibly corrected, or even more optimistically cured. He or she is not measles, rheumatic fever, asthma, diabetes mellitus, osteogenic sarcoma, an optic leoma, a detached retina, a convulsive disorder, nephrotic syndrome, or even a sore throat or a runny nose. That child, adolescent or adult is, indeed, an impressionable human being and a member of a family who are all very much interested not only in that patient's blood sugar curve, leukocyte count, or in the outcome of any EKG, EEG, echocardiogram, brain scan, electroretinogram, or indeed even a bone marrow aspiration or an aortic, mitral or tricuspid valve prosthetic replacement or correction, but very much more profoundly in the human being that that patient is.

Medical students and interns receive excellent instruction in the treatment of diseases and the examination of bodies. If some time and thought, however, could be given to teaching these students and young physicians how to deal with the child and adolescent patient, and, indeed, adult patient – themselves, as people – then our hospitals and medical schools, in addition to their very first-class contributions to the physical education and treatment of illness, would also contribute to the physical welfare of children and would render considerable service to the preservation and promotion of the future mental health of the patients entrusted to their care.

When this happens, and indeed we're now pleased to say that it is happening in some children's hospitals and adolescent medical units across this and other countries, then the child specialist, whether physician or surgeon, psychoanalyst, psychologist or other, will be able to announce with a sense of justifiable pride that pediatrics is for children. That, essentially, is the frame in which I would like to proceed.

From the cradle onward man is both blessed and burdened by his imagination. Compared to other species, he is a child longer than any member of the animal kingdom. If fantasy burgeons early, often outstripping and outdistancing his cognitive

* The present paper is an edited version of Dr. Becker's recorded presentation. Due to his untimely death, the original manuscript was unavailable.
Every effort was made to preserve Dr. Becker's exact words and style of writing. However full justice to his contribution was not possible since much of his lecture involved the presentation of slides.
The typescript was edited by Dr. Katz. The editor is grateful to Roerig Division, Pfizer, Inc. for facilitating publication of the paper.

Psychopathological and Neurological Dysfunctions Following Open-Heart Surgery Ed by Becker et al.

powers of articulation, in his early years the fruits may be of singular spontaneity and of naive beauty, but also of unbridled terror. Playgrounds become battlefields and battlefields playgrounds. Can we wonder that the shiny arsenal of the intensive care unit may become a chamber of horrors more unreal yet far more alarming than the dull, lifeless waxworks of Madame Tussaud's. In apprehension the unknown constitutes a powerful vacuum which, if not filled with reasonable, respectful, and honorable explanation, with a full disclosure of the truth, will soon fill up with the very worst imagination the child can supply, far worse than the actual encounter with reality.

We cannot dismiss the child's often unvoiced and unspoken fears as nonsense. In a world where man is still capable or perhaps even more capable of conceiving, publishing and manufacturing even more sophisticated forms of horror, then these issues do make sense and must be attended to. The child cannot be expected to know the ethics of the Hippocratic Oath. All of it means nothing to him. He sees the white-gowned – or should I say green-gowned – *Grande Person* as on omniscient phantom of authority with incomprehensible instruments of punishment. That may be a bit harsh, but I'm hopeful that this perception of child-in-hospital and child-facing-surgery will be reconsidered.

We have also heard a bit about the body image concept from a previous speaker. Let me just say a few words about this before we proceed to looking at some drawings which, I hope, will in further measure convince you that it makes sense.

The concept of the body image, though an illusive one, difficult to define operationally and to test empirically, is of obvious central and great significance to successful medical and surgical care. Serious distortion of the body image may mask psychopathological symptomatology. For the surgical patient, whether child, adolescent or adult, prospective surgery may threaten a change in body image so traumatic as to keep the adolescent or adult patient from an informed agreement to consent to a much needed, perhaps life-saving operation, and may indeed postsurgically interfere with recovery and rehabilitation in menacing fashion. When the therapeutic ideal, whether medical or surgical, is the restitution to a functional state of improved health, rather than just restoration of a healthy organ system or a laboratory result, then a body image problem, whenever present, must be taken into account in the overall treatment program. The concept of body image problems is sufficiently unfamiliar and complex, as applied to general medicine and cardiothoracic surgery in particular, that there may be need for instructive case reports. It is the purpose of this paper to present such a series of case reports which illustrate the effects of cardiac surgery on body image following surgery.

In this century major and significant developments and achievements within the science of medicine and its applications to the physical and therapeutic care of the hospitalized patient seem no more evident than in the specialized fields of pediatrics: pediatric surgery, cardiothoracic surgery, and indeed, increasingly, in adolescent medicine. The medical technology thus far advanced in this century has indeed been most impressive and we continue to make important innovative research and therapeutic strides and technical advances each year. It is, however, equally as clear from a close review of both the clinical and research findings thus far published that there has been a relative indifference to the sometimes subtle problems of pre-existing, concurrent, naturally emergent emotional needs of children and adolescents coming to hospital for reasons of illness or heroic operation. The emotional, psychological, and cognitive considerations may often extend quite beyond the modification, removal, or reversal of symptoms which may have accompanied the overt, presenting organic disease and may necessarily, therefore, include clinical management of problems which preceeded or followed the onset of illness as well as disturbances during convalescence.

In the pressing anxiety of contemporary life, in connection with many diagnostic, therapeutic and surgical procedures carried out obstensibly in routine fashion in the large modern university-connected medical teaching centers across this and other countries, physicians and surgeons have not always directed their attention, time, or interest to specific psychological issues now known and understood to be operative, which bear heavily upon illness and the speed, nature, quality, and extent of recovery in their youthful patients. Those charged with medical and surgical care of both children and adolescents must begin to understand and indeed treat disease – I might say more importantly to treat patients with disease – in the broadest and most comprehensive terms. Attention to such factors as the adolescent's concept of his illness or a child's perception of illness, the age of onset, the emotional prehospitalization history, the cognitive impact of disease, the surgical experience and convalescence, the degree to which the patient seems to have been honorably prepared for either illness, hospitalization of the accompanying instabilities which very often may preceed or follow impending surgery, and the level of sophistication, awareness, understanding and acceptance by the parents must each be sensitively and judiciously appraised when projecting the probable postsurgical emotional course. The child's and adolescent's response to illness, the adequacy of his adaptive emotional defensive forces, together with his unique ability or indeed inability to function without parents in a continuing stressful atmosphere of the hospital setting, the intensive care unit in particular, all need to be taken into account in advance of conducting any medical, diagnostic or surgical procedure, lest the youthful patient experience further predictable, potentially psychopathological insults.

Too often it has been shown that an adolescent's emotional response to his or her illness has either been totally or initially recognized, or responsibility for its management injudiciously, hastily, or more tragically and regrettably never arranged for in the first instance. Most patients of whatever age cannot always be expected to understand the nature of their illness or disability or in fact the reasons for its occurrence in the first place. It has been shown that children and adolescents often dramatically, though unconsciously, distort the actual reality of aspects of their illness and attendant surgical procedures which are brought forward to correction, for reasons which remain neatly idiosyncratic and unconscious in each child. These cognitive distortions require a systematic, comprehensive, patient, and sensitive clinical review at the very time of their onset or when clinically diagnosed and recognized. Physicians, nurses and others, in direct and intimate emotional and clinical medical contact with children and adolescents during the course of illness and convalescence, must be vigilant and perceptive equally to the quiet, uncomplaining, frightened, overwhelmed, mute, regressed patient who may be too panic-stricken and terrorized by his own fantasy inner-life experience to come forward with his many unarticulated, unspoken and hence quietly self-regulated fears and anxieties. Clinical attention must equally be paid to the hyperactive, misbehaving, dissocial patient whose anxiety gets differentially played out in impulsive, disorganized or manipulative, poorly-controlled action. Both types of emotional reactions require early recognition and direct, competent, early therapeutic intervention and management. Each of these patients will clearly remain highly at risk for a potentially traumatic psychological outcome postoperatively, even if the procedure was understood to have been medically and surgically, fully competently achieved, if these emotional indications of psychological status go unnoticed.

The massive and often proliferating anxieties, combined with the stress of medical and surgical crises, need not occur and are indeed in most instances able to be clearly avoided when appropriate therapeutic actions are taken to prepare a child or adolescent for what the expectancies realistically and honorably and faithfully are going to be. When adequate therapeutic safeguards are devised and sensitively respected, instituted, and faithfully observed by the whole comprehensive care team, the child or adolescent – and dare I say adult – who is potentially a candidate for experiencing dramatic emotional upset postoperatively or even before may be helped, and the psychopathological consequences almost fully averted if not minimized. Thus, the occasion of illness, hospitalization, or indeed surgery in this and other countries need not be the dehumanizing, humiliating, and anxiety-arousing ordeal or experience that it almost universally is for the unprepared child, adolescent, or adult, for that matter, coming to hospital.

In our experience the occasion of illness can equally assist in the process of mastery or individuation or provide occasion for emotional growth. These outcomes, however, have all too infrequently been demonstrated. The former and more tragic course seems to be the more predictable. Indeed, only on rare occasions can the experience of illness or the ordeal of surgery promote in the otherwise emotionally healthy individual prior to hospitalization a positive individuating response.

Let me return to the concept of the body image. The body image is not a body organ, a psychological picture, or a little person in the head. It is best described in terms of the functions it ostensibly and theoretically serves and the levels at which it is experienced. The body functions as a sensory register, an instrument for specific and unique cognitive action, a source of drives, a stimulus to the self and others, a private and unique inner universe, and as an expressive instrument. The four levels of body experience are schematic, self, fantasy and concept. A complete description of body image disorder that identifies the source of the disorder and its effect on the functions and levels of experience would probably be a reasonable theory. Behavioral treatment of body image disorders may develop basic sensory motor capacities, teach specific skills, promote interpersonal relationships with others having similar problems, or use traditional techniques depending on the needs of the individual patient.

Although the term body image has become increasingly more popular and well-coined in psychotherapeutic environments, even functioning within the intensive care unit in medical and psychological theory and practice particularly, its use has not always proved helpful. As a theoretical entity it leaves much to be desired. The body image has suffered the fate of many other similar constructs. It has become a thing rather than an abstraction. It has been defined in so many ways that it has lost its specific, intended, and unique special meaning. Its relation to other theoretical constructs has long been ignored, or described so imprecisely that its properties have been obfuscated rather than clarified. In clinical practice, the diagnostician who attaches the label "body image disorder" to the medical chart of the patient or the patient's condition may gain a sense of satisfaction that may block further inquiry into the acute nature of the cognitive malfunction or the techniques which may be later applied to assist the patient in overcoming it.

Two obvious possibilities are that a body image disorder is 1) a set of disruptive physiological processes, or 2) that it is a mantle, that is, symbolic, idiosyncratic, psychiatric, and a unique patient-specific psychiatric condition. If a body image disorder is wholly physiological in its origin and manifestation, the recommendation would seem to be obvious: restore healthy bodily function and it will disappear. Little but verbal convenience may be gained by calling a condition "body image disorder" when a description that identifies a physical cause and prescribes proper treatment is what is really required of us. Just as a physician or physiologist may regard body image disorders as physical disruptions, a psychiatrist or clinical psychologist working in this area may regard the body image as a mental projection, that is, a cognitive manifestation, and interpret its attendant disorders as symptomatic of basic personality dysfunction. Diagnostic and therapeutic attention will then be directed toward other aspects of a patient's life such as his emotional conflicts, psychosocial background and the unique and peculiar impact illness or surgically-induced trauma may have on his sense of self. Whatever one's orientation, the practitioner will search the scientific literature in vain for laws or principles to guide him in describing body image disorders unambiguously or in describing effective treatment. Authorities have attempted to solve these problems by proposing new definitions of terms, but none have thus far succeeded to my knowledge. Perhaps it is because definitions or distinctions are largely semantic and are only helpful if they lead to useful descriptions of actual processes and events, and lead us to believe that concurrent therapeutic interventions may be possible.

Editor's Remark

Dr. Becker then proceeded to show slides which illustrated the clinical value of the body image concept as interpreted from drawings made by children undergoing heart surgery. The wealth of information concerning the child's psychological status and understanding of the surgical procedure yielded by those drawings was demonstrated, and their importance in Dr. Becker's daily clinical work was emphasized.

Discussion of Session V

Answering different questions from the floor Clarkson pointed out in addition to her paper:

I think a lot of parents do release their hold and overprotectiveness to some extent once they have got a reasonably healthy child. On the other hand, some parents do require convincing and having this pointed out to them.

We did see seizural activity as an acute postoperative phenomenon in four patients, and this was a transient thing. They had some anticonvulsants at that time, but subsequently not beyond that, 24–48 h after the episode, so that these episodes are regarded as an acute response to a fairly acute insult and the patients were not maintained on long-term anticonvulsive therapy. The ones who had convulsions didn't seem to have any adverse permanent sequelae from that sort of episode.

Regarding critical limit of 60′ of circulatory arrest Clarkson answered:

This was based partly on available experimental work and partly on the clinical practice of Japanese surgeons who had used this technique and considered it satisfactory. This was the sort of limit I placed on the technique not knowing anything very much better at that stage. It didn't seem quite right that we should be able to go on indefinitely and this seemed to fit limits that would be expected to be safe.

Becker added to Jänsch's paper:

The number of times that we see acute psychotic reactions in childhood appears, on the basis of the observations presented to us now, to be relatively infrequent and hence a major crisis if they do occur and easily recognized by a surgical or nursing team.

Replying to the scepticism of some of the audience concerning the analyses of the childrens drawings Becker answered:

You will soon understand that we in no measure ever intend these drawings to be looked at in the same way a cardiologist would look at a series of X-rays taken during catheterization. The next point is that we are not applying fractional analysis to these drawings. We are looking at them from a macroscopic position. If we look at drawings sequentially, over a period of time, preoperatively, even before an acute phasial sets in and the prospect of open-heart surgery comes forward, I am quite convinced that one of the best psychological measures in predicting postoperative outcome with respect to psychological issues may well be the human figure drawing for a child. For an adolescent or an adult, clearly I would agree that there are very major differences. Human figure drawings are an absolutely vital part of the preoperative preparation in our work in Jerusalem, and in no small measure offer us the opportunity for what they call corrective emotional revisions and what could otherwise be projected as cognitive distortions of reality.

Thereafter Becker added some comments on signs of psychosis:

To call someone or something psychotic it has to represent a distortion of reality and an inability to correctly appraise and assess life situations adequately. Looking at these drawings blind, and not knowing the context within which they are produced is a wholly unethical and clearly counterproductive enterprise. But knowing the child and knowing the context of anxiety in which he produced that drawing. I still dont't think the knowledge of the forthcoming operative procedure on its own could have produced that picture. That, in combination with preexisting psychopathology, augmented the perception of illness.

Blacher added in this respect:

I have done drawing studies of adults both with commissurotomies and recently with other procedures. They are quite different being very disguised. For instance, what they used to see with the very sick rheumatics, for the first picture, would be a tree, a bare stump with nothing on it. After surgery, when they are better, they began to see the progression of drawings with the leaves coming out, and than the fruit coming out, and the people in the same sort of way. Adults' views of what we do to them in cardiac surgery are very different from your drawings pertaining to open-heart surgery in children.

VI

Postsurgical Adaptation: Issues and Experience

Recovery After Major Heart Surgery: Medical, Psychological, and Work Outcomes*

B.A. Stanton, St.J. Zyzanski, C.D. Jenkins, M.D. Klein

Introduction

Major heart surgical procedures have become some of the most common and fastest growing types of surgical procedures performed in referral hospitals in the Unites States. While no precise data appear to be available, federal authorities estimate that over 110 000 major heart surgical procedures were performed last year in the United States. While the future incidence of congenital and rheumatic heart disease requiring surgery is uncertain, there is little doubt that coronary artery bypass graft surgery has experienced explosive growth in the United States within the last 10 years and that the total numbers of procedures performed annually is increasing even though its efficacy has only partly been investigated.

Cardiac surgery has proliferated as a result of the prompt and dramtic relief of symptoms, and increase in physical capacity following surgery. The success of major cardiac surgery in adults has been measured in terms of reduction in mortality, rate of graft closure for bypass patients, and relief of symptoms [1]. Some of the earlier studies have focused on neurological sequelae of the surgical procedure, especially postcardiotomy delirium [2]. Psychological and behavioral factors have been investigated both as predictors of postoperative course [3–7] and as outcome measures [8–11]. In many instances, however, these studies were conducted with small numbers of patients, were limited to either cardiac valve or coronary artery bypass patients, or were generally restricted to a very narrow set of outcome variables.

The present study was designed to attempt to provide a more comprehensive understanding of the many factors which affect long-term recovery after major heart surgery. The specific aims of the study were to:

1. Identify the major social and psychological barriers to complete recovery in preparation for our current, more intensive, prospective study;
2. estimate the prevalence of psychosocial and biomedical problems in persons who have undergone different types of heart surgery;
3. search of variables which might prove to have important influences on recovery; and

---

* This research was supported in part by Mended Hearts, Inc., and by research grant HL 20637 from the National Heart, Lung and Blood Institute.

Psychopathological and Neurological Dysfunctions Following Open-Heart Surgery Ed. by Becker et al.

4. determine whether the frequency of psychosocial problems is strictly a function of the severity of biomedical problems or whether other "risk factors" could be identified.

Methods

A random sample, representing 25% of the active members of each chapter of Mended Hearts, Inc., a self-help group throughout the United States and Canada, was mailed a precoded, eight-page questionnaire, a letter explaining the study, and a stamped, return envelope. Of the 1400 questionnaires mailed, over 1100 were returned giving a response rate of 80.6%.

Only those patients having coronary artery bypass grafts or mitral or aortic valve surgery were included in the present analysis. Persons who had surgery to repair congentital anomalies were excluded as were those having rare or minor procedures (e.g., implantation of a pacemaker). This restricted the population of 949 adults of which approximately 75% were men and 75% were between the ages of 50 and 69 years. Only about 4% were under the age of 40 and another 4% were over the age of 70. The distribution of patients by sex, type of surgery, and the average age and years since surgery for each group are displayed in Table 1.

Overall, 76% of the respondents had bypass surgery, 16% had mitral valve surgery, and 8% had aortic valve surgery. The sex ratios for these various procedures were quite different. Six times as many men as women had coronary artery bypass surgery, twice as many men as women had aortic valve surgery, but less than half as many men as women had mitral valve surgery. A total of 8% of patients had two different surgical procedures performed at the time of their first surgery. The most common combination was repair to both the mitral and aortic valve. Repair of aneurysms was also a relatively common second procedure.

Table 1. Mean age and years since surgery by sex and type of surgery for 949 postoperative patients

Type of Surgery	Sex	%	Sample size	Age	Years since surgery
1-vessel	Males	10	98	56.7	3.7
bypass	Females	3	29	58.2	3.0
2-vessel	Males	26	245	56.9	3.5
bypass	Females	5	46	58.0	2.7
3-vessel	Males	29	278	57.1	2.9
bypass	Females	3	28	56.2	3.0
Mitral	Males	5	44	57.1	7.0
valve	Females	11	103	54.7	8.0
Aortic	Males	5	53	54.4	5.3
valve	Females	3	25	57.8	6.8
Totals		100	949	56.7	3.5

The survey questionnaire contained items covering basic sociodemographic characteristics, life circumstances before surgery, and the surgical experience. Occupational level before and after surgery was investigated as was the coronary-prone behavior pattern (Type A). Type A behavior was estimated by a condensed scale abstracted from the Jenkins Activity Survey [12]. The questionnaire also contained a broad array of questions dealing with changes before surgery to the present.

Three scales were developed from these clusters of questions of similar content asking patients to compare their circumstances before surgery with those 1 year after surgery. These scales dealt with psychological changes, social adjustment changes, and economic changes. Two scales were developed from items concerning current emotional state and current social network. Items on scales reflecting postoperative status had precoded descriptive alternatives which were then scored as reflecting good, average, or poor status. For each item, the responses which indicated a clearly negative outcome were assigned a point value of 0, while neutral or positive responses were assigned a value of 1. Mean scores for these dichotomously scored items were then computed for each person (adjusted for missing data when necessary) on each scale. All scale scores were then transformed to standard scores having a mean of 50 and a standard deviation of 20, to provide a common metric for comparing results across the various outcome measures. Greater mean values reflect positive outcomes, and scores less than 50 reflect negative outcomes. Four major psychosocial composite scales were computed in this fashion. Two deal with changes in interpersonal relationship and feelings compared before and after surgery, and two address current levels of psychosocial functioning. The first behavioral change scale is called "Emotional or Psychological Changes After Heart Surgery". An item total correlational analysis showed that the key items defining this six-item composite scale were those pertaining to feelings of depression, anxiety, pleasure in life, and optimism, which the patients perceived as having changed from 1 year prior to surgery to the present. The average item total correlation of these items was 0.79. The second behavioral change scale, based on ten items, is labeled "Social Adjustment Changes After Heart Surgery." Its key defining items, with an average item total correlation of 0.67, pertain to changes in interpersonal relationships between patient and spouse, (including sexual relations); relationships with children; relatives; and with co-workers. The third scale, "Current Emotional State," has 11 items with an average item total correlation for the stronger items of 0.60. The strongest items are those pertaining to feelings, during the past month, of anxiety, nervousness, restlessness, sadness, happiness, contentment, and feeling that psychological problems, such as discouragement or fearfulness are interfering with recovery. Also included in this cluster is the patient's use of tranquilizers or medication to aid in sleeping.

The fourth nine-item scale labeled "Current Social Network" (with an average item total correlation of 0.50) is based on current marital status; size of household; attendance at organizational meetings or religious services; perceived affection received from family members; and family's responses during the recovery period (i.e., overprotection, adequate support, isolation, or avoidance.) One final scale, "Economic Changes", contains two items: changes in family income and changes in standard of living since surgery. Here, positive outcomes were defined as having both an increase in income and standard of living since surgery. Worse outcomes were defined in terms of a reduced income and standard of living, in particular, excessive debts, depleted savings or having to move to less expensive housing.

Results

Between the time of initial surgery and the response to this survey, (an average of 3 years for bypass and 6 years for valve patients), these 949 patients experienced a variety of medical problems which are summarized in Table 2. Hospitalization since surgery was reported by 51% of the patients. Over half of the patients (65%) were hospitalized for various cardiovascular problems, including arrhythmias. This includes the 12% of all persons who reported being hospitalized for heart attack. Thirteen percent of all patients were admitted for gastrointestinal disorders and the remaining 23% were hospitalized for other reasons. A total of 8% of all respondents underwent a second major heart operation (5% of all bypass patients, 14% of aortic valve patients, and 22% of mitral valve patients). This may have been influenced by the longer average follow-up interval of the valve patients' surgery and this study.

The percentages of persons experiencing severe and recurring symptoms of their heart condition in the past month and those requiring 3 or more days of bed rest in the past month are gratifyingly low, suggesting an excellent therapeutic result of surgery, on the average. Among bypass patients, a higher percentage of women than men reported severe recurring chest pain or dyspnea. For all types of surgery, women were confined to bed in the past month twice as frequently as men.

Table 3 summarizes the distributions of the three change scales and two postoperative status scales for the entire population. For social adjustment and economic changes, the most common response was that things were the same before and after surgery. For the two psychological scales, however, the most common response was that psychologically and emotionally, patients were better now than before surgery and, in their own judgment, better than average. The very low frequencies of deteriorated social adjustment after surgery and poor emotional or social networks currently are quite encouraging. For the scale on economic changes, 36% of the patients did report that they were worse off after their surgery.

In general, however, family income went up at least a little for 47% of the patients, remained the same for 21%, and went down for 32% of the patients. Approximately 29% of the patients had at least a 25% decrease in income, had to give things up, or went into debt. This created hardships of varying degrees, with 21% having encountered periods of financial crisis. The probable reason why the surgery was not financially devastating for more of the patients is that insurance covered costs completely for 54% of patients and partially for 91% of patients.

Table 4 summarizes the results of a series of multivariate analyses of covariance which examine the relationships between six independent variables (age, sex, educational level, type of surgery, forced retirement, and Type A behavior) and the behavioral change scale "Emotional Changes After Heart Surgery". In Table 4, only those associations which were found to be statistically significant after controlling for nine medical covariates are presented. The medical covariates are: (1) total number of

Table 2. Rates of selected medical outcomes by sex and type of surgery

		Sample size	% With second surgery	% Who were hospitalized since surgery	Of hospitalized, % cardiovascular	% With current severe and recurring pain or dyspnea	Reporting 3 or more days in bed last month
1 vessel	Males	98	8	57	60	6	7
	Females	29	7	48	71	10	14
2 vessels	Males	245	4	50	58	3	4
	Females	46	7	54	72	9	15
3 vessels	Males	278	3	42	67	3	6
	Females	28	11	71	76	11	18
Mitral valve	Males	44	23	59	81	2	5
	Females	103	22	60	63	3	10
Aortic valve	Males	53	13	47	77	2	8
	Females	25	16	68	65	0	12
Total sample		949	8	51	65	4	7

Table 3. Percentage of patients doing better or worse after heart surgery for five psychosocial outcomes

Changes from presurgery to 1 year postsurgery	Better	Same	Worse	Total
Psychological changes	44%	40%	16%	100%
Social adjustment changes	14%	83%	3%	100%
Economic changes	9%	55%	36%	100%
Postoperative status	Good	Average	Poor	Total
Emotional state	51%	46%	3%	100%
Social network	48%	50%	2%	100%

Table 4. Factors affecting *emotional changes* after heart surgery. [Standard scores (mean = 50) adjusted for nine medical covariates]

		Sex				
Type of surgery	n	Male	Female			
1-vessel bypass	127	51.5	52.5		Interaction:	
2-vessel bypass	291	50.9	44.6		$F = 4.0$	
3-vessel bypass	306	48.5	39.1		$P < 0.003$	
Mitral valve	147	49.0	53.4			
Aortic valve	78	48.1	59.8			
Forced retirement	Forced to retire (n = 109)	Not forced, but not working (n = 50)		Currently working (n = 380)	F	P
(Limited to persons under 61 years)	44.7	47.4		51.9	6.9	0.001
Behavior type	Type A (n = 351)	Intermediate (n = 296)		Type B (n = 302)	F	P
	48.4	48.4		53.0	5.0	0.007

surgical procedures performed at time of initial surgery; (2) current age; (3) time since surgery; (4) rehospitalizations; (6) second heart surgery; (7) presence of continuing noncardiac health problems; (8) current severe and recurring pain, and (9) having spent 3 or more days sick in bed in the past month. Changes in levels of anxiety, depression, and general emotional state after heart surgery were significantly related to sex, type of surgery, forced retirement and type A behavior pattern. The significant "sex by type of surgery" interaction indicates that female multiple bypass patients more than male bypass or female valve surgery patients, were likely to report that emotionally they felt worse now than they did 1 year prior to surgery. For the "forced retirement" variable, statistical analysis was limited to those patients 60 years of age or younger to permit an adequate time period for returning to work which would not overlap with retirement ages. The results shown in Table 4 indicate that persons reporting forced retirement experienced significantly more negative emotional changes than either persons currently working or those not working but not forced to retire. Patients who were clearly Type A personalities or intermediate in behavior type also experienced significantly more negative emotional changes than those categorized as Type B. Although the mean values in Table 4 do not show large numeric differences, the standard errors of the mean differences are very small, and hence the statistical significance is high and the group differences are meaningful.

Some factors affecting social adjustment changes after heart surgery are shown in Table 5. The patients experiencing the most negative changes in personal relationships

Table 5. Factors affecting *social adjustment* changes after heart surgery [standard scores (mean = 50) adjusted for nine medical covariates]

		Sex				
Level of education	n	Male	Female			
Some H.S. or less	138	51.3	56.5		Interaction:	
H.S. grad or added Training	357	51.2	47.2		$F = 2.7$	
Some college	254	48.3	53.4		$P = 0.05$	
College grad or postgrad	200	47.9	52.1			
Forced retirement	Forced to retire (n = 109)	Not forced, but not working (n = 50)		Currently working (n = 380)	F	P
(Limited to persons under 61 years)	44.1	48.4		52.0	10.7	0.001

Table 6. Return to work after heart surgery for persons 60 years old or less at surgery

	% Employed before surgery	% Re-employed after surgery	Average no. months to return to work
Men			
Coronary bypass	92% (505)[a]	81% (467)	3.7 (379)
Cardiac valve	91% (86)	82% (78)	4.1 (64)
Women			
Coronary bypass	57% (77)	61% (44)	5.0 (27)
Cardiac valve	48% (111)	81% (53)	4.4 (43)
Total	82% (779)	80% (642)	3.9 (513)

[a]Numbers in parentheses indicate group size for each calculation

with spouse, family, and co-workers were persons of either sex reporting forced retirement, female high school graduates, and males with college education. These relationships with specific education subgroups may be associated with the type of disease bringing the patient to surgery. Small subsample sizes precluded more detailed analyses.

Table 6 illustrates the rates of return to work after surgery for patients who were 60 years of age or less at the time of surgery. Over 80% of both male and female valve surgery patients went back to work. A total of 81% of male, but only 61% of female bypass surgery patients went back to work after surgery.

Table 7 demonstrates that preoperative occupational level is strongly associated with return to work. The rate of return to work is highest in executives, professionals, administrative, and clerical positions. It appears that occupations with the highest rate of return to work require very little physical exertion. It may also be that people in higher level occupations have the most authority and flexibility in their work situation.

In the final scale "Current Social Network" low scores represent deficits in psychosocial supports including living alone, lack of participation in community activities, family withdrawal, and lack of affection. These deficits were most common in females ($P = 0.01$), Type A persons ($P = 0.03$), and those with lower levels of education ($P = 0.02$). Additionally, significantly more women then men reported that their families responded by expecting too much of them too soon during the recovery period.

Table 7. Preoperative occupation and return to work in preoperatively employed persons, 60 years of age and younger

Hollingshead classification	Percent of study group	Percent returning to work
1. Executives, major professionals, proprietors of large firms	15% (92)[a]	89%
2. Managers, lesser professionals proprietors of medium firms	29% (184)	83%
3. Administrative personnel, minor professionals and proprietors	20% (128)	84%
4. Clerical and sales workers, technicians, specialized services	18% (111)	81%
5. Skilled manual employees, provers of skilled services	11% (71)	66%
6. Machine operators, semiskilled employees, drivers	6% (41)	66%
7. Unskilled workers	1% (4)	(2/4)

[a]Number in parentheses indicate group size

Discussion

A number of the findings deserve additional attention. Inquiry regarding postoperative medical status revealed what seemed to be a rather high frequency of hospitalization. Over 50% of persons had been hospitalized one or more times in the average elapsed time of 3½ years. Chronic gastrointestinal problems seemed particularly common. This finding deserves further investigation to see whether the array of orally administered drugs commonly prescribed for these patients may be contributing factors. The frequency of severe dyspnea and angina was gratifyingly low, suggesting a high rate of continuing effectiveness of the surgical correction.

The findings that physical medical problems are correlated with poor psychosocial outcomes was expected. What was uncertain was whether additional indicators such as type of surgery, social characteristics, or the Type A behavior pattern would be associated with psychosocial outcomes after the impact of physical medical problems had been accounted for. Independent relationships with poor psychosocial outcomes were particularly strong for the variables: forced retirement, Type A behavior pattern, and the sex-by-type-of surgery interaction identifying females who received multiple bypass operations. The direct relationship of these three variables to poor recovery outcomes is further supported by the fact that these predictors were also significant in the subgroup of patients who had none of the seven major postoperative physical health problems covered by the study.

The rate of return to work of male patients (under 60 years of age) appears to be comparable to those rates reported in a more focused study of return to work after bypass surgery [13].

The extended period of convalescence after heart surgery would be expected to create more frustration in Type A than in Type B persons. Forced retirement can cause a severe loss of self-esteem and self-acceptance and interfere with emotional adjustment in persons, such as Type A's, for whom occupational role is central to self-concept. For many persons, employment provides much more than just a livelihood; it provides a social network and a variety of psychological gratifications.

Focused study is needed to discover the reasons why women undergoing multiple bypass procedures tend to experience worse medical and psychological outcomes than men undergoing the same procedures or women having valve surgery. It may be that a substantial fraction of these women have either small vessel disease or cardiospasm, neither of which was corrected by surgery or a different psychological profile.

In summary, these findings provide additional documentation of the problems faced by open-heart surgery patients. They show that the surgery did not cause a permanent change in the social or psychological situation of most patients. The observation that psychosocial outcomes were relatively independent of medical outcomes suggests that the postoperative medical care of heart patients should be augmented by attention to psychosocial factors in order to promote a more complete recovery.

References

1. McIntosh HD, Garcia JA (1978) The first decade of aortocoronary bypass grafting. Circulation 57:405–431
2. Elsberry NL (1972) Psychological responses to open-heart surgery. Nurs Res 21:220–227
3. Kimball CP (1969) A predictive study of adjustment to cardiac surgery. J Thorac Surg 58:891
4. Kimball CP (1969) Psychological responses to the experience of open-heart surgery. Part I. Am J Psychiatry 126:348–359
5. Tufo HM, Ostfeld AM (1968) A prospective study of open-heart surgery. Psychosom Med 30:552–553
6. Henrichs TF, McKenzie JW, Almond CH (1969) Psychological adjustment and acute response to open-heart surgery. J Nerv Ment Dis 148:158–164
7. Kilpatrick DG, Miller WC, Allain AN, Huggins MB, Lee WH (1975) The use of psychological test data do predict open-heart surgery outcome: A prospective study. Psychosom Med 37:62–73
8. Blachly PH, Blachly BJ (1968) Vocational and emotional status of 263 patients after heart surgery. Circulation 38:524–532
9. Lucia W, McGuire LB (1970) Rehabilitation and functional status after surgery for valvular heart disease. Arch Intern Med 126:995–999
10. Frank KA, Heller SS, Kornfeld DS (1972) A survey of adjustment to cardiac surgery. Arch Intern Med 130:735–738
11. Heller SS, Frank KA, Kornfeld DS, Malm FO (1974) Psychological outcome following open-heart surgery. Arch Intern Med 134:908–914
12. Zyzanski SJ, Jenkins CD, Ryan TJ, Flessas A, Everist M (1976) Psychological correlates of coronary angiographic findings. Arch Intern Med 136:1234–1237
13. Anderson AJ, Barboriak JJ, Hoffmann RG, Mullen DC (1980) Retention or resumption of employment after aortoconary bypass operations. JAMA 253:543–545

Psychosocial Situation of the Open-Heart Surgery Patient One Year After Operation

S. Davies-Osterkamp, G. Siefen, K. Möhlen, H. Müller, M. Schlepper

In follow-up studies the success of a major operation is often evaluated by several criteria besides the improvement in the patient's bodily condition. One of these additional criterion is whether the patient returns to work or not. Although rarely explicitly stated the use of this criterion would seem to rest on the following two arguments: (1) The surgeon feels a broad conception of health to be appropriate and consequently regards himself as being responsible not only for repairing the patient's bodily damage but also for helping him/her to restore his/her overall social functioning and well being, which includes the ability to work. (2) From a psychosomatic viewpoint it can be argued that retirement per se is a traumatic event, which implies the loss of important social functions and contacts and is considered as a threat to ego-identity and self-esteem.

Whereas the validity of the first argument depends only on the professional or personal conception of health which is adopted, the validity of the second argument could be tested empirically by studying the impact of retirement on health. There is however little evidence of deleterious effects of retirement on health and, in fact, some studies even suggest beneficial effects [5, 9]. Some authors even argue that much of the theoretical writings on the meaning of work in society are applicable only to workers who do highly skilled and creative work [9].

In some studies of open-heart surgery patients no significant correlations between the patient's employment status (whether a patient works or not) and bodily condition after the operation were obtained [8]. In fact in the case of heart patients there is in general a low correspondence between objective physical status and the patient's feeling of well-being [4]. However, it would be premature to conclude that the discrepancy between employment status and bodily condition is explained by the assumption that a relatively high proportion of patients, despite an improvement in their bodily condition, do not work because of a tendency to maintain a sick-role behavior pattern. It seems to be certain that the decision to go back to work is not primarily the patient's own decision. Several institutions, social security, health insurances, employers, etc. might influence this decision in the light of their own interests. These influences might be especially important in times of economic recession, particularly for older patients.

In this article we will present some results of a follow-up study of open-heart surgery patients 1 year after the operation. Our specific goal was to investigate whether patients who did not resume work are in a worse psychological condition than those who did. We were not in a position to determine which of the above-mentioned

Psychopathological and Neurological Dysfunctions
Following Open-Heart Surgery. Ed. by Becker et al

Table 1. Description of the sample

	Original sample			Follow-up sample[a] (1 year after the operation)		
Operative procedure	n	Age $\bar{x}$	Female/male	n	Age $\bar{x}$	Female/male
Mitral valve replacement	11	57	6/5	7	58	3/4
Aortic valve replacement	24	49	6/18	21	51	5/16
Multivalve replacement	4	53	2/2	2	47	1/1
Coronary bypass	21	50	1/20	15	50	1/14
Other	12	43	10/2	6	42	8/2
Total sample	72	50	25/47	55	50	18/37

[a] Nine patients died; eight patients could not be followed up for organizational reasons

reasons might be responsible for each patient's employment status after the operation. Our main question was whether there is any evidence that differences in patients' psychological well being are correlated with their employment status.

Table 1 contains a description of the sample. Of the 72 patients of the original sample [6] 55 could be followed up, nine died within 1 year after the operation, and eight could not be followed up because of organizational difficulties.

In 55 patients of the follow-up sample were classified into three groups: Group 1 (n = 13) consisted of patients who did not work or had already retired 1 year before the operation, mainly, but not always, because of their illness. As Blachly and Blachly [3] have shown, the chance of reemployment is poor if a person is unemployed for more than a year ("law of the year"). This was also true for our patients. Groups 2 (n = 19) and 3 (n = 23) consisted of patients whose work was interrupted by their illness and the operation but who had not made the decision to give up their work permanently. Whereas the patients in group 2 did not resume work after the operation those in group 3 did. Women who were housewives before and after the operation were allocated to group 1; housewives who held part- or fulltime jobs before the operation, which they gave up after the operation, were allocated to group 2. This procedure should not be interpreted as meaning that we do not regard housework as an occupation. It is simply a reflection of the fact that in the present investigation the classification of housework as an occupation could result in biases: If housewives are classified both before and after the operation as being employed then this will lead to the overall percentage of patients working after the operation being largely dependent on the number of women in the sample. This can furthermore lead to the (wrong) conclusion that the operation has less influence on the working status of women in general than on men, only because role expectations lead to a large percentage of housewives among women.

Significant differences between these three groups were found in the following areas: 1) There were significant differences in age: Group 1 had a median age of 57 years, group 2 had a median age of 52 years, and group 3 had a median age of 45 years. 2) The duration of bodily complaints due to their illness was longer for patients in group 1 than for patients in the other two groups. 3) There were significant differences between men and women. In accordance with role expectations more women than men gave up their work. The overall figures were as follows: 67% of the men as against 25% of the women resumed their work. This could at least partially be explained by the finding that the preoperative vocational status of women showed less continuity and financial reward. 4) There were differences between patients with different types of operations. None of the patients with mitral valve replacement went back to work in contrast to patients with aortic valve replacement or coronary bypass. 5) The preoperative financial income was higher for patients in group 3 than for patients in the other two groups which can partly be explained by the different number of women and pensioners in the three groups.

No differences between the three groups were found with respect to educational level or social class. With regard to social class the sample was homogeneous. Most patients were blue or white collar workers.

In the following we will present some results concerning the question of differences between these three groups with regard to their general psychological adaptation. In examining this question we compared the patients' scores on different personality tests and questionnaires which were given preoperatively and at different intervals postoperatively. All comparisons were made by analyses of variance.

Each of two personality tests were given twice: 1) The Giessen-Test (GT) [1] was given preoperatively and 1 year after the operation. 2) The Freiburger Personality Inventory (FPI) [7] was given preoperatively and in the first follow-up 3 months after the operation. A questionnaire of bodily complaints (Giessener Beschwerdebogen, GBB) [2] was completed three times: preoperatively, 3 months, and 1 year after the operation. This questionnaire consists of four scales which cover the following areas: a) exhaustion, b) gastric symptoms, c) pain in the limbs, and d) cardiovascular complaints. Finally, a specially designed questionnaire which asked for the patients' subjective attitude and experience concerning recovery was completed three times: shortly after, 3 months, and 1 year after the operation. This questionnaire consists of two scales: a) the tendency to adopt a sick-role behavior pattern, and b) a tendency to denial of illness and the operation.

In addition to these assessments the patients were interviewed during the follow-up. A semistructured interview was used with special emphasis being placed on the following areas: health behavior, contact with medical institutions and special rehabilitation programs, the patient's evaluation of the operation in terms of bodily and psychological recovery, his/her social contacts, leisure activities, work situation, and relation to the family.

Comparison of the three groups produced the following results:

1. With respect to general psychological and psychosomatic adaptation, as assessed by the personality tests and the inventory of bodily complaints, there were no differences between the three groups. All groups showed a marked decrease in depression (FPI) and a change from being more undercontrolled to being more overcontrolled (GT). Differential effects for the groups were only detected with regard to aggression (FPI). Whereas patients in group 2 and 3 (i.e., those patients who worked before the operation) showed a decrease in aggression, patients in group 1 showed an increase. Except for aggressiveness the profiles of the three groups were not different from the norms.

Concerning bodily complaints there was for all groups a significant decrease in cardiovascular complaints over the period of the follow-up. The amount of change was the same for the three groups. There was also an overall decrease with regard to gastric symptoms, but this was largely accounted for by patients in group 1, who had a higher preoperative level than the other two groups. At the time of the follow-up no significant differences had been obtained.

2. This finding of a relatively good psychological adaptation was confirmed by the interview data; there were no differences between the groups concerning different aspects of social activity, satisfaction with family life and emotional stability. Furthermore, we found no evidence that patients who did not resume work after the operation showed a more pronounced tendency to sick-role behavior, as assessed by the questionnaire three times postoperatively and during the follow-up interview, than patients who did go back to work.

Despite these overall positive findings there remained the fact that patients who retired after the operation were not content with their new status. Of the 19 patients only three viewed the fact of retirement positively. Compared with patients who went back to work retired patients did not consider their former work situation to be more negative and unsatisfying. In the light of this finding it is not surprising that patients who retired after the operation were less satisfied with its outcome concerning their health status than both other groups.

Their own expectation of being able to resume work because of the operation had obviously not been met. Despite the fact that factors other than health status and not lying within their control might have been responsible for their loss of work, their assessment of the outcome of the operation is influenced by the discrepancy between expectation and outcome concerning their ability to work. This patient group might therefore be in special need of rehabilitation programs which would either help them to regain work or to cope with retirement and the loss of work. The availability of rehabilitation programs for all patients' groups was, however, poor: None of the patients took part in special retraining courses after the operation and none of the patients had any psychiatric or psychological counseling, despite the fact that 20% were convinced that such a counseling might have helped them to cope with the postoperative period. This applies to patients in all three groups. The fact that 30% of patients who went back to work experienced their postoperative work situation as more unsatisfying and 50% as more strenuous than their preoperative vocational status clearly indicates that an individualized approach concerning the aim of rehabilitation programs is appropriate.

References

1. Beckmann D, Richter HE (1972) Der Giessen-Test (GT). Huber, Bern
2. Brähler E, Scheer JW (1979) Skalierung psychosomatischer Beschwerdenkomplexe mit dem Giessener Beschwerdebogen (GBB). Psychother Med Psychol 29:14–27
3. Blachly JS, Blachly HJ (1968) Vocational and emotional status of 263 patients after heart surgery. Circulation 38:524–532
4. Brown JS, Rawlinson M (1975) Relinquishing the sick role following open-heart surgery. J Health Soc Behav 16:12–27

5. Carp FM (1977) Retirement and physical health. Adv Psychosom Med 9:140–159
6. Davies-Osterkamp S, Möhlen K, Lademann HR, Scheld H (1980) Postoperative reactions in open-heart surgery patients. In: Speidel H, Rodewald G (eds) Psychic and neurological dysfunctions after open-heart surgery. Thieme, Stuttgart, INA 19:162–168
7. Fahrenberg J, Selg H, Hampel R (1973) Das Freiburger Persönlichkeitsinventar, 2nd edn. Hogrefe, Göttingen
8. Führer U, Both A, Fischer G, et al. (1977) Sozialanamnestische und hämodynamische Untersuchungen 4 bis 6 Jahre nach prothetischem Klappenersatz. Z Kardiol 66:251–256
9. Kasl SV (1977) Contributions of social epidemiology to studies in psychosomatic medicine. Adv Psychosom Med 9:160–223

Relationship Between Preoperative Coping Styles, Immediate Postoperative Reactions and Some Aspects of the Psychosocial Situation of Open-Heart Surgery Patients One Year After the Operation

K. Möhlen, S. Davies-Osterkamp, H. Müller, H.H. Scheld, G. Siefen

For patients undergoing open-heart surgery the operation is a stressful event. From other investigations on psychosomatic patients it is well-known that certain events, especially those which have the character of object loss, may trigger states of illness [7, 16]. In these cases not only the stressful event itself is discussed, but other circumstances of the patient's life are included as well [5, 12]. These are development of personality, object relationships, and his/her social condition. There are many investigations on open-heart surgery patients which in this sense look for special predictors for postoperative reactions [2, 6, 8, 11, 14, 15, 19].

One of our main questions was whether the object relationships, coping styles, and the general emotional behavior of patients, developed shortly before the operation, may be predictors for postoperative psychological reactions and certain aspects of bodily recovery. If this can be shown, the next question arises: is the long-term outcome of an open-heart surgery patient also dependent on these preoperative coping styles?

Method

Seventy two patients undergoing cardiac surgery were evaluated preoperatively and studied postoperatively for a period of 1 year. A description of the sample is given by Table 1.

For the investigation of the outlined questions the main preoperative instrument was a semistructured interview. All patients were seen 1 or 2 days before the operation for about three-quarters of an hour (by D.-O., Mö.). Following the interview the interviewer rated the patient's behavior on a 56-items questionnaire, which had been devised after a preliminary investigation. The questionnaire covered four topics:

1. The patient's general behavior during the interview, his or her emotional involvement, manner of speech and interaction.
2. The patient's method of coping with illness.
3. The patient's mood, feeling and coping mechanisms concerning the operation.
4. The patient's history concerning neurological and psychiatric disorders.

The other preoperative instruments we used were of lower or even of no interest for the results I will report on (details are given elsewhere, see [4]).

Psychopathological and Neurological Dysfunctions
Following Open-Heart Surgery. Ed. by Becker et al.

Table 1. Description of the sample

Operative procedure	n	Age $\bar{x}$	Female/Male
Mitral valve replacement	11	57	6/5
Aortic valve replacement	24	49	6/18
Multivalve replacement	4	53	2/2
Coronary bypass[a]	21	50	1/20
Other	12	43	10/2
Total sample	72	50	25/47

[a] includes two patients also with valve replacement
Sex: $\chi^2 = 24.15$; *df*, 4; $P < 0.01$
Age: $F = 3.14$; *df*, 4/67; $P < 0.05$

During the patient's stay in the intensive care unit, following the operation, his or her psychological condition was assessed daily. This was done by using a special rating scale which asked for psychopathological symptoms (a modified version of the AMP System, [18]) as well as observing changes in mood and affective behavior. Concerning postoperative bodily recovery during hospital stay, disturbances and complications were registered precisely. Each patient was awarded to total score for organic complications by rating the severity of complications on a three-point scale in eight different areas.

One year after operation 55 patients were included in the follow-up study. They had a cardiological check-up and all social and demographic data were collected. The patients completed a personality questionnaire (GT, [1]), an inventory of bodily complaints (GBB, [3]). and a questionnaire concerning their own estimation of recovery. Again the patient took part in a semistructured interview (Siefen). In this interview special emphasis was placed on the following areas: health behavior, contact with medical institutions, the patient's evaluation of the operation in terms of bodily and psychological recovery, social contacts, leisure activities, work situation, and relationship with the family.

Results

First I will report on correlations between the findings of the immediate postoperative phase and the preoperative interview.

We found four different groups of patients concerning their psychological reactions. Seventeen patients (23%) showed distinct psychiatric dysfunctions. This group was devided into two subgroups. Group I (n = 8) consisted of patients with anxiety and paranoid ideation, while Group II (n = 9) of those with more delirious symptoms. Out of these nine patients six showed some evidence of organic brain damage, whilst there was no such patient in Group I. Of the remaining 55 patients 34 were classified into three subgroups according to their scores on the dimensions aggression and depression. This resulted in a group of patients with a distinctly depressive-distressed reaction

Table 2. Postoperative psychological reaction

Type of reaction	n
Distinct psychiatric dysfunctions	17
delirium (9)	
paranoid ideation, anxiety (8)	
Depressive-distressed reaction	12
Aggressive-hostile reaction	12
Inconspicious reaction	10
Mixed reactions	21
Total	72

(n = 12), one group with an aggressive-hostile reaction (n = 12), and an inconspicious group (n = 10) (details in [4]). Table 2 shows the results of a survey. Concerning preoperative predictors for psychological reaction and the bodily recovery we found the following correlations:

The aspect of behavior and emotional involvement in the preoperative interview could be described by the following three scales which were derived by factor analysis:

1. Emotional withdrawal versus emotional openness.
2. Depressive inhibition versus hypomanic disinhibition.
3. Activity versus passivity.

A comparison of the four postoperative psychological groups on these scales showed the following: The aggressive-hostile group showed significantly higher emotional withdrawal on the first scale and a significantly higher depressive inhibition on the second scale. There were no differences between the groups on the last scale. Another result was that patients with a higher rate of emotional withdrawal before the operation had a low score of organic complications. In other words, those patients who reacted immediately after the operation in an aggressive, hostile manner and had a good bodily recovery could be identified as those who were emotionally withdrawn or depressedly inhibited in the preoperative interview.

For the distinct psychiatric dysfunctions, namely the paranoid ideation and heavy reaction of anxiety, predictors were found in that section of the interview which dealt with the coping processes with respect to the forthcoming operation. Using factor analysis again four dimensions in this area could be identified. The following two were relevant:

1. Conceiving the operation as a more or less technical event.
2. Optimistic versus pessimistic expectations for the future.

On both dimensions the psychiatric disturbed group had significantly higher scores than the other groups (i.e., more technical event, optimistic expectations for the future). An additional analysis showed that this was due only to Subgroup I, i.e., those patients with paranoid ideation and anxiety. In other words patients who conceived the operation as a more technical event, had clear plans and optimistic expectations for the future, and did not try to avoid discussing the forthcoming operation, had statistically the highest probability of reacting with paranoid ideation and anxiety after the operation.

The next step involved investigating the correlations between the preoperative and the follow-up interview. Almost the same dimensions (three out of four) which had a predicting value for the short-term outcome were found to be predictors for the long-term outcome. These were:

1. The emotional withdrawal before the operation.
2. The depressed-inhibited behavior in the preoperative interview.
3. The rationalizing and technically oriented coping style concerning the operation.

The correlations were not very high. They ranged between 0.30 ($P < 0.05$) and 0.44 ($P < 0.01$).

Patients who had a high emotional withdrawal preoperatively were statistically relatively more disappointed with their postoperative course 1 year after the operation. They had expected a greater improvement and assessed their health situation as being worse than before the operation. In the follow-up interview they talked little about their heart disease and that in a minimizing way. Patients who showed preoperatively a depressed-inhibited way of communication also tried to minimize the topic heart disease in the follow-up interview and talked little about it. On the other hand they considered themselves mentally well balanced, more tolerable, and less depressive than preoperatively.

A very different long-term outcome was found in those patients who preoperatively conceived the operation as a pure technical event. These patients judged themselves in the postoperative course more depressed, more restless, and mentally less stable. They also considered themselves to be medically and psychologically poorly supported by their family doctors.

Discussion

Our findings suggest that the coping styles concerning the operation and the emotional behavior shortly before the operation are dimensions which have a good predicting value for the immediate postoperative psychological and bodily reaction. They even have a certain value as predictors for the long-term outcome. The following three dimensions are particularly important:

1. The emotional withdrawal before the operation.
2. The depressed-inhibited behavior in the preoperative interview.
3. The rationalizing and technically orientated coping style concerning the operation.

These dimensions seem to be indicators for the patient's Ego functions, particularly his/her defense mechanisms.

Open-heart surgery is an extremely threatening and frightening event which mobilizes impulses of fight and flight. Because of the speciality of the event – the patient himself wants to be operated upon and hopes to recover as a result – both reactions – fight and flight – are futile. Our patients are in this conflict whilst anticipating the operation. In this situation extreme demands are placed on the patient's Ego functions and typical defense mechanisms are provoked. They are comparable to those provoked by an acute organic disease [9]. With this in mind our findings may be interpreted in the following way:

Patients who – concerning their Ego functions – are able to anticipate the operation in its whole meaning, show an emotional withdrawal before the operation. This withdrawal indicates a retreat of libido from the objects. By cathecting their own Self with more libido a stabilization is achieved. The arising impulses of fight and flight can be partly neutralized or repressed. Shortly after the operation these patients show an aggressive reaction. The aggressive impulses provoked by the operation are not repressed any longer and can be openly expressed. The bodily recovery of these patients is relatively good. One year after the operation the preoperatively emotionally withdrawn patients admit realistically that they still suffer from their heart disease and that they had expected more improvement. But they don't stress this. They talk little about their heart disease. This finding might also be an indication for relatively stable Ego functions. These patients have the ability to cope with their chronic disease. The realistic behavior may be an indication for a successful process of grieving. Especially after an operation which is usually the last hope for recovery grieving and coping with the chronic disease is necessary [13, 17].

A very similar way of coping with the operation and the chronic disease seems to be established by those patients who preoperatively show a depressed inhibited communication. In these cases the aggressive impulses seem to turn against the Self for a short period and to be followed by a depressive reaction. Soon after the operation – the acute stress which had to be mastered is over – the aggression becomes manifest for a short period. It is important to say that at no time after the operation – immediately or 1 year later – is depression assessable for these patients. They even judged themselves to be mentally well balanced, more tolerable, and less depressive than preoperatively. The defense mechanisms developed by these patients also seem to be adequate and helpful.

Patients who show, before the operation, a rationalizing and technically orientated coping style seem to differ in their Ego functions. They try to cope with the threatening event by avoiding an emotional involvement with this event. The anticipation of the operation is deficient and the threat by the event is denied. They deal with the operation in a contraphobic way and conceive it as a pure technical event. Shortly after the operation they show unrestrained anxiety and paranoid ideation. The impulses of flight accompanied by anxiety which were split off before the operation now seem to flood the patient. The Ego functions of these patients are overtaxed by the operation.

Assuming that the preoperative rationalizing is an unsuccessful attempt at coping with the operation – because of overtaxing the patient's Ego functions – the correlations with the dimensions assessed 1 year after the operation are accountable. Depression, restlessness, and mental lability might be indicators for the inability to cope with the chronic disease. Emphasizing that they are psychologically poorly supported by their family doctors might be an indicator for dependency on objects by the patients.

For these patients a supportive psychotherapy [10] might have been helpful.

References

1. Beckmann D, Richter HE (1972) Der Giessen-Test (GT). Huber, Bern
2. Blachy PH, Starr A (1964) Post-cardiotomy delirium. Am J Psychiatry 121:371
3. Brähler E, Scheer JW (1979) Skalierung psychosomatischer Beschwerdenkomplexe mit dem Giessener Beschwerdebogen (GBB). Psychother Med Psychol 29:14–27
4. Davies-Osterkamp S, Möhlen K, Lademann HR, Scheld H (1980) Postoperative reactions in open-heart surgery patients. In: Speidel H, Rodewald G (eds) Psychic and neurological dysfunctions after open-heart surgery. INA 19:162–168. Thieme, Stuttgart
5. Dührssen A, Jores A, Schwidder W (1965) Zum Streßbegriff in der psycho-somatischen Medizin. Z Psychosom Med Psychol 11:234
6. Egerton N, Kay JH (1964) Psychological disturbances associated with open-heart surgery. Br J Psychiatry 110:433
7. Engel GL, Schmale AH Jr (1967) Psychoanalytic theory of somatic disorder-conversion, specificity, and disease on set situation. J Am Psychoanal Assoc 15:344
8. Flemming B, Meffert H-J (1980) The role of personality traits for psychic disturbances after open-heart surgery. In: Speidel H, Rodewald G (eds) Psychic and neurological dysfunctions after open-heart surgery. INA 19:169–180. Thieme, Stuttgart
9. Freud S (1946) Zur Einführung des Narzißmus (1914). Imago, London. (Gesammelte Werke, vol X)
10. Freyberger H, Speidel H (1976) Die supportive Psychotherapie in der klinischen Medizin. Bibl Psychiatr 152:141
11. Henrichs TF, McKenzie JM, Almond CH (1971) Psychological adjustment and psychiatric complications following open-heart surgery. J Nerv Ment Dis 152:332
12. Joraschky P, Köhle K (1979) Maladaptation und Krankheitsmanifestation. Das Streßkonzept in der psychosomatischen Medizin. In: von Uexküll T (ed) Lehrbuch der psychosomatischen Medizin. Urban & Schwarzenberg, Munich
13. Kimball CP (1975) Medical psychotherapy. Psychother Psychosom 25:193
14. Kimball CP, Quinlan D, Osborne F, Woodward B (1973) The experience of cardiac surgery. Psychother Psychosom 22:310
15. Kornfeld DS, Heller SS, Frank KA, Moskowitz R (1974) Personality and psychological factors in postcardiotomy delirium. Arch Gen Psychiatry 31:248
16. Mitscherlich A (1961) Anmerkungen über die Chronifizierung psychosomatischen Geschehens. Psyche (Stuttg) 15:1
17. Möhlen K (1979) Trauer um das verlorene Herz – Psychosomatische Aspekte bei chronischen organischen Herzerkrankungen. Euromed 19:744
18. Scharfetter C (ed) (1972) Das AMP-System. Manual zur Dokumentation psychiatrischer Befunde, 2nd edn. Springer, Berlin Heidelberg New York
19. Speidel H, Dahme B, Flemming B, Götze D, Huse-Kleinstoll G, Meffert HJ, Rodewald G, Spehr W (1978) Psychosomatische Probleme in der Herzchirurgie. Therapiewoche 28:8191

Psychological and Behavioral Responses Following Coronary Artery Bypass Surgery*

St. S. Heller, K.A. Frank, D.S. Kornfeld, S.N. Wilson, J.R. Malm

Introduction

Although reduction in angina has been confirmed following coronary artery bypass surgery, long-term studies of longevity have showed equivocal findings, requiring further time to provide definitive conclusions [1–3]. Until such medical data are available, postoperative quality of life studies remain of particular importance in justifying the use of this costly procedure.

Several studies have not shown sufficient improvement in postoperative employment rates to justify the surgery on the basis of cost benefit analysis [4–6]. Moreover, Lamendola and Pelligrini [7] reported that employment fell off for all age groups. Nevertheless, even older patients were highly satisfied and felt physically improved, leading the authors to suggest a study of broader criteria of quality of life.

Rabiner and Willner [8] have studied long-term psychological outcome in both cardiac valvular and coronary artery bypass surgery patients. Their primary focus was on the role of preoperative organicity as a predictor of outcome. They found that while valvular surgery patients postoperatively showed improved psychosocial adaptation, they did not achieve the level attained by coronary bypass patients. Both groups tended to improve in leisure and activity levels, while the bypass group showed a significant reduction in what the authors termed preoperative "hyperactivity".

Studies of long-term psychological and behavioral outcome after valvular surgery are available [9–13] but have limited comparability to outcome after coronary artery bypass surgery. The patients involved are substantially different both medically and psychologically. Coronary bypass patients are, for the most part, unburdened by the physical limitations and associated psychological adaptation of patients with long-standing chronic illness. Quite the contrary, many are typically hard driving and competitive individuals showing type A behavior patterns. However, little is currently known about the persistence of these behaviors in the face of illness and surgical intervention.

This study undertook to trace the postoperative psychosocial and behavioral course of patients following coronary artery bypass surgery. Particular attention was paid to the quality of life issue and the postoperative stability of the coronary prone behavior pattern. Medical outcome variables were concurrently examined.

---

* This work was supported in part by Alcohol, Drug Abuse, and Mental Health Administration Grant MH-12756 from the National Institute of Mental Health

Psychopathological and Neurological Dysfunctions Following Open-Heart Surgery. Ed. by Becker et al

Method

One hundred consecutive patients who underwent coronary artery bypass surgery at the Columbia-Presbyterian Medical Center from December, 1972 to February, 1975 were evaluated at the time of their surgery and then followed for as long as 4 1/2 years in order to study their postoperative psychosocial and behavioral course. There was one death within the first 30 postoperative days (1%).

Fifty-four patients returned for a personal follow-up visit at 9 months postoperatively. Fifty-seven patients returned a follow-up questionnaire administered 3 1/2 years postoperatively on the average. Thirty of them had also been seen at the 9-month visit. The medical outcome at approximately 4 1/2 years for 92 patients was obtained by questionnaire or telephone follow-up.

Data were analyzed statistically by correlation analysis, with the criterion of statistical significance at the 0.05 level (two tailed).

Sample

The mean age of the operative sample was 52.1 years with a S.D. of 7.1 years, and ranged from 35 to 65 years. Ninety-three percent were male, and 91% married. The sample was relatively well-educated with half having attended college. The group was primarily middle-class with 74% in Social Classes 3 and 4 [14]. Classes 1, 2 and 5 had 7%, 9%, and 11% sample membership respectively.

Chest pain was the usual indication for surgery and it was extreme in 44%, mild to moderate in 45%. Only 11% had no preoperative anginal pain. Fifty three percent had sustained at least one preoperative myocardial infarction, 13% more than one, and 20% had a history of congestive heart failure. The mean NYHA functional class was 3.21 at operation, 28% had one coronary artery bypassed, 56% two, and 16% three. Nine percent sustained a preoperative myocardial infarct.

The patients evaluated at the 9 month and 3 1/2 year evaluations were compared statistically. They did not differ significantly from one another or from the overall sample in terms of age, sex, marital status, or New York Heart Association Functional Classification [15].

Preoperative Data

Semistructured psychiatric interviews totalling 1 1/2–3 h were conducted prior to surgery. Psychosocial and behavioral data were scaled using: The Psychiatric Evaluation Form (PEF) [16]; the Adaptive Balance Profile (ABP) [16]; the Hackett-Cassem Denial Scale [17]; and the 16 Personality Factor Questionnaire (16PF) [18]. The Rosenman-Friedman Standardized Interview [19] to measure Type A coronary prone behavior was administered, and a rating was made of overall type A along with subratings of aggressive content, vocal stylistics, job commitment, and sense of time urgency. Our research team was trained in the use of the interview technique by Dr. Rosenman.

Medical data recorded included history of angina or myocardial infarction, number of coronary arteries occluded by more than 50% at angiography, and New York Heart Association Functional Classification.

Surgical data recorded included: the number of arteries bypassed, time on cardiopulmonary bypass and intraoperative myocardial infarction.

Postoperative Data

Interview (9 Month)

The semistructured psychiatric interview was repeated at approximately 9 months postoperatively, along with the standardized interview for the coronary-prone behavior pattern. The presence of angina and its severity, myocardial infarction, and reoperation were coded.

Questionnaire (3 1/2 Years)

At 3 1/2 years postoperatively, on the average, patients were asked to complete a questionnaire requesting demographic, psychosocial, behavioral, and medical data including retrospective ratings of change. Patients were asked to compare pre- and postoperative variables such as extent of anginal pain and their response to it, physical limitations, weight, smoking, exercise, and manifestations of coronary-prone behavior. They were asked to estimate their compliance with their doctor's advice with regard to smoking, diet, exercise, behavior, and medication.

Medical Follow-Up (4 1/2 Years)

After 4 1/2 years, on the average, the patients' postoperative medical course was studied by contacting them and/or their physicians. Among the data recorded were fatalities, and cardiovascular events such as episodes of arrhythmia, congestive heart failure, myocardial infarction, and cerebrovascular accidents. Additional coronary bypass surgery and pacemaker operations were also noted. Severity of angina and extent of activity limitation were quantified.

Results

Medical Outcome. Questionnaire subjects, 3 1/2 years postoperatively, were usually pleased that they had undergone the operation, 60% extremely so. Only 4% were displeased. Postoperatively, chest pain had been dramatically reduced; now it was rated extreme by only 4%, moderate by 16%, minimal by 28%, while 53% were pain free. There were commensurate activity improvements in the number of blocks walked and flights of stairs climbed. The response among those patients who still had pain was identical to that preoperatively: 57% stopped activity, 34% slowed down, and 9% continued.

Twenty-eight percent had been hospitalized at least once since surgery for cardiac disease and 11% had sustained a myocardial infarction. Sixteen percent had been reoperated upon.

Data was obtained on 92 patients (92%) at the time of the 4 1/2 year medical follow-up. Twenty-three (23%) were reported as deceased. Fifteen of the 23 fatalities were clearly due to cardiac causes, and in only three patients was a non cardiac cause known. When the relationship between type A behavior and mortality was studied, it was found that 87% of the fatalities were in individuals rated type A preoperatively, with 67% AI; while the overall sample was 84% Type A and 61% AI.

Data on angina assessment was available for 64 survivors. Thirty-five patients (55%) had no angina, in ten (16%) it was rated mild, 7 (11%) moderate, and 12 (19%) extreme.

Return to work. Seventy-seven percent of the patients were working at the time of surgery. Seventy-six percent of the patients were working at the time of the 9-month evaluation. As would be expected failure to return to work correlated with measures of cardiac disease severity.

Patients who returned to work were significantly younger ($P = 0.05$), showed more improvement in angina ($P = 0.01$), and were more likely to be type A preoperatively ($P = 0.05$) and postoperatively ($P = 0.001$).

Sixty-five percent were employed, 3 1/2 years postoperatively, with 65% having more than one job. Of those working, 62% worked full time. As noted in Table 1, two-thirds of the patients reported improved satisfaction in their work.

Return to Sexual Activity. Preoperatively, 67% were sexually active at least once a week, 22% were less active and 11% abstained. Nine months postoperatively, sexual acitivity had decreased. Thirty-eight percent were sexually active at least once a week, 29% were less active, and 31% abstained. Postoperatively, frequent sexual activity correlated with pre- and postoperative type A ratings ($P = 0.05$) and with a tendency to an active adaptation ($P = 0.01$). Return to work and frequent sexual activity were correlated ($P = 0.01$). Reduced frequency of sexual activity correlated with preoperative cardiac impairment (New York Heart Association Functional Class [$P = 0.001$]).

Quality of Life. There was substantial improvement in all areas studied 3 1/2 years postoperatively: pleasure in life, nervousness, mood, and job, family and sexual satisfaction (Table 1). Pleasure in life was the most improved (77%), while sexual

Table 1. Change in life adjustment 3 1/2 years after surgery (n = 57)

	% Change					
	Pleasure	Nervousness	Mood	Job satisfaction	Family relations	Sexual satisfaction
Much better	65	30	42	41	48	22
Slightly better	12	23	24	21	22	22
No change	12	32	24	22	25	33
Slightly worse	9	11	5	10	10	10
Much worse	2	4	5	6	2	13

satisfaction improved least (44%). Conversely, only a minority reported worsening in these areas, with family relationships worsening least (4%) and sexual satisfaction most (23%).

Behavior Risk Factors

Smoking. Thirty-nine percent were smokers when they came to surgery, 30% consuming a pack or more every day. At 9 months postoperatively, only 13% smoking.

Persistent smoking correlated with 16PF Factor I, "sensitive and dependent" as opposed to "tough and realistic" ($P = 0.05$) and negatively with 16PF Q4 "tension" (P 0.001), indicating that "fearful" persons smoked less.

At 3 1/2 years, 57% of the sample had been advised not to smoke. Sixty percent rated their compliance as full; 28% said they had complied fairly well, 9% poorly, and 3% not at all.

Weight. At 9 months, smoking correlated inversely with postoperative weight gain, ($P = 0.05$). The mean preoperative weight had been 156 lb. Postoperative weight was generally little changed with only 7% having a marked increase. Postoperative weight gain correlated negatively with preoperative 16PF factor Q3 "will power" ($P = 0.01$).

At 3 1/2 years, 62% had been advised to change their diet; of those only 22% had done so fully. Sixty-eight percent rated their compliance as fairly good and 11% as poor.

Exercise. At 9 months, exercise level correlated inversely with the preoperative NYHA Functional Class ($P = 0.05$) indicating that sicker patients exercised less. There was a positive correlation with preoperative anxiety ($P = 0.05$).

At 3 1/2 years, 67% had been advised to change their exercise pattern, primarily to increase it. Thirty-eight percent did so fully, 47% fairly well, and 15% poorly.

There was generally good compliance with advice related to cardiac medications, 86% complying fully, and 11% fairly well. Three percent did not comply at all.

Type A. Preoperatively 64% were rated A1, 24% A2, 11% B3, and 2% B4. Postoperatively 55% were rated A1, 29% A2, 15% B3, and 2% B4. Table 2 shows preoperative and 9 months postoperative behavior type ratings, and changes within each type. Following surgery, 41 (75%) were unchanged in overall A rating. Four patients (7%) had changed in a more type A direction, while ten patients (18%) were less so. Only three patients (5%) changed from A to B.

Of the components of Type A, vocal stylistics and aggressive content were extremely stable, while job commitment and time urgency showed some change (Table 3). Less than half (12 of 27 = 44%) of the type A1 job commitment group remained A1. Thirteen (48%) became A2 level of job commitment while one each became B3 or B4. Preoperative A2 job commitment ratings were more stable. Nine (60%) of the fifteen A2 preoperative patients remained unchanged. The change for them was slightly more toward type A1, while 2 (13%) became B3. Six of the eight (75%) preoperative B3 patients were unchanged while one each became A1 and B4. Again, few

Table 2. Pre- and postoperative behavior type ratings

Preoperative type	Postoperative type		
A1	A1	26	(74%)
n = 35	A2	7	(20%)
	B3	2	(4%)
	B4	0	
A2	A1	3	(23%)
n = 13	A2	9	(69%)
	B3	1	(8%)
	B4	0	
B3	A1	1	(17%)
n = 6	A2	0	
	B3	5	(83%)
	B4	0	

Table 3. Comparison of pre- and postoperative type A ratings (Pearson product-moment correlation coefficients) (n = 54)

Rating	*r*	*P*
Overall	0.67	0.001
Vocalistics	0.93	0.001
Aggressive content	0.86	0.001
Time urgency	0.71	0.001
Job commitment	0.76	0.001

patients, only 4 (7%) changed from A to B types. The results for time urgency were similar.

Preoperative correlates of persistent Type A behavior at 9 months included denial of illness (Hackett-Cassem Denial Scale) ($P = 0.001$), 16PF Factor A, "outgoingness" ($P = 0.05$) and activity (Adaptive Blance Profile), ($P = 0.001$). Postoperative angina correlated with pre- and postoperative type A behavior traits, ($P = 0.05$).

Patients reported that they had generally been told by their physicians to slow down. Seventeen percent were told to do so strongly, 50% moderately, 13% mildly, and 20% not at all. At 3 1/2 years postoperatively, only 31% thought they had actually slowed down a great deal, 21% somewhat, 25% a little, 16% not at all, and 7% pushed themselves more.

Ten patients who had died by the time of the 4 1/2 years follow-up had been seen at the 9-month interview. Preoperatively, seven of these patients had been rated A1, and one each A2, B3 and B4. Nine of the ten remained unchanged in Overall score, one A1 becoming A2, while type A Vocalistics, Time Urgency, and Job Involvement were unchanged. Aggressive Content had diminished in four and increased in one. Six patients with extreme angina at 4 1/2 years, who had been rated A1 preoperatively, were still rated A1. However, over time, severe angina apparently led to a change in behavior patterns since six of the eight patients who reported extreme angina on the 3 1/2 year questionnaire, had slowed down substantially.

Discussion

The majority of patients who are long-term survivors of coronary artery bypass surgery reported substantial improvement in angina and exercise capacity. The operation also led to substantial improvements in quality of life, including general pleasure, reduction of anxiety and depression, and reported improvement in job and family roles. However, it did not increase the number employed. Sexual adjustment improved less than the other measures. In fact, at 9 months frequency of sexual activity had been reduced for approximately one-third of the sample, while at 3 1/2 years one-quarter continued to report a worsened sexual adjustment compared to their preoperative status. Although the sicker patients have less sex, it is not clear if that is related to physical impairment, or anxiety in the patient or spouse.

"Placebo" benefits have been found in up to 80% of patients treated for angina by medical and surgical methods which were later abandoned [20]. However, the persistence of improvement for almost 5 years suggests that this is a valid therapeutic effect.

Compliance with medical recommendation was relatively good for smoking and exercise but not for weight control. Follow-up psychological assessments revealed the persistence over time of the type A behavior pattern in a heavily type A group. Although severe angina over time was associated with reduction in hard-driving behavior, postoperative physical improvement typically allowed for resumption of activity.

In contrast to cardiac valve repair patients whose psychopathology tended to be in the direction of postoperative passivity, it would appear that most type A patients continue to be overly active, although there is a trend to change in job involvement from A1 to A2. Among the type A-related behaviors, job involvement was most reduced; perhaps because of all the behaviors measured, it is most subject to volitional modification. The majority of postcoronary artery bypass surgery patients are not characterized by inhibition in work or sex after surgery, but by persistence of type A behavior patterns, which may lead to coronary disease recurrence [21].

The study suggests the need for physicians to discuss sexual activity with their patients following surgery to relieve postoperative misconceptions and inhibitions. Further efforts are also needed to modify type A behavior in the postoperative period. Motivation for change should be highest at that critical time. Further research is needed into the effectiveness of such intervention efforts [22]. Until definitive studies are completed, physicians are urged to periodically remind patients of the probable need to reduce type A behavior.

References

1. Braunwald E (1978) Evaluation of the efficacy of coronary bypass surgery II. Am J Cardiol 42:161–162
2. Loop FD, Proudjit WL, Sheldon WC (1978) Coronary bypass surgery weighed in the balance. Am J Cardiol 42:154–156

3. Huldgren HN, Taucaro T, Detrie KN, et al. (1978) Evaluation of the efficacy of coronary bypass surgery I. Am J Cardiol 42:157–160
4. Barnes G, Ray MJ, Oberman A, et al. (1977) Changes in working status of patients following coronary bypass surgery. JAMA 238:1259–1262
5. English MT, Logan GA, Eyer KM, et al. (1975) Employment following coronary artery bypass graft surgery. Circulation [Suppl 2] 52:144
6. Rimm AA, Barboriak JJ, Anderson AJ (1976) Changes in occupation after aorto-coronary vein-bypass graft surgery. JAMA 236:361–364
7. LaMendola WF, Pelligrini RV (1979) Quality of life and coronary artery bypass surgery patients. Soc Sci Med 13A(4):457–461
8. Rabiner CJ, Willner AF (1980) Differential psychopathology and organic mental disorder at follow-up, five years after coronary bypass and cardiac valvular surgery. In: Speidel H, Rodewald G (eds) Psychopathological and neurological dysfunctions following open heart surgery. Thieme, Stuttgart
9. Heller SS, Frank KA, Kornfeld DS, et al. (1974) Psychological outcome following open-heart surgery. Arch Intern Med 134:908–914
10. Frank KA, Heller SS, Kornfeld DS (1972) A survey of adjustment to cardiac surgery. Arch Intern Med 130:735–738
11. Kimball CP (1969) Psychological responses to the experience of open-heart surgery I. Am J Psychiatry 126:348–349
12. Lucia W, McGuire LB (1970) Rehabilitation and functional status after surgery for valvular heart disease. Arch Intern Med 126:995–999
13. Blachly PH, Blachly BJ (1968) Vocational and emotional status of 263 patients after heart surgery. Circulation 38:524–533
14. Hollingshead A, Redlich FC (1978) Social class and mental illness. Wiley, New York
15. Spitzer R, Endicott J (1966) Progress report biometric research. New York State Department of Mental Hygiene, Research Division, Washington Heights Community Service, New York State Psychiatric Institute, Dept of Psychiatry, New York
16. Karish A, Easer BR, et al. (1964) The evaluation of ego strength I: A profile of adaptive balance. J Nerv Ment Dis 139:332–349
17. Hackett TP, Cassem NH (1974) Development of a quantitative rating scale to assess denial. J Psychosomat Res 18:93–100
18. Cattell RB, Eber HW (1962) Handbook for the 16PF questionnaire. Institute for Personality and Ability Testing, Urbana
19. Rosenman RH, Friedman M, Straus R, et al. (1964) A predictive study of coronary heart disease. JAMA 189:15–26
20. Benson H, McCallie D (1979) Angina pectoris and the placebo effect. N Engl J Med 300: 1424–1429
21. Jenkins CD, Zyzanski SJ, Rosenman RH (1976) Rise of new myocardial infarction in middle-aged men with manifest coronary heart disease. Circulation 53:342–347
22. Frank KA, Heller SS, Kornfeld DS (1979) Psychological intervention in coronary heart disease: A review. Gen Hosp Psychiatry 1:18–23

Effects of Environmental Stress Upon the Long-Term Outcome of Open-Heart Surgery: A Five-Year Follow-up Study

Ch. J. Rabiner, A.E. Willner, K. Detmer

Introduction

There have been previous reports on the incidence of psychopathology and cognitive disorder following open-heart surgery, but to date little is known about the quality of life patients enjoy in the postoperative period. This paper explores the quality of life during the 5-year period following surgery and examines areas of occupational adjustment, leisure time interests, socialization, activity level, sexual activity, and family adjustment. The patients studied have been interviewed at several points along the 5-year period.

The Psychopathology and Cognitive Disorder (PCD) syndrome has been defined, and its implications for high mortality risk after open-heart surgery have been reported [14]. The specific phenomenology of the PCD patients has been described elsewhere in this symposium. In view of the fact that our patients fall into four groups, we have chosen to compare these groups in terms of adjustment to life's stresses following surgery. These groups then are those patients having both psychopathology and a cognitive disorder, patients with a cognitive disorder only, patients with psychopathology only, and those patients free of disorder.

Materials and Methods

The patients followed are 51 patients of the 69 reported by Willner and Rabiner. Of the 18 subjects not reported, 16 died and two were quite ill, and quality of life data could not be obtained.

Eighteen patients had cardiac valvular surgery, 29 had coronary bypass, and four had both types of surgery. Of the 51 patients in our sample, six had PCD, 14 a cognitive disorder but no psychopathology, eight psychopathology but no cognitive disorder, and 23 had neither a cognitive disorder nor psychopathology. The quality of life ratings were filled out by the interviewer, a psychiatrist or a psychologist, after a clinical interview. An overall clinical impression was recorded, the patients' employment status was noted, and six ratings of quality of life variables were done. These ratings were done at seven periods of time: immediately preoperatively, best functioning in the 6 months preoperatively, and 1, 2, 3, 4, and 5 years postoperatively. Both immediate preoperative functioning and best functioning in the 6-month pre-

Psychopathological and Neurological Dysfunctions
Following Open-Heart Surgery Ed. by Becker et al

operative period were rated, to permit differentiation between those patients who had a sudden worsening in their condition just prior to surgery from those who had little change in their condition preoperatively.

Employment status was designated as employed full-time, part-time, unemployed, retired, and housewife. Although the first three variables obviously form an employment scale, it is difficult to place the retired patients and housewives within this scale.

The patient's level of functioning in carrying out his (her) role-expected behavior was assessed. The interviewer rated employed people according to how well he believed they functioned in their job, housewives on how well they carried out their daily activities, and retired people on how effectively they spent their time during retirement. On this scale (Table 1), as on all the quality of life scales, the interviewer not only rated the patient, but also described, in brief narrative form, changes in behavior which took place and the reasons the patient gave for these changes. The seven points on the scale were excellent, very good, good, fair, poor, very poor, and terrible:

Leisure time activities were assessed. The interviewer determined how involved the patient was in hobbies or other interests. Socialization was rated in terms of how many times per month the patient left his home and visited other people. The interviewer rated the patients' general level of activity with optimal activity being the mid point of the scale, and the two ends of the scale labeled very hyperactive and very underactive. The frequency of the patients' sexual activity was noted in terms of the number of sexual contacts per month. Finally, the interviewer rated how well the patient got along with other members of the family.

Results

Figure 1 shows the mean occupational adjustment scores of the four patient groups at seven points in time from preoperative performance to 5 years postoperatively. The group having neither psychopathology nor cognitive disorder has the best occupa-

Table 1. Chart for the assessment of occupational role adjustment (the patient's level of functioning in carrying out his role expected behavior)

	Immediately preoperation	Best in 6 months preoperation	1 Yr	2 Yr	3 Yr	4 Yr	5 Yr
1. Excellent							
2. Very good							
3. Good							
4. Fair (average)							
5. Poor							
6. Very poor							
7. Terrible							

Please describe as fully as possible the exact changes in behavior which took place, the reasons given for these changes, and your feelings as to their validity.

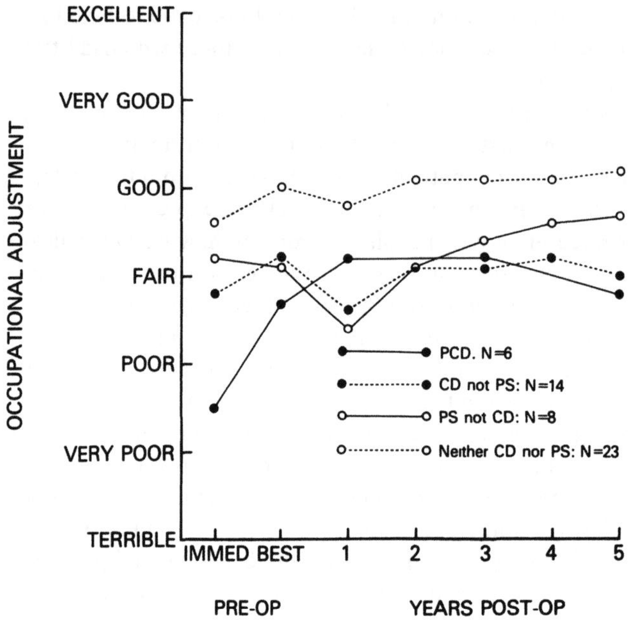

Fig. 1. Occupational adjustment of open-heart surgery patients over a 5-year period

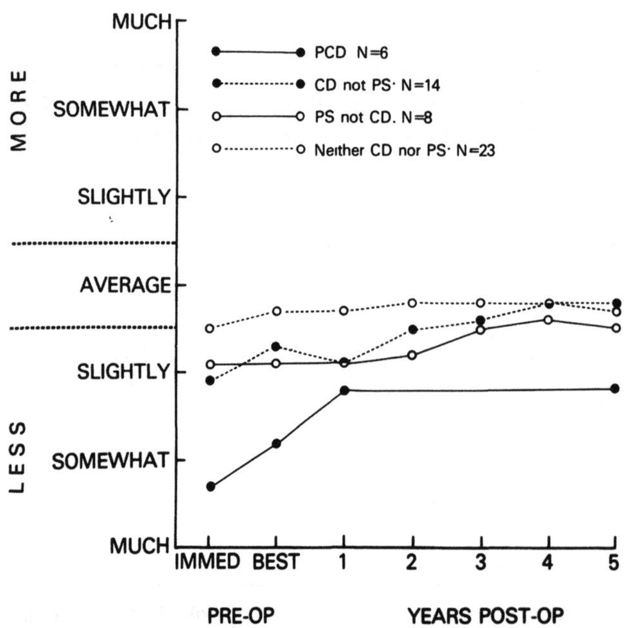

Fig. 2. Range of interests of open-heart surgery patients over a 5-year period

tional adjustment ratings at all seven time intervals (P between < 0.05 and 0.005 at five of the seven intervals). The PCD group has the worst occupational adjustment ratings in the last 2 years ($P < 0.05$, 5th year).

Figure 2 shows that the PCD group has the most restricted range of interests at all seven time intervals ($P < 0.005$ preoperatively only). The group with neither disorder has the broadest range of interests at six of the seven intervals (significant preoperatively only).

Figure 3 shows that at all seven intervals, the PCD group has the most limited social activity and the group with neither disorder has the most extensive social activity (P between < 0.05 and 0.005 preoperatively and at 2 and 3 years postoperatively). The psychopathology only and cognitive disorder only groups appear rather similar.

Figure 4 shows that the group with neither disorder has the closest to optimal activity level at all seven time intervals (P between < 0.05 and 0.005 preoperatively and at 2 years postoperatively), and the PCD and cognitive disorder groups tend to be most active.

Figure 5 indicates that the PCD group has the least sexual activity at all seven time intervals (P from < 0.025 to 0.005 at all intervals), and the psychopathology only group has the most at all seven intervals. The higher degree of sexual activity for the psychopathology only group as compared with the patients having no disorder is significant at none of the seven intervals.

There is no discernable difference between the groups when rated on family adjustment.

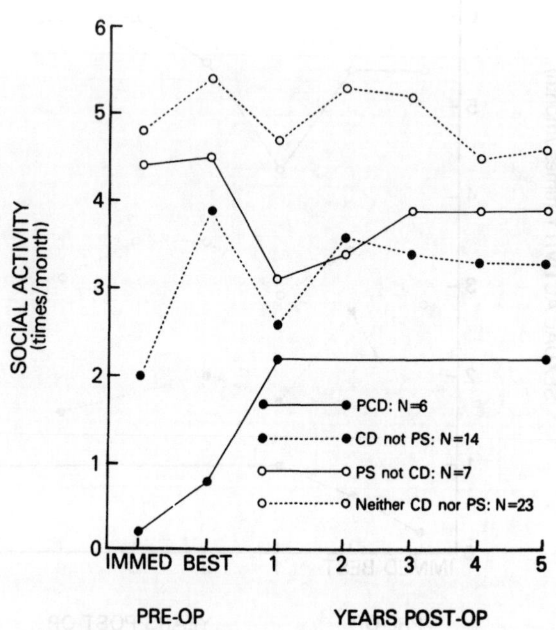

Fig. 3. Social activity of open-heart surgery patients over a 5-year period

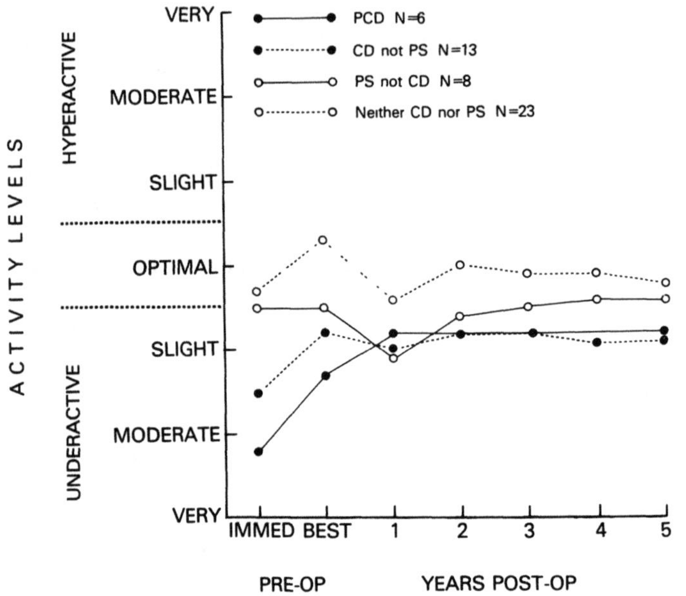

Fig. 4. Activity of open-heart surgery patients over a 5-year period

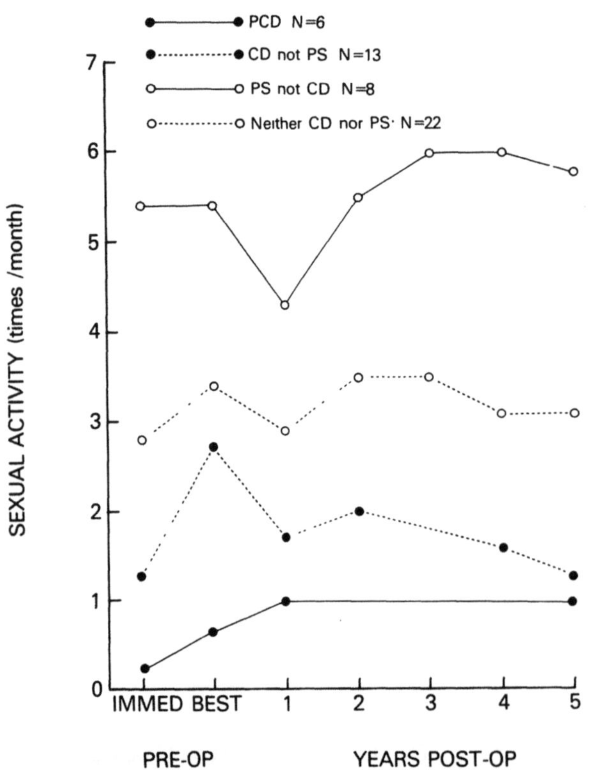

Fig. 5. Sexual activity levels of open-heart surgery patients over a 5-year period

Case Vignettes

Three case vignettes are presented. The first two are from the study, and indicate that in spite of the presence of either psychopathology or a cognitive disorder, it is still possible to effectively cope with life's stresses in the years following surgery. A third case is taken from our cardiac clinic, a clinic set up to treat patients with emotional difficulties associated with cardiac disease, and shows the difficulties faced by a patient with PCD.

Mr. R.D., now aged 61, was found to have a cognitive disorder, but no psychopathology at the time of surgery. When interviewed at the 5-year follow-up visit, he stated that he was doing very well. He was working long hours as a cook, a job he enjoyed, and functioned very well in the job. His position did not require overtime, but he often volunteered to fill in when other people were absent. His wife had died 3 years ago, and he stated that he missed her. However, he remained close to other members of his family, and since his wife's death, he and his daughter managed the house. He found time to be active in civic organizations such as veterans' organizations and his church. He appeared to be living a full and productive life.

Mrs. B.F., aged 64 at the time of the 5-year follow-up visit, was leading an active life in Florida. She was working in a ladies' shop on a part-time basis and doing well there. She described an active social life which included driving, dancing, and going out in the evening with friends. She had been living with her sister who had recently died. She missed her sister, had to decide whether or not to move when her current lease expired, but seemed perfectly capable of dealing with the problem.

At the time of surgery, she had developed psychopathology but no cognitive disorder. The symptoms included a postoperative mild depression and a brief period of hallucinosis. Her CLAT score at the time was 8, indicating the absence of a cognitive disorder. At 18-month follow-up, she was doing very well despite many problems. She dealt with her husband's illness and subsequent death without developing any psychiatric symptoms, and appeared to be coping equally well with the loss of her sister.

A much different picture was presented by Mr. D.A., a 57-year-old retired bank officer who applied to the cardiac clinic because he was feeling "depressed" 3 1/2 years following surgery. After his aortic valve surgery he was "phased out" of his job at the bank and he found himself with markedly diminished physical capacity and a reduced income. In spite of cardiograms that failed to reveal any extension of the illness he felt "unable to do things". He limited his activities to reading, watching T.V., and walking one to two blocks only when necessary. His wife stated that he exaggerates and has recently cost them "double in doctors' bills" by continuing to complain after initial tests were negative.

Mental status revealed a soft-spoken man who appeared depressed and chronically ill. He was oriented but had trouble with serial sevens, could recall only five digits toward and could not recall three digits backward. Proverbs were interpreted concretely. His CLAT score of 2 was consistent with a cognitive disorder.

During the treatment he quickly developed a dependent attachment to the therapist, and used the session to ventilate and complain. He did not have the intellectual skills to work with abstractions or to develop insight. The therapist did not believe there was much change as a result of the weekly sessions, but the patient expressed gratitude for the help he received.

Discussion

All patients face considerable stress in the years following open-heart surgery. These stresses include the stress related to the surgical procedure itself, the stress related to a change in job, and the stress related to a change in family role. Some patients have the additional stress of psychopathology and/or reduced coping abilities due to a cognitive disorder. In addition to the above, patients frequently encounter stress in later years such as loss of spouse or loved ones, and the onset of additional illness.

The results from the study clearly indicate substantial differences between the four patient groups preoperatively, and that these differences persist during the 5-year postoperative period. The PCD group almost always had the most impaired, and the group with neither psychopathology nor cognitive disorder, the least impaired functioning. These results are consistent with the hypothesis that the PCD syndrome is a manifestation of an often unsuspected preoperative organic brain syndrome. This condition is assumed to leave the patient especially vulnerable to the effects of stress, both in the hospital and during the years after discharge. The case vignettes are presented to indicate that patients with PCD fare poorly, not only when compared with patients with neither disorder but also when compared with patients with either psychopathology or a cognitive disorder.

It would appear that when patients display both psychopathology and a cognitive disorder they are more vulnerable to environmental stress prior to surgery, and continue to do poorly throughout the years following surgery.

References

1. Blachly P, Blachly B (1968) Vocational and emotional status of 263 patients after heart surgery. Circulation 38:524
2. Cochran WG (1954) Some methods for strengthening the common chisquare tests. Biometrics 10:417–541
3. Frank K, Heller S, Kornfeld D (1972) A survey of adjustment to cardiac surgery. Arch Intern Med 130:735–738
4. Freyhan FA, Gianelli S Jr, O'Connell RA, et al. (1971) Psychiatric complications following open heart surgery. Compr Psychiatry 12:181
5. Heller S, Frank K, Malm JR, et al. (1970) Psychiatric complications of open heart surgery: A re-examination. N Engl J Med 283:1015
6. Heller S, Frank K, Kornfeld D, et al. (1974) Psychological outcome following open heart surgery. Arch Intern Med 134:908
7. Heller S, Kornfeld D, Frank D, Hoar PF (1979) Postcardiotomy delirium and cardiac output. Am J Psychiatry 136:337
8. Kilpatric D, Miller W, Allain A, et al. (1975) The use of psychological test data to predict open heart surgery outcome: A prospective study. Psychosom Med 37:62
9. Kimball CP (1969) Psychological responses to the experience of open heart surgery I. Am J Psychiatry 126:348

10. Kimball CP (1972) The experience of open heart surgery. III. Toward a definition and understanding of postcardiotomy delirium. Arch Gen Psychiatry 27:57
11. Kornfeld D, Heller S, Frank K, et al. (1974) Personality and psychological factors in postcardiotomy delirium. Arch Gen Psychiatry 31:249
12. Meyendorf R (1980) Psychopathology in heart disease aside from cardiac surgery. In: Speidel H, Rodewald G (eds) Psychopathological and neurological dysfunction following open heart surgery. INA 19:14–18, Thieme, Stuttgart
13. Quinlan DM, Kimball CP, Osborne F (1974) The experience of open heart surgery. IV. Assessment of disorientation and dysphoria following cardiac surgery. Arch Gen Psychiatry 31:241
14. Rabiner CJ, Willner AE (1976) Psychopathology observed on follow up after coronary bypass surgery. J Nerv Ment Dis 163:295
15. Willner AE (1970) Towards development of more sensitive clinical tests of abstraction: The analogy test. Proc Annu Conv Am Psychol Assoc 78:553–554
16. Willner AE (1971) Conceptual level analogy test. Cognitive Testing Service, New York
17. Willner AE, Struve FA (1970) An analogy test that predicts EEG abnormality: Use with hospitalized psychiatric patients. Arch Gen Psychiatry 23:428
18. Willner AE, Rabiner CJ, Wisoff BG, et al. (1976) Analogical reasoning and postoperative outcome in patients scheduled for open heart surgery. Arch Gen Psychiatry 33:255
19. Willner AE, Rabiner CJ, Wisoff BG, et al. (1976) Analogy tests and psychopathology at follow-up after open heart surgery. Biol Psychiatry 11:687

Discussion of Session VI

Kimball pointed out:

Much of what happens in terms of patients occurs after they are out of the hospital, once the acute stage in the convalescent stage is over and they go into what I call the rehabilitative phase. We know less about how patients cope and adapt. We are now beginning to get some data in terms of some of the outcome, some of the follow-up, which is getting increasingly impressive because it goes up to 5 years. We will still have a lot of work to do because we will need to tease out the specific, and what I call particulate factors that make for good or poor adaptation and coping. We need to define our terms in this area over the next decade or so.

Heller added to his presentation:

Type A should be overrepresented in any group of coronary artery disease since the incidence of coronary artery disease in patients between 39 and 59 did double in Type A as opposed to Type B. Then there would be a further increase in the Type A's in that more would come to operation. Type B would be more willing to settle for a restricted life, restricted by their angina, whereas Type A, because of the need for activity and dominance, would seek the surgery. Then, too, there was a kind of filtering process in that the more progressive patients ought out Columbia Presbyterian Hospital in New York City.

Other studies have shown that there is a preponderance of Type A's also in that of sudden death in people who also never came to surgery sample, because the pool of coronary artery disease in Type A is greater.

The amplitude of speech, the variation in speech, the repetitiveness of response, and the speed of response after a question was asked were all consistent and differed from the Type B patients who has a much more lackadaisical speech, allows others to interrupt him, and rarely interrupts others.

Finally, concerning the reason for reduced sexual activity I must say there are a variety of factors, one of which is of course the stress of surgery, and that has both physical and psychological consequences. I believe that the psychological ones in this instance are the most predominant, since for many persons sexuality is a luxury and a dangerous one at that, and if the person is willing the spouse often will not be. A year after myocardial infarction there is greater anxiety and depression in the spouse than in the victim, and the spouses probably are noncontributory. In a person who would tend to have sexual problems and to demonstrate impotence or premature ejaculation, surgery would be a magnifying glass which would tend to exacerbate it. Also one of the problems is that during the period of inability to perform due to severe angina during intercourse, either the spouse has lost interest or found other lovers.

Asked about the problem of statistical significance Stanton answered:

For some of these things it is not the statistical significance that we are the most concerned with, although we have good statistical significance. There are certainly significant numbers of people who do not go back to work, who are forced to retire, and who personally feel that they have not done well. However, even who have severe psychological problems do not seek counseling. There is not one patient in this sample of 949 people who sought counseling from a psychiatrist or a psychologist. There were a few people who sought counseling from a marriage counselor or a priest, religious type of counseling. In the prospective study which we are doing now with the current technology, we are at the point of the 1-year follow-ups on the patients looking at the 6-month follow-up data. Some of these findings look as though they will be replicated even with the new technology, even though type of oxygenator that is used is different, with different surgical teams, but some of the problems apparently still exist.

Kimball added from his own experiences:

At least in the extensive histories that I obtained on patients prior to surgery in my studies, sexual complaints were one of the leading reasons for people coming for surgery, particularly in the male population, to a lesser extent in the female population.

VII

General Psychological Issues

Achievement Motivation After Chronic Disease

G. Dahme

Introduction

It is a well-known fact in the field of rehabilitation, that less people go back to work after successful medical treatment than could be expected for medical reasons. For instance, in a group of patients after successful open-heart surgery we found that from the patients with valvular replacements and shunts one-quarter had not yet resumed work in the span between 6 and 32 months after surgery [2].

The psychological reasons that account for this phenomenon are probably not specific for specific diseases. Therefore, it should be fruitful to analyze how chronic diseases could affect the achievement motivational process. The main thesis of this paper is that changes in the process of achievement motivation, that have been functional during the time of illness, tend to persist dysfunctionally even after successful treatment.

Further analysis is based on the theory of achievement motivation in the version of Heckhausen [10]. This version is an extension of Atkinson's well-known Expectancy X Value theory of achievment motivation [1] combined with elements of cognitive attribution theory [24]. More than 20 years of intensive research in the realm of this theory have yielded an impressive body of theoretical and empirical findings, which should be used to analyze and solve problems in applied fields.

In the first section the model will be explained, followed by a description of those parameters of the theory that could be affected by chronic disease. Which of them are affected, is an empirical question that should be answered by future research. In the final section some suggestions will be made about therapeutic implications in the rehabilitative process.

A Cognitive Model of Achievement Motivation

A motivational process can be described, according to Heckhausen [10], as a mental anticipation of the possible outcomes of activities one can carryout and of the consequences of these activities. An individual will perform the activity, out of several possible ones, that leads to the most favorable anticipated outcomes. Favorability in this sense depends (1) on the perceived probability, that an activity will lead to an outcome, (2) on the degree of perceived instrumentality of an outcome for the consequences, and (3) on the incentive value of the consequences.

Psychopathological and Neurological Dysfunctions Following Open-Heart Surgery. Ed by Becker et al

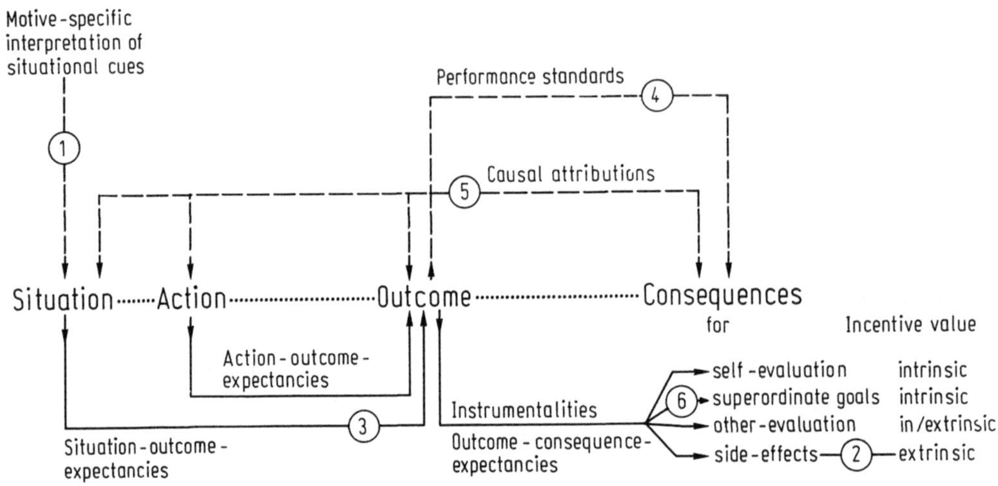

Fig. 1. A process model of achievement motivation. 1–6, parameters that could be affected by chronic disease

Strength and persistence of achievement motivation thus depend on three subjective variables: expectancies, instrumentalities, and incentive values. Interindividual differences in the achievement motive influence these three parameters.

Heckhausen [10] has shown that an acitivity outcome brings about, as a rule, several kinds of consequences, that one outcome has different instrumentalities for different consequences, and that the same outcome has different consequences for different individuals. Figure 1 shows the main parameters in the temporal sequence of a motivational process (adapted from 10).

It starts with a situation that contains cues that could be relevant for different motives (achievement, power, affiliation, aggression etc.). If an individual appraises them as achievement-demanding, he will try to anticipate the possible outcomes of his possible activities (action-outcome-expectancies). Furthermore, he can expect that the situation will lead to a desired outcome apart from his own contributions (situation-outcome-expectancies).

An outcome may have immediate or delayed consequences: self-evaluative consequences are immediate, consequences for superordinate goals, for other-evaluation, and for other motives (extrinsic side effects) are delayed.

The incentive values of consequences depend (1) – in the case of self-evaluation and superordinate goals – on comparisons between the actual outcome of one's striving and performance standards, which are derived from the person's self-concept of own abilities, (2) on mediating cognitive processes which determine if an individual attributes the outcome to internal/external, stable/variable, and intentional/unintentional causes; these processes of causal attribution determine the incentive values of consequences, and (3) on their instrumentality for attaining superordinate goals.

For instance, if an outcome, compared with subjective performance standards, is classified as a failure, and if this failure is attributed internally, that is, as caused by the actor himself, and variable, that means to insufficient effort, it will elicit unfavorable self-evaluations and the affective reaction of shame, but will not affect performance standards for further trials. The incentive value of these consequences, moderated by the individual's achievement motive, will motivate further achievement striving.

Influences of Chronic Disease on Parameters of the Motivational Process (Theoretical Analysis)

It is suggested that achievement motivational differences between patients with chronic diseases and healthy persons could be anchored in one or several of the following six parameters of the motivation process:

1. motive-thematic interpretation of situational cues,
2. incentive weight of extrinsic side effects,
3. situation-outcome-expectancies,
4. performance standards, depending on self-concept of abilities,
5. causal attributions and,
6. instrumentality for attaining superordinate goals.

Motive-Thematic Interpretation of Situational Cues

People differ in their interpretation of situational cues according to their dominant motivational value dispositions. A strongly achievement-motivated person may interpret situational cues as achievement-thematic, while another, high in need for affiliation, may appraise the same situation as a release for affiliative activities.

The individual hierarchy of motives determines to which type of cues an individual is especially sensitive.

It is suggested here that chronic disease can affect this hierarchy in such a way that the achievement motive loses importance mainly for the benefit of the affiliative motive.

In the life of healthy persons achievement behavior plays an important role in assuring adequate living conditions. For an impaired chronic patient affiliative behavior may often be a better guarantee for attaining this goal. Thus, attaining social support could become functionally equivalent to achievement striving.

This would explain a decrease in achievement-motivates behavior.

Incentive Weight of Extrinsic Side Effects

This parameter is related to the first one and refers-to the individual's susceptibility to incentives of other than achievement-related motive classes.

A performance in a task has not only achievement-relevant, i.e. intrinsic consequences, but also extrinsic ones. Depending on the individual's hierarchy of motives, these extrinsic side effects can get higher incentive weights than the achievement-related effects. This effect is not detrimental to achievement behavior since it associates performance with the individual's dominant motive class. As Kleinbeck and Schmidt [13] have shown, achievement behavior can be elicited by other than achievement-thematic incentives [22]. People can work hard in their job, not because they want information about their own ability (self-evaluative consequence) or because they are striving for an occupational career (consequence for superordinate goal), but because they want to be accepted (affiliative goal) by their colleagues or because they want to gain power over them. This effect should be used in interventional programs.

Situation – Outcome – Expectancies

Situation – outcome – expectancy refers to the perceived probabilty that the situation will lead to a desired goal without any action on the actors' side.

A patient who expects to earn his living without own achievement activities but by benefit, will not be very motivated to go back to work.

Performance Standards, Depending on Self-Concept of Abilities

Performance standards are defined as subjective probabilities of success in the light of the individual's previous performance history. They act as norms for self-evaluation. Success or failure in an achievement task are defined as perceived discrepancy between the individual's aspiration level or norm standard and the achieved outcome.

Performance standards are derived from self-evaluation of one's competence for a task in question.

It can be assumed that a chronic disease lowers the probability of success for tasks in many areas. To avoid constant experience of failure and its tremendeous self-diagnostic implications most patients will adapt their aspiration level and the corresponding concepts of own competence [18]. As Hallermann and Meyer [8] have shown empirically, the individual's persistence after continuous failure – (an indicator of strength of motivation) is lower, the lower the individual's perceived competence for the task is. The theory of achievement motivation, especially in the version of Meyer [17], further predicts that individuals in the situation of free choice will prefer tasks of intermediate *subjective* difficulty. That means that a person with a low concept of own abilities will prefer tasks of very low *consensual* difficulty [18].

It is evident that occupational rehabilitation after successful medical treatment requires a rise in standards of comparison for own performance, paralleled by alternations of the self-concept of own abilities.

Alterations of the self-concept are not automatic consequences of changed performance. If a performance affects a self-concept at all it depends on mediating cognitions, by which the individual decides if it has diagnostic relevance for the self-concept (and has not occurred randomly for instance).

Epstein [3, 4] has proposed seeing the self-concept as part of an individual's theory about reality. The self-concept contains theories about one's own traits and abilities. Persons with high self-esteem are characterized by favorable theories about themselves.

The individual treats empirical informations about his own abilities like a scientist: he tries to save his theory even in the light of opposing evidence. A person with high self-esteem who fails in an important examination will try to save his favorable self-concept and therefore attribute his failure to external circumstances.

Laymen as well as researchers will try to assimilate theory-inconsistent information before they are willing to change their theories. This mechanism explains the self-reinforcing properties of the motivational process. They immunize the self-concept partly against change and thus make therapeutical interventions so difficult [9, 21].

Causal Attributions

The incorporation of attribution theory into the theory of achievement motivation by Weiner [23] resulted in a cognitive reinterpretation and specification of the two main parameters of the Atkinson model: expectancy and incentive value.

The basic idea of this attributional version is not that the mere achievement outcome determines incentive values and expectancies of future outcomes, but that these effects are mediated by causal attributions.

The mere discrepancy between a performance standard and an achievement outcome does not lead to specific responses: What is important though is how the individual ascribes these discrepancies. Individuals allocate the causes of success and failure mainly to four sources: ability, effort, task difficulty, and luck or random occurrences. These sources are contained within two causal dimensions: locus of control (internal vs external) and stability (fixed vs variable).

This systematization is well-accepted, but produces difficulties if the question is asked regarding how attributions of failure on chronic disease could be classified.

In Weiner's as well as in Heckhausen's and Gergen's publications hints can be found that at least one further (nonorthogonal) dimension should be added. Heckhausen [11] calls it international vs nonintentional, Gergen [7] voluntary vs non-voluntary. According to Heckhausen [11] attributions to disease are attributions to variable and nonintentional factors, but it is unclear whether they are internally or externally ascribed.

If a disease is not transitory but chronic, it should be regarded as a stable factor.

Attribution theory makes clear predictions only about the effects of attributions to the locus of control as well as to the stability dimension.

Table 1. Perceived determinants of success and failure. (24, p. 240)

	Locus of control	
Stability	Internal	External
Fixed	Ability	Task difficulty
Variable	Effort	Luck

Stability Dimension

Attributions to this dimension affect the individual's proneness to shift expectancies of success following success or failure. Since attribution to chronic disease means attribution to a relatively stable factor, the individual will have to change his expectancies. In the case of failure that means to lower them.

Locus-of-Control Dimension

Attributions to this dimension have self-evaluative consequences. These cognitive consequences are accompanied by or lead to [26] affects of shame and pride.

Internal causal attributions influence the individual's self-concept. According to Stroebe [21] an individual has a tendency to ascribe those experiences internally that are consistent with his self-esteem (thus stabilizing it).

External causal attributions have no relevance for the self-concept and may prevent an individual from lowering his appraisal of own abilities.

What does it mean, if a patient attributes his failure to his chronic disease? Is that an internal or an external attribution?

The answer depends on the patient's view of his disease. The patient who feels that the disease has partly changed his identity, and who is identified with the role of a chronic patient, will interpret attributions to disease as internal attributions and correspondingly will develop the self-concept of a 'disabled'.

On the other hand, if a patient sees himself as exposed to a disease, to something that is beyond own influence and control, and that does not affect his 'real self', he will attribute failure to an external factor and not derive self-evaluative consequences.

Probably, the duration of illness plays a decisive role in the perception of diseases as stable and internal. Congenital diseases, for instance, should lead to internal ascriptions, since a concept of 'real healthy self' could not be built up.

Dimension of Internationality

Attribution of an outcome to this dimension means to attribute responsibility for an activity to the actor.

In our culture most diseases are thought to be caused unintentionally; the patient is not regarded as being responsible for performance impairments attributed to the disease (psychoanalytical interpretations of diseases are exceptions to this rule: with the construct of unconscious intentionality they attribute responsibility and possibility of control).

Weiner et al. [26] suggested that ascription of responsibility is associated with a feeling of control over the situation. That means that intentionality is not orthogonal to the other two dimensions but could have a moderating effect on them. Ascription of unintentionality probably means that internally attributed outcomes do not elicit the usual feeling of shame after failure. Weiner's datas are not inconsistent with this conception [26, p. 163].

If attribution on unintentionality and internality impedes feelings of shame, the assumed dependency of affect from cognitions is much more complicated that Weiner et al. [26] assumed.

What effect does an attribution of failure have on disease if disease is perceived as an internal, stable, and unintentional cause?

The patient perceives himself to be the cause of failure and will therefore develop a very unfavorable concept of own abilities, without perceiving any possibility of change accompanied by the feeling of having no control over the situation.

As Weiner et al. [26] have shown, affects like hopelessness, helplessness, and depression are elicited when failure is attributed to stable and internal causes.

According to Klein et al. [12] this attributional pattern produces the well-known constellation of learned helplessness [20]. Frese [5] has described (for patients after infarctions) passivity as a reaction to the perception that activity and outcome of activity are unrelated.

Both types of possible conceptions of chronic disease as a cause of failure (internal, stable, unintentional or external, stable, unintentional) lead to a low level of achievement motivation.

Instrumentality of Outcome for Attaining Superordinate Goals

Individual differences in achievement motivation are associated with differences in the structuredness and time span of future orientation.

Raynor [19] has developed the concept of contingent vs noncontingent action paths to superordinate goals. He assumes that individuals who perceive their path as contingent will exhibit higher levels of motivation for each task on the way, than those who perceive it as noncontingent. A path is called contingent when immediate success is known to guarantee the opportunity for further striving for the end goal, and immediate failure is known to mean loss of opportunity to continue in the path. A prerequisite for the establishment of contingent paths is the feeling of control over the factors relevant for goal attainment.

Obviously, patients will be objectively and will feel subjectively impeded by their disease regarding the development of a structured and contingent future orientation. The factors that determine goal attainment are partly or totally out of their control and less dependent on their competence or effort expenditure than on their illness-dependent physical state.

According to the Heckhausen model this will affect the perceived instrumentality of an outcome for superordinate goals. Decrease in instrumentality lowers the resultant action valence (that means: the achievement motivation for a task).

Directions for Interventional Strategies

Interventions could be necessary in the case where a patient does not change his achievement-motivational behavior in an appropriate time span after successful medical treatment. As was outlined earlier in this paper, people do not automatically accommodate their theories about their abilities to take into account new experiences.

In these cases the parameter that is responsible for this effect should be identified. The final section gives some suggestions as to how it could be influenced.

1. Insensitivity to situational cues that are achievement relevant should be influenced by techniques that McClelland [16] used to train entrepreneurs in India. In one part of the complex training procedure they learned to recognize achievement-related ideas in their own TAT stories, to score them according to the nAch key, and to write stories higher in nAch. Furthermore they learned to discriminate between achievement and otherthematic fantasies. The aim of this part of the program was to influence the individual to think in achievement-thematic terms.
2. An attempt should be made to identify which is or has become the dominant motive in the individual's hierarchy. During the process of development – together with the patient – of a contingent path (see 6.), special attention should be given to the question of how the different steps in the path could be chosen in order to maximize satisfaction by extrinsic side effects.
   This is especially important for the development of occupational end goals.
3. If high situation-outcome expectancies lead to a decrease in achievement-related activities, and if these expectancies are realistic, the only measure that promises success lies in destroying them.
   This is especially relevant if a patient realistically perceives his chances of getting his old age pension prematurely.
   Doctors should be careful not to grant a certificate stating that the patient is not able to work, too easily.
4. and 5. The literature on training programs to change a person's achievement motive from a dominance of fear of failure to hope of success is sumarized by Krug and Hanel [14]. All successful programs tried to influence at least these three parameters:
   - Goal setting
   - Causal attribution
   - Self-reinforcement.

Realistic goal setting has to do with performance standards (parameter 4) and the development of contingent achievement paths (parameter 6), while causal attribution refers to the fifth parameter and self-reinforcement strategies refer to the self-evaluative consequences of performance.

Since these concepts are closely related, they will be discussed here together.

The three parameters should be altered by interventional programs in the direction of realistic performance standards, appropriate causal attributions and proper administration of self-reinforcement [14]. The goal of all interventional activities should be the establishment of a changed self-regulatory system.

It is not the place here to describe special techniques. The general approach should be guided by conceptions which were developed in the frame of cognitive behavior therapy. Mahoney [15] characterizes the main idea of this approach: a patient should be equipped with the same tool to solve his personal problems that we as empirical scientists have to solve ours. The patient should be trained to observe his behavior as well as his intermediating cognitions, to analyze them in terms of aspiration levels, patterns of causal attribution etc., to formulate hypotheses about his abilities, to test them by achievement striving, to compare the outcome with appropriate standards of comparison, to alter or to revise his self-theory etc. The aim should be to make him an expert for his own achievement problems. Special techniques for this device can be adapted from cognitive therapies. Krug and Hanel [13] have applied them successfully and attained changes in all three parameters.

6. How could psychotherapeutic assistance facilitate the acquisition of appropriate future orientation?
   From Raynor's model can be derived the fact that achievement motivation for a task rises with the number of steps in a contingent path, that success motivation is associated with long, contingent paths, and that at the beginning of a path high prohabilities of success should be preferred. Thus, strategies should be derived to formulate or recognize paths that fulfill these requirements and to assess the instrumentalities of a single outcome for a superordinate goal.
   Raynor [11] believes that it is more important to know the general structure of such a plan than to fill it with concrete content.

As Krug and Hanel [14] in his review of therapeutic programs concluded, only those programs that could be embedded in the daily life of the individuals had lasting influences on real-life behavior. But before the suggested interventions should be applied, more research is necessary to clarify (1) the empirical question of which of the six parameters plays the most important role in insufficient achievement striving, and (2) the theoretical question of how premorbid motivational differences superpose the parameters discussed here.

References

1. Atkinson JW, Feather NT (eds) (1964) A theory of achievement motivation. Wiley, New York
2. Dahme G, Dahme B, Kornemann J, Vollers A, Huse-Kleinstoll G (1980) Fulfillment of patient's expectation concerning outcome of open heart surgery. In: Speidel H, Rodewald G, (eds) Psychic and neurological dysfunctions after open-heart surgery. Thieme, Stuttgart pp 228–236
3. Epstein S (1973) The self-concept revisited, or a theory of a theory. Am Psychol 28:404–416
4. Epstein S (1979) Entwurf einer integrativen Persönlichkeitstheorie. In: Filipp S-H (ed) Selbstkonzeptforschung. Klett-Cotta, Stuttgart, pp 15–46
5. Frese M (1978) Coping strategies in work and illness: A pilot study. Bielefelder Arbeiten zur Sozialpsychologie, no 36
6. Gergen KG (1979) Selbsterkenntnis und die wissenschaftliche Erkenntnis des sozialen Handelns. In: Filipp S-H (ed) Selbstkonzeptforschung. Klett-Cotta, Stuttgart, pp 75–96
7. Gergen KJ, Gergen MM (1978) Attribution im Kontext sozialer Erklärungen. In: Görlitz D, Meyer W-U, Weiner B (eds) Bielefelder Symposium über Attribution. Klett-Cotta, Stuttgart, pp 221–238
8. Hallermann B, Meyer WU (1978) Persistenz in Abhängigkeit von wahrgenommener Begabung und Aufgabenschwierigkeit. Arch Psychol (Frankf.) 130 (4):335–341 (Ehs Abstr.)
9. Heckhausen H (1972) Die Interaktion der Sozialisationsvariablen in der Genese des Leistungsmotivs. In: Gaumann CF (ed) (Handbuch der Psychologie, Sozialpsychologie. Hogrefe, Göttingen vol 7/2, pp 955–1092)
10. Heckhausen H (1977) Achievement motivation and its constructs: A cognitive model. Motivation, Emotion 1:284–329
11. Heckhausen H (1978) Kommentar zum Beitrag von Weiner, Russell u. Lermann. In: Görlitz D, Meyer W-U, Weiner B (eds) Bielefelder Symposium über Attribution. Klett-Cotta, Stuttgart, pp 175–180
12. Klein DC, Fencil-Morse E, Seligman MEP (1976) Learned helplessness, depression and the attribution of failure. J Pers Soc Psych 33:508–516

13. Kleinbeck U, Schmidt K-H (1976) Die Analyse leistungsbezogener Verhaltenssequenzen: Der Instrumentalitätsaspekt. In: Schmalt H-D, Meyer W-U (eds) Leistungsmotivation und Verhalten. Klett, Stuttgart, pp 61–80
14. Krug S, Hanel J (1976) Motivänderung: Erprobung eines theoriegeleiteten Trainingsprogramms. Z Entwicklungspsychol Päd Psychol 8:274–287
15. Mahoney MJ (1974) Cognition and behavior modification. Ballinger, Cambridge/Mass
16. McClelland DC (1965) Toward a theory of motive acquisition. Am Psychol 20:321–333
17. Meyer W-U (1976) Leistungsorientiertes Verhalten als Funktion von wahrgenommener eigener Begabung und wahrgenommener Aufgabenschwierigkeit. In: Schmalt H-D, Meyer W-U (eds) Leistungsmotivation und Verhalten. Klett, Stuttgart pp 101–136
18. Moulton RW (1974) Motivational implications of individual differences in competence. In: Atkinson JW, Raynor JO (eds) Motivation and achievement. Winston, Washington pp 77–82
19. Raynor JO (1974) Future orientation in the study of achievement motivation. In: Atkinson JW, Raynor JO (eds) Motivation and achievement. Winston, Washington pp 121–154
20. Seligman MEP (1975) Helplessness. Freeman, San Francisco
21. Stroebe W (1978) Selbstwertgefühl und Attribution: Individuelle Unterschiede in der Ursachenerklärung von Erfolg und Mißerfolg. In: Görlitz D, Meyer W-U, Weiner B (eds) Bielefelder Symposium über Attribution. Klett-Cotta, Stuttgart pp 93–104
22. Vroom VH (1964) Work and motivation. Wiley, New York
23. Weiner B (1972) Theories of motivation. Markham, Chicago
24. Weiner B (1974) Achievement motivation and attribution theory. General Learning, Morristown
25. Weiner B, Heckhausen H, Meyer W-U, Cook RE (1972) Causal ascription and achievement behavior: Conceptual analysis of effort and reanalysis of locus of control. J Pers Soc Psychol 21:239–248
26. Weiner B, Russell D, Lerman D (1978) Affektive Auswirkungen von Attributionen. In: Görlitz D, Meyer W-U, Weiner B (eds) Bielefelder Symposium über Attribution. Klett-Cotta, Stuttgart pp 139–174

The Fantasy of Resurrection and Rebirth in Cardiac Surgery Patients

R.S. Blacher

Introduction

Every culture considers death as an altered state of life. It is striking that in no recorded society, whether primitive or advanced, is death thought of as an actual termination of being. Some cultures conceptualize an afterlife as occurring in a geographical heaven or hell; others picture the dead as becoming free-dwelling spirits. Death may also be thought of as an eternal sleep or other altered state of consciousness, at times pleasant, at times uncomfortable.

Man's interest in death, immortality, resurrection, and afterlife, was always considered the realm of the theologican and philosopher, and later the anthropologist, until Freud's *Totem and Taboo* [5] and *Thoughts for the Times on War and Death* [6] brought the study of these matters into the psychological field. Freud stated: "It is indeed impossible to imagine our own death; and whenever we attempt to do so, we can perceive that we are in fact still present as spectators . . . in the unconscious everyone of us is convinced of his own immortality." [6, p. 289] Freud traced the sense of immortality to man's need to retain the people lost to death. Man accepted the reality of death but denied its significance as annihilation. Thus, Freud speculated, did man invent spirits. Other writers [9] have suggested that the idea of immortality is an adaptive attempt to deal with a major anxiety, that of dying. The idea of heaven is seen as a regressive symbiotic reunion with the archaic mother, as a defense against loss.

An afterlife is one form of immortality. Another variant is seen in the ability to return from death, either through reincarnation or from a geographical afterworld. Reincarnation is usually open to anyone in a culture, whether in Asian religions or in the beliefs of South Pacific islanders. Here the soul returns by being born in the body of a new baby. A form of resurrection open usually only to mythological heroes is that of returning from the afterworld. For example, in Greek mythology, Orpheus was almost able to rescue his beloved Euridyce by descending into the underworld to bring her back. Certain Oceanian groups believe that *all* the dead have a choice of returning or not at certain stages in their afterlife. [7, p. 461]. The New Testament anticipates the day of judgement when all souls will return from heaven to join their earthly bodies, but this must be considered a special case, since it is not considered an ongoing process.

The direct return of the dead to life is a most dramatic form of resurrection. The raising of Lazarus by Jesus and Jesus' own resurrection are among the most vivid

Psychopathological and Neurological Dysfunctions Following Open-Heart Surgery Ed. by Becker et al.

episodes in the Bible. They affirm to the believer the immense power of a god and especially his power to grant immortality.

Resurrection in the form of rebirth, that is, being born again in the same body, is a phenomenon noted in most cultures. In primitive societies, puberty initiation rites are often marked by the children being symbolically killed, mourned by their parents, and then reborn as adults who know the ritual secrets of the group. They may even emerge from a womb-like structure as part of the ceremony. [3, pp. 9, 36] These rites and other forms of rebirth noted in the religious, anthropological, or psychological literature refer to *symbolic* rebirth. A lifting of a grief or depression, resulting in a revival of interests, may be referred to as a psychological rebirth. A revival of interests, may be referred to as a psychological rebirth. A revival of religious fervor may result in someone becoming a "born-again Christian".

The story of Jonah and the Whale, wherein the hero is disgorged from the belly of a monster, is reflected in stories from many cultures – several ancient Finnish myths involve this same theme, as do widespread variations in myths of Oceania. These stories seem to express both a descending into the netherworld and into the womb, and of course, a rebirth.

We can see a recurrent, universal preoccupation with life after death and resurrection, which is, as noted, assigned to myth, religious belief, and symbolism. In recent years, we have encountered a new phenomenon, namely resuscitation after cardiac arrest. Modern techniques have made such a procedure a common place in our hospitals, but it continues to be a dramatic episode and the usual newspaper report of such an event states, "Person dies – is brought back to life". Here we see the conceptualization of the situation as actual death, since death is equated with the cessation of the heartbeat. Nor is this restricted to the naive. A sophisticated surgeon brought this to my attention when he could not sleep the night before cardiac surgery. He knew that they would stop his heart and maintain his circulation with a pump. "I know that they keep your vital functions going, but with your heart stopped, you're really dead," he said. This vignette also illustrates how heart surgery adds another dimension to cardiac arrest. In surgery, the stopping of the heart is anticipated and contemplated. Rather than having to deal with a sudden, massive trauma, that of cardiac arrest, the surgical patient has a chance to anticipate the situation and leisurely elaborate his fantasies.

For reasons to be discussed below, such patients often show elements of rebirth fantasies as well as thoughts of resurrection. In my experience, sudden-arrest patients deal almost exclusively with thoughts of resurrection with only a rare reference to rebirth phenomena. I will discuss both resurrection and rebirth together, since they usually overlap. References to the fantasy of rebirth are usually not, in these patients, directly expressed, whereas the idea of return from death is explicitly stated. There have been some exceptions, of patients referring to themselves as "reborn", especially in the early days of cardiac surgery. Fox et al. [4, p. 205] described a very dependent man who sent the surgeon a card on Mother's Day, signed, "Your reborn son". We also noted a patient who referred to the day of operation as his "birthday". [8] But most references are indirect as the following examples will indicate.

In discussing his concept of surgery, a man was asked how he thought the surgeon restarted his heart. He replied: "Well, I know they don't pick you up by the heels and spank you."

A 55-year-old woman with a valve replacement spontaneously remarked after surgery: "I hope the operation lasts and doesn't need redoing every 9 months."

A 62-year-old man was temporarily confused after surgery and wasn't sure where he was. When I asked him to guess, he remarked: "I'm either in Children's Hospital or the Boston Lying-In" (a maternity hospital).

References to *giving* birth are seen in the following cases.

A 65-year-old woman turned to me as soon as she could speak after surgery, and asked: "Was it natural or did I need a Caesarean?"

"How many children did I have?" asked a 60-year-old woman after a mitral valve replacement.

A 58-year-old woman became psychotic shortly after a valve replacement. Her family pointed out that the psychotic state closely resembled the picture she presented during two postpartum breakdowns. Following the deliveries, and before the heart operation, she had weathered several major general surgical procedures without psychological difficulty, so the mere fact of surgery in general did not seem the precipitating factor. Here one may speculate that the patient represented both the mother who delivered and the reborn baby itself.

The first three of the above cases suggest a fantasy of being reborn after dying during the operation and being brought back to life. The task of the cardiac surgery patient is unique. In general surgery, the patient fears that his heart will stop and he will therefore die. The cardiac patient accepts the idea of his heart being stopped; his worry concerns whether it can be started again. By his lights, he will die and be resurrected in *reality*, not symbolically. Patients commonly point out that, "when you're being operated on and your heart is stopped, you're dead."

Most patients do not spontaneously voice their fears before surgery, but instead employ the useful mechanism of denial. When one man referred to several incidents of preoperative cardiac arrest as "dying and being brought back to life", I suggested he sounded afraid of dying. His reply was: "Why should you worry about something that may never happen." Some patients, however, find that their fears of dying make it impossible for them to accept the operation.

A 46-year-old chemist came for consultation because of her disabling ambivalence over a suggested coronary bypass procedure. Her severe angina pectoris made an active life impossible, yet for reasons she could not understand, she was sure she would die during the surgery she so eagerly desired.

Raised a Catholic, she had given up her religion during her middle teens over her father's objections. Her mother had died of heart disease when she was 10, and she spoke warmly of the close relationship with her. An only child, she was doted on by both parents, but the father was never able to be the special person her mother had been.

She talked of her knowledge of the surgical procedure and kept returning to the stopping and starting of the heart. "When the heart stops, it's dead. Not you, but your heart." When, in the second hour, she began to reminisce about the wonderful early experiences with her mother, I suggested that her fear of surgery was due to the fantasy that when her heart was stopped, her soul would leave her body, go to heaven, and join her dead mother; then when the surgeon restarted the heart, she would be in conflict between staying in heaven with the mother or returning to life. To this rather wild-sounding interpretation, she responded with an eager nod and stated: "You hit it on the head." She was relieved that it was something one could talk about, and after this discussion, she could accept the operation calmly.

In a later interview with students and residents, the patient volunteered: "I'll tell you what Dr. Blacher thinks – that I'll die when my heart stops, and I'll rejoin my mother in her womb."

Here, my statement about the reunion with her mother in heaven was revised to her returning to the womb and thus being born again on the return from surgery. The patient's statement supports the concept of heaven as a symbiotic reunion with the archaic mother. Here the rejoining is at an earlier intrauterine level.

A 53-year-old businessman scheduled for a mitral valve replacement was so anxious prior to surgery that cancellation of the procedure was contemplated. On interview, he revealed that he had avoided the operation for over a year despite increasingly disabling symptoms and was certain that he would not survive, despite reassureances from his physician that the risk was small. He began talking spontaneously of his father who had died when the patient was 12. As he spoke of still missing him, his eyes filled with tears. He had been dreaming of his father for the past several nights. When I told him that he felt he would go to heaven during surgery and then would not know whether he wanted to stay with his father or rejoin his own close-knit family, he immediately responded: "That's *exactly* what I've been thinking." As we discussed his fantasy, the anxiety began to diminish.

A 50-year-old woman had discussed her concern that she would be dead during the time her heart was stopped for a valve replacement. After the operation, she stated that she would have had much less anxiety had the doctors emphasized that she would be oblivious to everything during the surgery. She was quite surprised that she had experienced nothing. "I can't stand the sight of gory things," she noted. Since she had been completely anesthetized during previous operations, her concern about being aware while on the table was puzzling until she then told of a friend who had "died during a heart attack." During an episode of apparent cardiac arrest, he had experienced a sensation of floating above his bed and looking at himself from above. She could verify that with her anticipation that she would die when her heart was stopped, her expectation was of floating above the operating table and being upset by the gory things she would see.

These cases illustrate the medical importance of an awareness of the fantasy of "dying" during cardiac surgery. Because of the biochemical disruption brought on by anxiety, such patients can very well be at a higher risk during any major procedure, since they require more anesthesia and since their increased catecholamine production may create cardiac arrhythmias. For some, the anxiety may even prevent their acceptance of necessary surgery.

Discussion

Cardiac surgery provides an experiment in nature whereby patients are confronted with what the average expectable person would interpret as dying – namely a situation where the heart is stopped and operated upon. Usually, the patient has an opportunity to anticipate and think about the situation. Unlike people who are dying of a chronic illness, these patients are subjected to what I have called "acute dying" [1]. Because they know there is a good chance of recovery, such patients can contemplate death and resurrection, and thus provide an opportunity for us to glimpse the formation of a defensive concept of immortality. Since these patients come from a stable culture with a strong theological outline for life-after-death, one may say that they bring nothing to the situation except their religious backgrounds. However, there are enough idiosyncratic emendations and additions to make one realize that their religious backgrounds may be used in the service of rationalizing a new set of spirits and demons along the lines Freud described in *Thoughts of the Times on War and Death* [6]. Thus the chemist who planned to see her mother in heaven had no intellectual belief in religious ideas, including an afterlife, until confronted with surgery. She reminds us of the wartime comment about there being "no atheists in foxholes" – when faced with the danger of death, the process of immortality formation begins anew. The form it takes is understandably in keeping with one's culture, but also of course in keeping with one's individual development. It is no coincidence that those who talk most concretely about heaven come from a religious tradition where an afterworld is considered a geographical entity, but nevertheless, everyone seems to invent a personalized *dramatis personae* to people that world.

There has been an increasing interest recently in life after death both in the popular literature and, interestingly, in the scientific literature as well [10]. While the devout believer accepts religious dogma concerning heaven and hell on the basis of faith, we find an attempt on the part of some people to prove the existence of an afterlife as a scientific fact. This is not a new endeavor on the part of scientists who *believe* in their religion but at the same time require proof for what they accept in their scientific work. Difficulty in obtaining evidence in this area stems from the fact that return from death is not possible, or wasn't thought so until cardiac resuscitation was developed. Using the old standard for death – of cardiac standstill – one then could say that these patients had died and had been resurrected and thus one could study the effects of the experience. That this "return" represents a wish fulfillment for the examiner is obvious, but it is a wish congruent with our mythology and thus is doubly reinforced. That proof of an afterlife would lower the anxiety concerning death is undoubtedly true. No longer would the playwright have to ponder the questions implicit in: "To sleep, perchance to dream . . ."

The "out-of-body" experiences described so often in the lay literature and illustrated by the patient's friend with cardiac arrest clearly represents a soul leaving the body, and is remiscent of Freud's comment about the invention of spirits [6, p. 294].

The fascination with resurrection goes beyond the question of immortality. It also involves elements of masochistic revenge – "they'll be sorry for how they've treated me" is an underlying theme among certain suicidal patients. This is also an important focus of one of the most intriguing episodes in American literature. In Mark Twain's

Tom Sawyer [11], Tom and his friends have gone off and are presumed dead. At one point, he sneaks home and eavesdrops on his aunt's pain at his loss. The next day, a funeral service is held for the boys and in the midst of hearing their virtues extolled, they stand up in the rear of the church and are joyfully welcomed back. The prohibition against speaking negatively of the dead – *de mortuis nihil nisi bonum* – practically ensured that the deceased would be praised. Those who have felt unappreciated at times – namely all readers – can enjoy vicariously the boys' having everyone feel sorry for their putative deaths.

When Freud wrote that no one can contemplate his own death [6], he was referring to the very mechanisms one sees in the cardiac surgery patients. These patients can think of death because they contemplate a life after dying – either a return to their regular lives or an immortality.

Why, one must wonder, do some surgical patients refer to rebirth rather than resurrection? Many writers in both psychoanalytic and anthropological literature refer to rebirth when the term resurrection would seem to be more precise. In using the term rebirth, I limit myself specifically to references to being or having a newborn child rather than having another chance at living.

I would make some speculative suggestions. The word rebirth suggests something more than a return from the dead. A newborn starts life with a clean slate, and is hopefully free of defects. A resurrected person has another chance, but with the same defective body and organs. Thus, the surgical patient feels about his cardiac repair that he has a new heart, and is therefore as good as new and with the chance of a long life. The surgery becomes for these patients a form of initiation and their return to life parallels the rebirth of the initiate in primitive cultures.

References to rebirth are certainly not limited to cardiac surgery. Other forms of surgery may occasionally elicit such reactions, but not to the same extent. Basch (personal communication) reports two kidney transplant patients who took on new birthdays – one, the date of the surgery, and the other, the date of the donor's birthday. Here, too, the patient starts life anew.

The situation in the intensive care unit following surgery may secondarily reinforce a sense of rebirth. Completely dependent on the ministrations of the nurses, and connected to seemingly magical equipment, the patient may regress beyond the usual state expected with serious illness. We have described elsewhere [2, p. 396] the duplication in the intensive care unit of the early mother-child relationship – with the nurse-mother responding to the patient's needs, even before the patient himself is aware of them. The feeling of being completely taken care of, in a real as well as symbolic sense, enhances a regression to an early symbiotic period of development. Such a state in turn may encourage a sense of immortality. Pollock [9, p. 341] has suggested that: "Paradise, heaven, or the ideal state of the afterlife may thus refer to the idealized initial state of existence. It may be that the regression to this beginning state of symbiosis forms the basis for the immortality belief ..." An opportunity to relive the archaic infantile relationship, despite the pain attendant upon the experience, can thus reinforce a sense of both immortality and starting life anew.

We have been struck by how readily cardiac surgery patients will talk about their ideas of dying and resurrection once they are led to believe that these topics are proper ones for discussion. It is not unusual for our patients to state bluntly that they will be dead, during the operation. Previous observers have focused on the *fear* of dying under these circumstances, and this is quite understandable since these operations seem so much more dangerous than they actually are. While the actual mortality rate in an uncomplicated coronary bypass operation, for example, is less than 1%, most cardiac patients will estimate that they have a 50:50 chance for survival. This represents not only the emotional importance of the heart, but also the unique on-off quality of the organ; it either beats and one lives, or it stops and one dies. Thus, the fear is based more on the special position of the heart in the psychic life of man than on the surgical hazards.

It is not easy at first to listen to these fantasies, and the natural impulse is to reassure the patient when he begins to talk of the mortal dangers of surgery. If the patient is allowed to continue however, he will provide the listener with a glimpse of an immortality-fantasy in the process of formation.

This fantasy of death is the central issue for many, if not most of our patients undergoing cardiac surgery. Improved techniques will hopefully diminish the cerebral insults imposed by surgery and by-pass. Yet the fantasies concerning this central organ, the heart, may not be amenable to our limited interventions and such surgery will therefore be a continuing naturalistic experiment in psychic stress of a particular nature – namely dying and resuscitation.

References

1. Blacher RS (1977) The student physician and 'acute' dying. Archives of the Foundation of Thantology, vol 6, no 3
2. Blacher RS, Joseph ED (1972) Psychological reactions to a cardiac monitor. M Sinai J Med 39/4:390–396
3. Eliade M (1958) Birth and rebirth. Harper & Row, New York
4. Fox HM, Rizzo N, Gifford S (1954) Psychological observations of patients undergoing mitral surgery. Psychosom Med 16/3:186–208
5. Freud S (1912–1913) Totem and taboo. Standard edition 13:1–161. Hogarth, London, 1955
6. Freud S (1915) Thoughts for the times on war and death. Standard edition 14:274–300. Hogarth, London, 1957
7. Luquet G-H (1959) Mythology of oceania. In: Larousse encyclopedia of mythology. Prometheus, New York, pp 457–479
8. Meyer BC, Blacher RS, Brown F (1961) A clinical study of psychiatric and psychological aspects of mitral surgery. Psychosom Med 23:194–218
9. Pollock GH (1975) On mourning, immortality, and utopia. J Psychoanal Assoc 23/2:334–362
10. Stevenson I, Greyson B (1979) Near-death experiences, JAMA 242:265–267
11. Twain Mark (1876) The adventures of Tom Sawyer. Harper & Row, New York, London, 1917

Psychodynamic Considerations and Findings About Patient Adjustment to Heart Operations*

Ch. Reimer, B. Flemming, P. Götze, G. Huse-Kleinstoll, H.-J. Meffert, H. Speidel

Introduction

After our year-long experience in the examination of patients shortly before and after open-heart surgery within the framework of the Hamburg research project, we turned our interest toward the patients' long-term responses to the operation. This interest was aroused by the observation that the operation almost always posed a decisive turning point in the patient's life. The concern of the present paper is psychodynamic study of the long-term response to surgery, and the role that the preoperative patient history and the individual psychological structure has played in determining that response. Specifically, in a study *still in progress*, we are seeking to determine whether and to what degree the operation offered the patient a possibility to "live out" his particular neuroses. Furthermore, we were interested in the dynamic parameters of the often strikingly poor psychic rehabilitation and the somatic factors related to it.

Methods and Subjects Under Study

The *preliminary* data presented here come from a still continuing study of patients, who have undergone a somatic as well as a psychological examination 2–4 years after open-heart surgery. The sample under consideration included 30 patients (20 men and 10 women) from 23–63 years of age. The surgical intervention consisted of the replacement of one or more valves in the case of 18 patients (nine men and nine women), and in the case of 12 other patients (11 men and 1 woman) it consisted of the insertion of one or more bypasses. Each of these patients was interviewed within the framework of this study by a psychoanalyst for approximately 90 minutes, with the intention of determining the degree of psycho-social rehabilitation and of ascertaining their personality structure. These interviews were divided among four psychoanalysts working on the investigation. They attempted to conduct the interviews in a casual and nondirected manner, while, at the same time, always taking into consider-

* With the aid of the Deutsche Forschungsgemeinschaft, Sonderforschungsbereich 115, Teilprojekt A3

Psychopathological and Neurological Dysfunctions
Following Open-Heart Surgery. Ed. by Becker et al.

ation certain aspects and problems of primary importance in this study. An essential aspect was the patients' experience of the pre- and postoperative period and those factors closely related to it. These include: specific reactions to the illness, the patient's own perception of his illness, and his feeling of physical well-being. Additionally, we found it important to focus our study on the patients' attitude toward his job, his behavior while doing the job, and his work motivation. Other important factors taken into consideration during interview were any changes in interpersonal relationships, especially those concerning the marriage partner and the immediate family. Early socialization of the patient and his present psycho-social environment were also matters of special concern during the interview. We projected the patients' relationships to the doctors and nurses largely against the background of this data. Of further consideration were the patient's orientation toward his future possibilities and his attitude toward aging and death.

In the course of this study the participating psychoanalysts met weekly to present each new patient and to discuss his or her personality structure and psychodynamics.

Preliminary Results

At first we would like to present two patients, one female valvular patient and one male coronary patient, as exemplary cases and to sketch briefly what seemed to us as two, with regard to sex and diagnosis, relatively typical courses of rehabilitation. To a great extent, these two case histories provide a documentary résumé of this study's results.

Firstly, we will consider the female valvular patient, who is now 62 years of age, and who underwent an operation for a ventricle-septum defect in 1976. A heart defect had already been diagnosed in early childhood, and for this reason her mother strongly instructed her to take extra care of herself. Due to this necessary self-restraint she was unable to participate in many of the activities of her peers, and she felt correspondingly impaired, although she had not yet perceived any of the physical symptoms of her heart ailment. Following a prescribed routine of extra care, she only worked at a half-day job. She had been under the care of a physician from her 25th year of age and had received medicine to strengthen her heart and her circulation, but she experienced the first subjective symptoms of her illness at 45 when she began menopause. At that time she had a cardiac rhythm disturbance and felt impaired in carrying out her everyday household tasks. The deterioration of her heart condition led to a special diagnosis in the university clinic that indicated the need for an operation. The patient had much difficulty in deciding to have the operation, but she informed herself about it and allowed herself to be encouraged by another female heart patient. She recovered from the operation well; after a short period of rehabilitation in a sanatorium, and 5 months after the operation, she was ready to return to her half-day job, where she worked until normal retirement age. She reported that the operation had helped her and that she was in this respect satisfied.

The life history of this patient displays a series of stable interpersonal relationships beginning in her childhood and continuing through her marriage in the relationship with her husband and her daughter. Despite the caution that she had to exercise throughout her life, she valued an exacting job and, in end effect, was able to establish a good compromise between a cautious restraint and a normal working life. Her achievement motivation can be documented with her statement that she never allowed anyone to do her work for her. She was reconciled to herself and to her fate, and she regarded herself as satisfied. As for her psychological structure – she made a friendly impression and exhibited no remarkable neuroses. At times she seemed to avoid conflict situations and to restrain all aggressive impulses, but this can certainly be ascribed to her strict upbringing, which had also left her a bit anxious; these traits were, however, in no way pronounced.

The second case-history which I would like to present to you deals with a 60-year-old man who underwent surgery for coronary stenosis in 1977. Ten years before the operation the patient had already had heart difficulty, of which he refused to take notice. In the year of the operation he suffered a cardiac infarction. Four months after this infarction he was operated on, and after an additional 4 months he returned to his job; for a short period, however, he was forced by a case of hepatitis to discontinue work. Thereafter he was fully employed again, but at a lower position. Before the operation he had held the post of plant director in a small company that employed one-hundred and fifty people, and after the operation he was demoted to the head of plant security. Incidental to his heart infarction had been a period of change within the company that had also affected his position and angered him terribly. He stated that he had been without any particular anxieties previous to the operation, but postoperatively he experienced a temporary psychotic episode. After the operation he noticed some long-term and subjectively, very unpleasant side-effects: especially at the end of a working day he had a feeling of emptiness in his head, and he increasingly avoided unpleasant confrontations and withdrew quickly from tense situations, even from those quite familiar to him. He regarded himself as having become irascible and thin-skinned after the operation, whereas he had viewed himself as cantankerous, direct, hefty, and as one who did not know the meaning of anxiety before the operation. Postoperatively, he was not troubled by occasional heart complications any longer, because he was physically healthy as the result of several follow-up checkups had shown. The operation was not viewed as disappointing in regard to it's organic outcome, but rather in regard to it's psychological outcome, which had surprised the patient and for which he could provide no explanation. In the initial postoperative period the patient attempted to dismiss his nervous symptoms by attributing them to the pain from the wound, but as this pain continued he could no longer hold to this explanation. He reported to us what he had heard about the operation from the other heart patients: that it caused instability and depression, and resulted in a growing intolerance and irascibility.

This patient had been brought up by parents who stressed achievement and motivation, and accordingly he was ambitious in his profession and had been able to draw a great deal of confirmation for his high self-esteem from his success in this area. In light of this achievement, one can easily understand his disappointment with his rehabilitation, because after the operation it resulted in a demotion, a negation of his earlier achievement, and to steady psychological disturbances. During the interview the nervous irritation exhibited by the patient appeared so severe that an emergency ambulant psychiatric treatment was advised. This patient displayed no remarkable neuroses, and his high motivation to succeed derives most certainly from one of the educational ideals of his generation. The heart infarction occurred during an emotion-packed dispute in his area of high achievement, and after the heart infarction a period of low achievement and a lack of confirmation set in, which led to the psychological difficulties that the patient has experienced for the first time in his life.

What the two case-reports discussed here should serve to demonstrate is some of the general differences between valvular and coronary patients in the psychological and professional rehabilitation success. Of 18 valvular patients only five were fully rehabilitated so that they could resume their old working positions; these were, without exception, women. Five other patients, three women and two men, were partially rehabilitated, enabling them to work at least part-time, and eight other patients from this group were not rehabilitated at all. This last group was composed of seven men and one woman. Only half of the coronary patients, one woman among them, was fully rehabilitated, while three were partially rehabilitated, and a final three were not rehabilitated at all.

Regarding only this data one might presume that coronary patients are more satisfied with the outcome of the operation with respect to postoperative rehabilitation. Our interview, however, speaks against this presumption. The majority of the valvular patients expressed satisfaction with the outcome of the operation, while only 1 of the 12 coronary patients expressed a similar satisfaction. Two-fifths of the coronary patients were not satisfied and another two-fifths expressed partial satisfaction. This tendency became even more evident as we proceeded to ask the patients about their contentment with postoperative life in comparison with their preoperative life. Only one coronary patient expressed contentment with his life after the operation, whereas almost all the valvular patients viewed themselves as content postoperatively.

More closely considered this data would seem to indicate that especially the coronary patients saw themselves negatively affected by the long-lasting complications that resulted from the operation. Complaints about continuous cerebro-organic and/or psychic disturbances were registered by the majority of the coronary patients after the operation; only a small part of the valvular patient group registered similar complaints. Among the most commonly reported disturbances was psychic instability characterized by depression, hyper-sensitivity, and general irritability. Especially some of the coronary patients were so dismayed by this development, that during the interview they even suggested that someone should have informed them of the possible side-effects before the operation. Another disturbing aspect, especially for the coronary patients, was seen in the area of sexuality. More than half of the male coronary patients reported chronic sexual problems after the operation. Either they had become impotent, or they had experienced a diminution of their libido. Corresponding sexual problems were reported by a third of the valvular patients mainly among the men.

Another problem that faced mainly the coronary patients was demotion at their place of work after the operation: Half of them had to experience this degradation, while almost all of the valvular patients had no experience with any similar degradation. A large part of our patients were granted an early retirement after the operation. More than half of the valvular patients retired early, two-thirds of them men. Only a quarter of coronary patients were willing to go into retirement. In examining the coronary patients it struck us that almost all of them possessed an extraordinarily high achievement motivation. They had generally rejected the proposal of an early retirement and insisted on returning to work after the operation.

From all the aforementioned factors, it becomes clear that disturbances and complications materialized especially among the male patients, and more especially among the male coronary patients. Unlike the female patients, the male patients often had to experience a degradation on the job; they more frequently received an early retirement, and complained more of long-term psychic, sexual, and/or cerebro-organic disturbances. They were also generally less satisfied with the outcome of the operation than their female counterparts.

Some Final Considerations

One should bear in mind that the data presented here are simply the initial findings of a study which requires a more throughgoing and complete psychoanalytic treatment. Nevertheless some preliminary conclusions can be made on the basis of the data gathered until now: The fact is that men especially have a difficult problem in coping with heart-damage and surgery, and that this problem of coping is more pronounced in the case of coronary patients. Apparently, these men have developed a feeling of uncertainty and insecurity in the understanding of their sex-role due to the serious symptomatic or to the surgical intervention itself. Considering the stress placed on achievement motivation in the socialization of men, it seems understandable that the narcissistic regulation is expected mainly through the gratification offered by achievement "on the job". Correspondingly, the heart symptomatic and the resulting operation present a narcissistic instability in the sense of a crisis in the patients' system of self-evaluation, which can be recognized in his general dissatisfaction with the operation, and in the chronic psychic irritations (for example; depressivity and hyper-sensitivity) and in various sexual disturbances. The fact that after the operation many men are not able to regain 100% of their previous achievement capabilities, seems to present a severe psychological offense to them. This offense appears to be coped with in two manners. Either the patient attempts to reach his old level of achievement as quickly as possible, in order to stabilize himself in the old routine, or the offense is enlarged in scope and dealt with regressively, a procedure followed by those who accept an early retirement. (That is by those who strive for a primary process-oriented, state-mother support as compensation for the psychological offense.)

Unfortunately, it appears to us that our system of social welfare seems to support such efforts by prematurely offering an early retirement to heart patients, which invites even the work-motivated patients to regress and to become resigned.

Acknowledgment. Translation was by E. Hüttenhain.

Patients' Fear of Cardiosurgery and Its Significance for the Pre- and Postoperative State*

B. Flemming, B. Dahme, P. Götze, G. Huse-Kleinstoll, H.-J. Meffert, L. Müller, Ch. Reimer, H. Speidel

Introduction

An imminent operation is, for the patients, an extremely stressful situation which, because of its ominous nature, gives rise to intensive feelings, such as fear of separation or bodily injury and fear of death, but, on the other hand, also the hope of a better future.

We shall report on patients who are about to undergo a heart operation entailing extracorporeal circulation. One particular aspect of this group is that the physical phenomena of the chronic diseases of the heart are allied to severe anxiety in their psychic experience. We are thinking in particular of heart rhythm disturbances, tachycardias, asthma cardiale, effects of angina pectoris and, above all, past infarctions.

In the following, the influence of the variable anxiety on the preoperative state of the patient in the intensive care unit and the surgical ward is to be investigated. This part of the investigation took place within the scope of our Hamburg research project, in which the factors influencing psychic and neurological circulation are investigated.

Two viewpoints led to the investigation of precisely this question:

The first is quite pragmatic: the psychologists and psychiatrists in our team are called into the wards in particular when preoperative patients give the impression to doctors and nurses of being especially anxious.

Apart from the aspect of the additional nursing required, there is the implicit assumption that it is precisely these patients who more frequently become conspicuous in the intensive care unit.

The second is to check the result of Janis·[7], who published one of the first svstematic papers about psychic processes in surgical patients: he found that postoperative psychic disturbances are determined by the extent of preoperative anxiety, although he did not find a linear correlation. In the case of patients with a medium level of preoperative anxiety, the disturbances were fewer than in patients with particularly high and low-anxiety levels.

This corresponds largely to Byrne's [2, 3] concept of anxiety, which represents an attempt to empirically classify anxiety defence mechanisms.

* With the aid of the Deutsche Forschungsgemeinschaft, Sonderforschungsbereich 115, Teilprojekt A3

Psychopathological and Neurological Dysfunctions Following Open-Heart Surgery Ed by Becker et al.

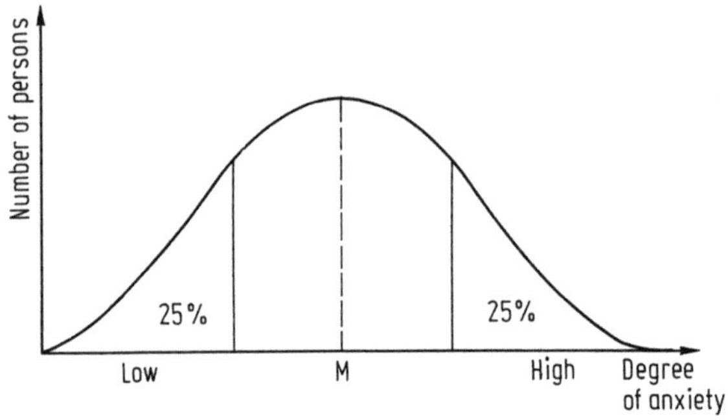

Fig. 1. Separation of low and high anxious patients

Byrne postulated that at every pole of the continuum anxiety, persons are localized who practice an extreme form of anxiety defence: repressers or low-anxiety patients who take as little notice as possible of the stimulus, that is to say, more or less ignore it, and sensitizers who perceive precisely numerous stimuli as a threat and in most cases verbally express the feeling of anxiety thus induced. It is assumed that both coping strategies lead to a reduction in anxiety.

In keeping with this concept, the patients were classified for this investigation, according to the postoperative extent of their anxiety, into extreme groups, after allocation to quartiles. Of a total of 228 persons, 114 patients of boths sexes between the ages of 20 and 65 were subjected to this investigation.

Allocation to extreme groups was made on the strength of the figures in the German translation of the Taylor Manifest Anxiety Scale [13]. A total of 63 patients were qualified as being low-anxiety or repressers, and 51 as high-anxiety or sensitizers.

There were no differences regarding age, sex, and diagnosis group distribution, the duration of the heart disease, and the socio-economic status between the groups. The last mentioned was ascertained with the aid of the details of the patients' schooling, occupation, and the partner's occupation.

The following *procedures* were used to record the pre- and postoperative states of the patients.

Two or three days before the operation, the patients completed the anxiety scale, a personality test (FPI), a mood list, and a complaints list. In addition, they were given a questionnaire on the psycho-social situation drawn up within the scope of the project.

About 10 days after the operation, the patients completed another questionnaire, also drawn up within the scope of the project, about how the intensive care unit was experienced and, for the second time, the complaints list, which is handed out for a third time just before the patient is discharged.

The psychologists assessed the patients before the operation, after an interview lasting 30–60 min, which was semistructured, that is to say, open in the first half, in the second, with the help of key words. The attitude to the operation and the illness as well as the emotional state were the main subject matter.

A corresponding interview, which dealt with, above all, experiences in the intensive care unit, took place about 10 days after the operation.

In the intensive care unit, daily contacts were established on at least 4 days, and the conversation lasted 5–15 min, depending on how much strain the patient could bear. Afterwards the psychologist or psychiatrist completed the psychic findings sheet of the AMDP system [12].

Some Results

Based on results quoted in the literature, for example, Byrne [3], Feder [5], Altrocchi et al. [1], Merbaum [11], and Krohne [8], who say that repressers represent themselves in the sense of social desirability, the following results were obtained with the help of the *t*-test with unilateral questioning.

In the *Personality Questionnaire*, the two groups differ in 11 or 12 scales, in ten of them highly significantly at the 0.1% level, in the scale "Sociability" at the 1% level, and in the scale "aggression" not at all.

The extremely anxious describe themselves as more nervous, more depressive, more excitable, less sociable, more irritable, more dominant, more inhibited, more introverted, more labile and more in keeping with a typically female self-description than the less anxious.

As the FPI measures traits, i.e., personality factors which are relatively stable permanently, the result formulated by Janis leads to the assumption that in most patients the extremely intensive preoperative anxiety can be regarded as an expression of a chronic psychoneurotic disposition and that it is situatively affected only in a few.

The result of the *Mood List*, which measures states, i.e., situative influences on certain personality characteristics, corresponds with the previous result.

The highly anxious describe themselves as more depressed, more anxious, and more passive than low-anxiety patients. This result is significant at the 0.1% level.

In the scale "annoyance" both groups differ at the 1% level. Repressers describe themselves as more irritable, a result which opposes the other description in the sense of social desirability.

In the *Psychologists' preoperative rating* after the interview, which was used with the help of a semantic differential to evaluate personality traits both groups differ in the scale "anxiety" and "disturbability" at the 0.1% level in the trend of their self-descriptions. In addition, the highly anxious are assessed as having less initiative and being less critical and more pessimistic than persons with a low-anxiety score. This difference is significant at the 1% level.

The result shows that the assessment of anxiety by the psychologists and presumably the medical staff, concurs to a large extent with the self-assessment of the patients.

In the *HHM Complaints List*, which like other preoperative procedures, was carried out 2–3 days before the operation, the highly anxious name 29 complaints out of a possible total of 60, i.e., almost half, whereas the low-anxiety patients listed only 12, a result which is noteworthy in view of the even distribution of the somatic data. Some 6–8 days after the operation, the number of complaints by the high-anxiety patients drops from 29 to 20 and rises shortly before discharge to 22, whilst with the

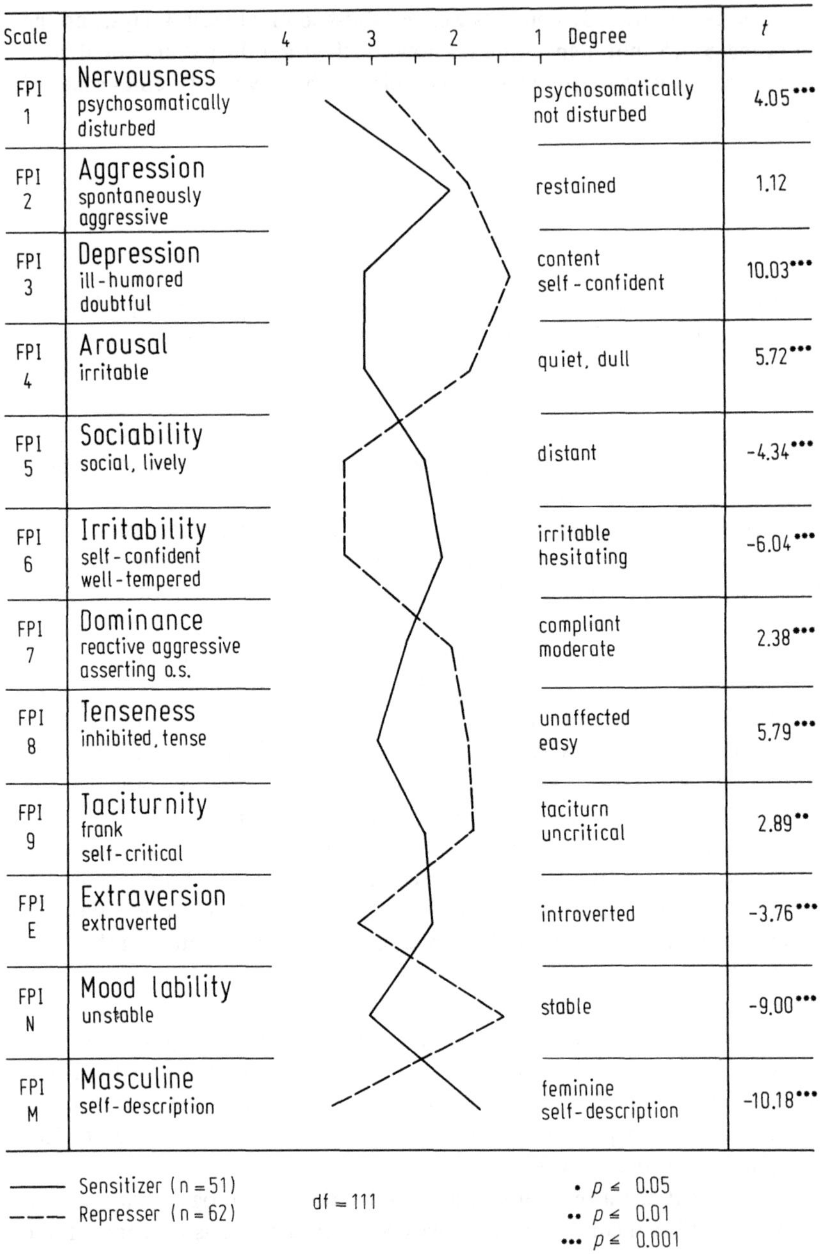

Fig. 2. Mean preoperative FPI profile of sensitizers and repressers. One-tailed t-test of significant differences

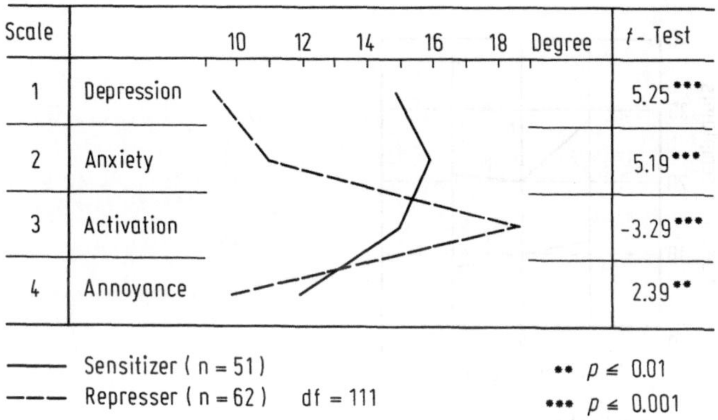

Fig. 3. Mean preoperative mood-list values of sensitizers and repressers. One-tailed t-test of significant differences

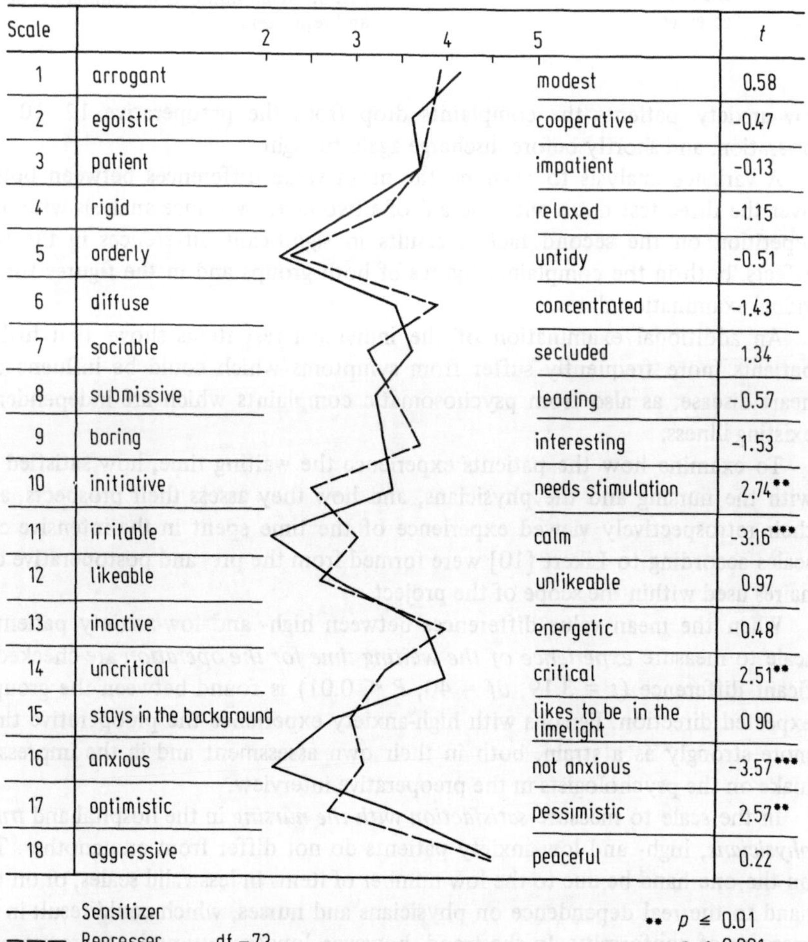

Fig. 4. Mean operative personality-profile (semantic differential) values of sensitizers and repressers. One-tailed t-test of significant differences

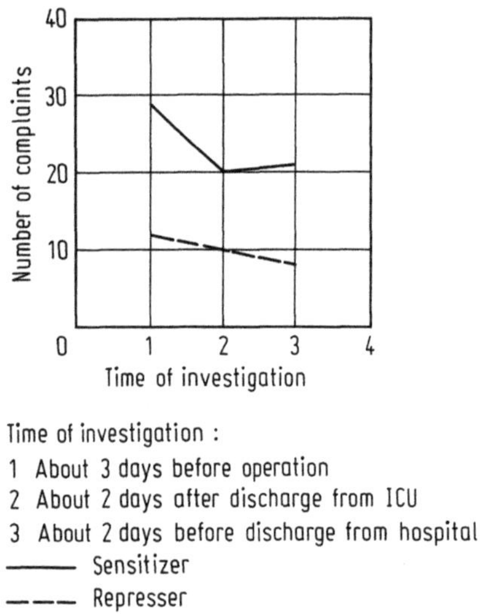

Fig. 5. Mean numbers of complaints of sensitizers and repressers

low-anxiety patients the complaints drop from the preoperative 12–10 after the operation, and shortly before discharge again to eight.

A variance analysis to examine the mean value differences between both groups over the three test dates with the aid of a two factor variance analysis with measuring repetition on the second factor, results in significant differences in the two main effects, both in the complaints figures of both groups and in the figures for the individual examination dates.

An additional examination of the individual test items shows that high-anxiety patients more frequently suffer from symptoms which could be influenced by the heart disease, as also from psychosomatic complaints which are independent of the existing illness.

To examine how the patients experience the waiting time, how satisfied they are with the nursing and the physicians, and how they assess their prospects, as well as their retrospectively viewed experience of the time spent in the intensive care unit, scales according to Likert [10] were formed from the pre- and postoperative questionnaires used within the scope of the project.

When the mean value differences between high- and low-anxiety patients in the scale to measure *experience of the waiting time for the operation* are checked, a significant difference ($t = 3.19$, $df = 40$, $P < 0.01$) is found between the groups in the expected direction. Persons with high-anxiety experience the preoperative time much more strongly as a strain, both in their own assessment and in the impression they make on the psychologists in the preoperative interview.

In the scale to measure *satisfaction with the nursing* in the hospital and *trust in the physicians*, high- and low-anxiety patients do not differ from one another. This may on the one hand be due to the low number of items in less valid scales, or on the other hand to the real dependence on physicians and nurses, which could result in a certain measure of conformity. In the trend, however, low-anxiety patients are more satisfied with the nursing and the physicians than are patients who score higher figures in the anxiety test.

In the scale, *assessment of the future*, it transpires that low-anxiety patients have more detailed plans, the fulfillment of which they look forward to with pleasure, than the high-anxiety patients, who hardly like to think beyond the operation ($t = 3.86$, $df = 33$, $P < 0.001$). This result confirms the expectation that low-anxiety patients assess the future more positively.

Investigation of the *frequency of psychic disturbances* in the intensive care unit showed no significant difference between both groups, contrary to various results in the literature [e.g., 9] according to which these disturbances were more severe in anxious patients.

Comparison of the extent or degree of psychic disturbances does show, however, that in 10 of 11 scales the psychic findings sheet of the AMDP the highly anxious display more severe disturbances than the low-anxiety patients.

For calculation, the highest scale figures, independently of the day on which a disturbance reached its maximum manifestation [4], were used. In the scale "psychomotoric" the two groups differ at the 5% level from each other, in the scales "disturbances of attention", "hypochondriac moods", "paranoia", and "depersonalization", at the 1% level and in the scale "mood disturbances" at the 0.1% level.

This result shows that in the highly anxious in the intensive care unit the disturbances are generally much more obvious, i.e., in 10 of the 11 scales, and this difference becomes significant in six scales.

The retrospective investigation of *how the intensive care unit is experienced*, again with the aid of a scale drawn up like Likert's [10], results in no obvious differences between high- and low-anxiety patients. That the degree of gravity of the various qualities of disturbances is reflected to such a low extent, can possibly be explained by the fact that severe phenomena in the intensive care unit quite frequently go hand in hand with amnesia about this period [6].

When summarizing the results, it becomes obvious that one should approve of or, in fact, encourage the pragmatical viewpoint of the therapeutic interventions in the case of preoperative patients who are particularly anxious, as they appear to be particularly subject to stress both before and after the operation. They suffer from more complaints, experience waiting for the operation more strongly as a strain, are more pessimistic when assessing their future, and display more severe disturbances in the intensive care unit than patients with low-anxiety.

Contrary to the sensitization-repression concept, but concurring with the observations made by Janis, the results suggest that, from an ego-psychological point of view, the highly anxious, or the sensitizers, have less developed ego-functions, that is to say, an unstable defence mechanism, whereas in the case of the low-anxiety patients, or the repressers, although a low level in the sense of the defence organization does in fact exist, they do have, contrary to the sensitizers, a functioning defence mechanism which is suggested by a number of correlations mentioned above concerning ego-functions and special defence mechanisms. The greater ability of the low-anxiety patients to steadfastly adhere to their own points of view is shown by their being less satisfied with the nursing and less trusting in the doctors, as well as having the greater initiative, and a more critical attitude in unilateral rating and this, because of their object-independent capability of reducing anxiety, points apparently to a well internalized early object relationship. The higher figure in the scale "annoyance" in the mood list and their ability to form autonomous concepts for the future point to this. In the case of the highly anxious by contrast, one can expect that, because of the greater object dependence, their anxiety can be reduced by early, personal therapeutic contacts.

Acknowledgments. Translation was by Kathleen Behnke and Richard A. Bird.

References

1. Altrocchi J, Parsons OA, Dickhoff H (1960) Changes in selfideal discrepancy in repressors and sensitizers. J Abnorm Soc Psychol 61:67–72
2. Byrne D (1961) The Repression-Sensitization Scale: rationale, reliability and validity. J Pers 29:334–349
3. Byrne D (1964) Repression-sensitization as a dimension of personality. In: Maker BA (ed) Progress in experimental personality research. Academic Press, New York, 1, pp 170–220
4. Dahme B, Achilles I, Götze P, et al. (1977) Klassifikation psychopathologischer Auffälligkeiten nach Herzoperationen. Thoraxchirurgie 25:245–249
5. Feder CZ (1968) Relationship between self acceptance and adjustment, repression-sensitization and social competence. J Abnorm Soc Psychol 73:317–322
6. Götze P, Dahme B (1980) Psychopathological syndromes and neurological disturbances after open-heart surgery. In: Speidel H, Rodewald G (eds) Psychic and neurological dysfunctions after open-heart surgery. Thieme, Stuttgart (INA vol 19)
7. Janis IL (1958) Psychological stress. Wiley, New York
8. Krohne HW (1975) Angst und Angstverarbeitung. Studientext. Standards Psychologie. Kohlhammer, Stuttgart
9. Layne OL, Yudofsky SL (1971) Postoperative psychosis in cardiotomy patients: The role of organic and psychiatric factors. New Engl J Med 284:518–520
10. Mayntz Th, Holm K, Hübner P (1972) Einführung in die Methode der empirischen Soziologie. Westdeutscher Verlag, Opladen
11. Merbaum M, Badia P (1967) Tolerance of repressors and sensitizers to noxious stimulations. J Abnorm Psychol 72:349–353
12. Scharfetter Ch (1972) Das AMP-System: Manual zur Dokumentation psychiatrischer Befunde. Springer, Heidelberg Berlin New York
13. Taylor JA (1957) A personality scale of manifest anxiety. J Abnorm Soc Psychol 48:285–290

Discussion of Session VII

Blacher and Spiro commented on the significance and incidence of autoscopic phenomena. In these instances the patients will see themselves lying on the operating table, dissociate from themselves and rise up, whether it be in a dream or in a visual hallucination. Neither had ever seen a patient who has had such an experience in the postoperative period after open-heart surgery.

Blacher stressed the need to be very careful about such phenomena because they are often referred to as "out of body" experiences and have been mostly described in the popular press. After cardiac arrest, however, these experiences exist. They are then called near-death experiences. One sees them occurring in cases of loss of consciousness due to slowly induced hypoxia and in large measures in patients who have had open drop ether in surgery.

Spiro's experience with these phenomena is confined to people who have suffered severe cerebral anoxia for some reason and this way apparently the beginnings of brain death. He commented on what occurred on the operating table analyzing dream material of patients post cardiotomy. He thinks that the out of body experience is much closer to derealization and depersonalization. In these one runs into with patients which were constructed around a denying, so-called "hysterical" character structure which he had frequently encountered. Especially if the preoperative management has been poor the patient experiencing a great deal of denial suddenly has to cope with distress and subsequently goes through a period of depersonalization.

Kimball pointed to the significance of the cardiac patient's dream. These dreams were compared to those from other groups of patients as they are as easily obtainable as the patient's life history and provide very important insight into the mind of the patient. Many dreams pre- and postoperatively relate to sexuality. The most common dream in men following successful surgery is that of sexual intercourse. Certainly the motivation of many men in having surgical procedures on their heart is with the hope – sometimes even fantasy – of improving their sexual life and performance. Women frequenly have dreams of pregnancy or giving birth. Kimball suggested that it would be important to look at the dreams of the caretakers, nurses, and surgeons, too, because from his experience he does not know a group of individuals who on the whole are more conscientious, more dedicated, and more involved with their patients than many cardiovascular surgeons.

Concerning the surgeons' courage, their sometimes excessive involvement with their patients, and their constant exposure to stress, Spiro recommended the development of more effective support systems, in terms of nursing staff and special staffing arrangements, as protection not only for the patient but also for the surgeon, who cannot possibly be there to manage all the advice coming from this conference.

As a second topic the resistance to showing patients prior to surgery the equipment, especially pacemakers, which is going to be implanted, was discussed. In Spiro's experience the primary issue was really to do with the surgeons' or any of the technicians, including psychiatrists, segregation of the techniqual aspects, and the scientific aspects from the human side, and one can sort of clip into one mode or the other. When one tries to link the two together it would appear as an impenetrable and perhaps very damaging barrier. Spiro suggested that it also has to do with mysticism, the high-priesthood of the doctors' profession, and that in a way these are his sacred symbols. They tend to overinvest them with the type of fears that patients are going to have of them and show an unwillingness to demystify what it is they do, and yet that very process of demystification, is essential. Therefore, the impressive denial is not in the patients but in the doctor.

Blacher commented on the anxiety about a lot of this equipment, but stated that the surgeons at his university do generally show some of it. The patients are also taken into the ICU before surgery, as with children. He suggested that the anxiety that these things evoke in people beforehand is really very much balanced by the sense of relief that they have afterwards when they know what is going to happen.

Kindling suggested that patients do better if they receive excellent information preoperatively, during the operative procedures, and postoperatively, as is the case in his clinic. All the patients in whom he implanted pacemakers will have held one in the hand or very often will have held one in the hand during the operation, and very often will look at the screen while the electrodes are being positioned.

VIII

Influence of Surgical Technique on Postoperative Neuropsychiatric Complications

Intracranial Hemorrhage and Hematoma Following Open-Heart Surgery

S. Hungxi, Hu Xiaoqin, Li Kongsoon, Guo Jiaquiang, Xu Letien

Introduction

Neurological damage following open heart surgery has been a subject of much concern ever since the employment of cardiopulmonary bypass in cardiac operations. Various lesions including cerebral edema, petechial hemorrhage, focal infarcts, areas of encephalomalacia, and various kinds of emboli [1, 2, 8] have received considerable attention while intracranial hemorrhage and hematoma, especially the large ones, have been comparatively neglected. Only a limited number of cases has been reported [3–7].

In October 1974, we had a patient who developed neurological signs and then became comatose 14 h after open heart surgery. A cerebral embolism was suspected and the patient was kept under close observation; however, the condition worsened and localizing neurological signs became more apparent. When we finally decided to do exploratory craniotomy a huge epidural hematoma was found and evacuated. Owing to extensive brain damage, it was too late to save the patient's life. This incident served to alert both the cardiac and neurosurgeons so that when similar complications arose in further cases we were able to make an earlier diagnosis and institute immediate surgical intervention.

From October 1974 to December 1979, we collected pertinent data on 20 cases of the same kind, two of which were found at autopsy and 18 diagnosed early enough to permit surgical treatment. Their clinical and pathological records have been analyzed, and the pathogenesis, diagnosis, and preventive measures formulated.

Case Analysis

In this series, all except three patients are under the age of 15, the average being 12.9. Their heart diseases and operations are indicated in Table 1. Mild hypothermia alone was employed in one case and hemodilution perfusion technique combined with mild or moderate hypothermia was used in 19; varying amounts of 20% mannitol were added to the perfusate in 16 cases. Moderate to high flow rates were chosen and the recorded perfusion times in 17 cases were not unduly long, averaging 53′19″. At the time of decannulation, the heparin was neutralized with protamine.

The clinical manifestations in 20 cases of intracranial hemorrhage and hematoma can be classified into three groups (Table 2). Group I: five patients failed to awaken

Psychopathological and Neurological Dysfunctions Following Open-Heart Surgery Ed by Becker et al.

Table 1. Types of heart disease and open heart operations in 20 patients

Types of diseases	Operations	No. of cases
A.S.D.	Repair	5
A.S.D. & P.D.A.	Repair & ligation	1
V.S.D.	Repair	9
V.S.D. & P.D.A.	Repair & ligation	1
Tetralogy of fallot	Radical operation	2
M.S. & M.I.	Valve replacement	2

Table 2. Classification of the clinical manifestations of intracranial hemorrhage and hematoma in 20 patients following open heart surgery

Group	Mental state	No. of cases	Clinical manifestations					
			Convulsion	Hemiplegia	Lethargy	Headache	Pupillary changes	Aphasia
I	Comatose	5	4	0	0	0	3	0
II	Semicomatose	3	2	2	3	0	2	0
III	Clear	12	7	6	6[a]	2	10	1

[a] Mentally clear for few hours then became lethargic

from anesthesia; Group II: three patients did not fully regain consciousness but were able to respond to simple requests by nodding or blinking, but they fell into coma rather quickly; Group III: 12 patients fully recovered from anesthesia, but showed neurological signs characterized by lethargy accompanied by progressive deterioration of consciousness and went into coma anywhere from 4–24 h after operation. Lateralizing signs such as focal or generalized seizures, hemiplegia, and unilateral dilatation of pupil appeared (Table 2). Ultrasonic scanning of the cranium was done in seven cases, five of which showed cerebral falx deviated toward the sound side. The spinal puncture done in two cases revealed bloody or blood-tinged cerebrospinal fluid.

During exploratory craniotomy in 18 cases, hematomas and hemorrhage were found in 14 and focal or diffuse hemorrhage in three cases. In another case the hematoma was only found at autopsy. The anatomical distribution of the sites of the intracranial hemorrhage and hematomas, including two cases found at autopsy and in which no craniotomy was performed, is well documented. It is important to notice that in 17 cases (85%), the hemorrhage and hematomas occurred either epidurally or subdurally or both. In only two cases (10%), was the hemorrhage in the brain substance, and in one case (5%) in the subarachnoid space (Table 3). This selective distribution of the hematomas near the dura mater may give some hint as to the pathogenesis of hemorrhage in those particular areas. When we look at the anatomical distribution of the hemorrhage and hematomas, in relation to the geographic areas of the cranium and cerebral hemispheres, we find that it is the frontal part which is

Table 3. Anatomical distribution of the sites of intracranial hemorrhage and hematoma in 20 patients following open heart surgery

Location	No. of cases
Epidural	9
Subdural	4
Both epidural & subdural	3
Subdural & intracerebral	1
Subarachnoid	1
Intracerebral	2

Table 4. Geographic distribution of the sites of intracranial hemorrhage and hematoma in 20 cases following open heart surgery

Geographic area	Left	Right	Bilateral	Total
Frontal	0	7	0	7
Parietal	1	0	0	1
Temple	0	1	0	1
Temple & parietal	2	1	0	3
Temple & frontal	0	1	0	1
Parietal & occipital	1	0	0	1
Temple, frontal & parietal	1	2	0	3
Temple, frontal, parietal & occipital	0	1	1	2
Undescribed	0	1	0	1
Total	5	14	1	20

most often involved in cases where only one area is affected. However, in those cases where hematomas occupy more than one area, the temple and parietal regions are involved in most instances (Table 4).

The size of the hematomas recorded in five cases varied from $5 \times 4 \times 4$ cm^3 to $15 \times 3 \times 3$ cm^3. The recorded weight of blood clots evacuated in eight cases was from 60–200 g, averaging 105 g. In one case the blood clot evacuated from two hematomas, one on each side of the superior sagittal sinus, weighed 300 g altogether.

After thorough evacuation, the site of the hematoma was examined carefully for the presence of active bleeders; tearing of the superior sagittal sinus was observed in three cases, bleeding from the engorged anomalous veins near the superior sagittal sinus in one, oozing from the vessels of the dura mater in two, and active spurting from the anterior branch of the left middle meningeal artery in one.

The recorded data of eight cases during surgery indicated marked brain edema in five, encephalomalacia in three, extensive petechial hemorrhage in one and severe cerebral dehydration in one. Autopsies in four cases revealed extensive subarachnoid hemorrhage in two cases, and extensive patchy and petechial hemorrhage scattered in the brain tissue, more pronounced in the basal ganglia, internal capsule, and hypothalamus in one. In another case, the intracerebral hematoma ruptured into the ventricle.

Table 5. The results of exploratory craniotomy in 18 patients with intracranial hemorrhage and hematoma following open heart surgery

Group	No. of cases	Results	
		Survival	Death
I	3	0	3
II	3	3	0
III	12	7	5

It is not likely that coagulopathy is the cause in most cases although oozing from the surgical wounds occurred in three cases. In one case, a huge hematoma formed in the mediastinum and the adjacent extrapleural space immediately after open-heart surgery. Faulty perfusion, i.e., inadequate flow rate, was suspected in two patients in Group I.

Results of neurosurgical treatment: of the 18 neurosurgically treated patients, ten survived and eight died. From Table 5 one can see the grave prognosis of this complication especially in Group I. The survivals gradually regained consciousness within a 1–2-week-period. The most common cause of death was the extensive and serious brain damage which resulted mostly from delayed surgical treatment.

Discussion

The pathogenesis of the intracranial hemorrhage and hematoma formation remains as yet an unsolved problem. The traditional concept which puts the blame mainly on cerebral embolism is not appropriate to explain the whole clinical picture of this particular complication. We, as other authors [6, 7], believe that some other factors play an important role in the production of this neurological complication, namely: intraoperative anticoagulation, hypertonic perfusion, excessive diuresis, preoperative, intraoperative and postoperative head trauma, venous or/and arterial hypertension during or after perfusion, etc.

Intraoperative anticoagulation: the administration of heparin during cardiopulmonary bypass is probably the basic factor that renders the vascular system more vulnerable to extensive bleeding and hematoma formation in the event of vascular damage. In this series of cases, however, one patient was operated upon under mild hypothermia and no anticoagulant was given. We, therefore, presume that intracranial hemorrhage following open-heart surgery is not due to anticoagulation alone.

Perfusion with hypertonic perfusate: in 1974, we usually added varying amounts of 20% mannitol to the perfusate during most of the open-heart operations both in children and adults. It is quite possible that this caused to some extent dehydration and shrinkage of the brain tissue. In addition, owing to a falling of the blood pressure, the intracranial pressure was lowered further. The figures in Table 6 illustrate the interrelationship between the incidence of intracranial hemorrhage and hematomas and

Table 6. The interrelationship between the incidence of intracranial hemorrhage and hematoma and the usage of mannitol in the perfusate

20% Mannitol	No. of cases	No. (%) of intracranial hemorrhage & hematoma
Used	245	10 (4.08)
Not used	207	2 (0.97)
Total	452	12 (2.66)

mannitol used in the perfusate, and seem to indicate that the usage of mannitol may be a contributory factor in the pathogenesis of intracranial hemorrhage in the vast majority of cases. On these grounds, we have restricted the use of mannitol in the perfusate since the occurrence of a third case of intracranial hemorrhage.

Excessive diuresis and dehydration: for a short period of time in 1974, we routinely retransfused the blood containing perfusate which was left in the heart-lung machine at the end of bypass. Therefore, a large amount of diuretics was administered just before or right after the termination of perfusion. Excessive diuresis resulted in a negative fluid balance in four of the five patients who developed intracranial hemorrhage and hematoma in one of our hospitals. We assume that shrinkage of the brain volume exerts a stretching force on the subdural structures and the dura mater, resulting either in tearing of the dural bridging veins on the uppermost part of the cerebral hemisphere, or in separation of the dura mater from the inner table of the cranium at the same place. A typical example will illustrate this event. In a 7-year-old girl, a V.S.D. was repaired during a 36-min cardiopulmonary bypass. Just prior to the conclusion of the operation, 200 ml of 50% glucose was given intravenously to counteract hypotension. She never woke up and soon developed generalized convulsion and the pupils were fully dilated on both sides. Exploratory craniotomy revealed two huge hematomas, one on each side of the superior sagittal sinus, and tearing of the sinus and large dural bridging veins bilaterally. It was also noticed that the brain tissue was so much dehydrated that it resembled a piece of dried bean curd. It seems to be justified in this case, to blame the intravenous injection of a large amount of concentrated glucose for her neurological complication.

History of head trauma and possible trauma during and after surgery: any head trauma before operation may initiate some bleeding which may subsequently lead to the formation of an acute or chronic intracranial hematoma. The hematoma may be dormant until it reaches a sufficient size. Intraoperative heparinization creates an ideal condition to hasten its development. In one of our cases, the patient slipped off the bed striking the upper frontal region on the cement ground 3 days before surgery. She became comatose 23 h after intracardiac surgery. Emergency craniotomy disclosed a big epidural and a small subdural hematoma right underneath the frontal bone. Unfortunately, the history of head trauma was not obtained preoperatively, otherwise, we would certainly have postponed her operation, since we never operate upon any patient who has suffered a recent head injury, no matter how minor.

With shrinkage of brain substance and reduction of its volume as a result of hypertonic perfusion and excessive diuresis, the brain tends to gravitate away from the frontal region toward the dependent part of the skull, as the patient lies face upward during bypass. However, when the anesthetist, to facilitate his duties, keeps the patient's head turned to one side, usually to the left, the brain tends to gravitate away from the frontal, temple and parietal bones which are on the upper side. This may explain why the frontal, temple and parietal regions were more often involved, and 70% on the right side. Under the same condition, any swift or sudden movement of the head from side to side, initiated either by the anesthetist or by the patient himself could cause the brain to shift back and forth inside the cranium. When this occurs the dural bridging veins may tear.

Venous hypertension in the superior vena cava system due to poor drainage during bypass can result in cerebral edema or capillary rupture. It is also dangerous to have the mean arterial perfusion pressure over 100 mmHg as it may provoke cerebral hemorrhage. Unfortunately, we do not have enough monitoring data either to deny or to support this assumption. Nevertheless, both conditions should be avoided by all means.

We have no intention of denying the possibility of some kind of cerebral embolism causing the hemorrhage in some of the cases.

Diagnosis of intracranial hemorrhage and hematoma is not difficult if the cardiac and neurosurgeons are fully aware of this dreadful complication and watch the patient carefully for neurological signs in the immediate postoperative period. Should a patient who has undergone open-heart surgery with satisfactory perfusion record fail to regain consciousness, besides cerebral embolism, an intracranial hemorrhage and hematoma should be also suspected until it is proved otherwise. In a patient with good respiratory and circulatory function, postoperative lethargy should be considered as a warning sign, and preparation for emergency craniotomy be made. Ultrasonic scanning for deviation of the cerebral falx has proved to be of much value as a diagnostic aid in instances of space-occupying intracranial lesions. In this series of cases, five of seven examined showed positive findings. It was this fact, together with the pupillary changes, that led to the decision of conducting early exploratory craniotomy. In addition, spinal puncture may be helpful in detecting intracranial hemorrhage, but negative findings obtained from these two procedures offer no guarantee. It has, however, been our experience that no time should be lost in trying to determine the exact location of the hemorrhage or hematoma once lateralizing signs appear or the patient becomes comatose, unless there is immediate access to gamma camera scanning, cerebral angiography, or computerized tomography.

It is vitally important to explore different parts of the cranial cavity thoroughly. Intraoperative cerebral angiography to locate the deeply hidden or intracerebral hematoma is advisable in case the surgeon is unable to pinpoint it.

References

1. Aguilar MJ, Gerbode F, Hill JD (1971) Neuropathological complications of cardiac surgery. J Thorac Cardiovasc Surg 61:676
2. Brierley JB (1963) Neuropathological findings in patients dying after open-heart surgery. Thorax 18:291

3. Department of Neurosurgery (1978) The General Hospital of Chinese People's Liberation Army: Intracranial hematoma complicating open heart operation. Chin J Surg 78:98
4. Department of Thoracic Surgery (1977) The General Hospital of Chinese People's Liberation Army: Summarization of 3 cases of epidural hematoma following intracardiac surgery under extracorporeal circulation. Unpublished paper presented at the Chang Chun Meeting of Cardiovascular Surgery, September 1977
5. Hu Xiao-qin, Shang De-yan (1979) Epidural and subdural hematomas following open heart surgery. Chin J Cardiovasc Dis 7:1
6. Humphreys RP, Hoffman HJ, Mustard WT, Trusler GA (1975) Cerebral hemorrhage following heart surgery. J Neurosurg 43:671
7. Krous HF, Tenckhoff L, Gould NS, Stamm SJ (1975) Subdural hematoma following open-heart operations. Ann Thorac Surg 19:269–276
8. Thomassen RW, Howbert JP, Winn DF Jr, Thompson SW (1961) The occurrence and characterization of emboli associated with the use of a silicone antifoaming agent. J Thorac Cardiovasc Surg 41:611

Focal Neurological Lesions and Diffuse Organic Brain Damage in Open-Heart Surgery Patients

Postoperative Thrombocytosis and Platelet Aggregation – A Possible Aetiological Factor in the Causation of Organic Brain Dysfunction

D.W. Bethune

Summary

Neuropsychiatric dysfunction occurring after open-heart surgery is usually considered to be related to intraoperative events.

A case history is presented which suggests that marked changes in neuropsychiatric function can occur in the immediate postoperative period with a history and time course which is incompatible with a direct intraoperative cause. The evidence from psychometric testing indicated a disturbance of delayed memory recall which would suggest an organic basis for the symptoms. Analysis of the records of a group of patients who were studied in detail with pre- and postoperative interviewing, identified a significant incidence of changes suggestive of organic neuropsychiatric dysfunction occurring remote from the immediate operative period.

Introduction

The role of platelets in the causation of arterial thromboembolic disorders is becoming increasingly recognised [1] and platelet aggregation may be important in the causation of organic brain dysfunction in the early postoperative period.

Following open-heart surgery there is an incidence of neurological dysfunction which is undoubtedly related to intraoperative events [2–3]. These symptoms and signs are present immediately after operation and then tend to become less obvious. In a number of patients there is no immediate evidence of neurological dysfunction but signs and symptoms develop later in the postoperative period [4].

In the management of patients with prosthetic valves embolic events have been recognised as a long-term potential complication and life-long anticoagulation is commonly used to reduce the incidence of such complications. The situation in the early postoperative period is conducive to the formation of platelet aggregates and these may play an important role in causing reversible organic neuropsychiatric dysfunction.

Psychopathological and Neurological Dysfunctions
Following Open-Heart Surgery Ed. by Becker et al

Patients and Methods

Two groups of patients were considered. One group of eight patients were scheduled for coronary artery bypass grafting; seven patients received between two and four coronary artery grafts, the eighth patient received three coronary artery grafts and in addition a small ventricular aneurysm was resected. Cardiopulmonary bypass support was provided with the assistance of Sci Med Kolobow membrane oxygenators for these eight patients. These patients were tested before operation and on the 3rd and 6th day after operation using a test of delayed memory function for visual stimuli with progressive prompting [5]. The test procedure used was similar to that described in previous studies [6–7]. Only the results of the delayed memory recall test are presented in this report and the associated questionnaire was extended to allow determination by direct questioning of any sensory or motor disturbance in the postoperative period.

A second group of 30 patients were being studied in detail as part of the clinical evaluation of three bubble oxygenators (Shiley S100A, Rygg VT5,000 (without arterial reservoir filters), and the Belco Oxibel D600). These patients were assessed in a similar way before operation and on the 6th day after operation. Following valve replacement the patients were anticoagulated with Warfarin. Therapeutic levels being achieved by day 3 after operation.

Results

In Fig. 1 the results of the delayed memory recall test is shown for the seven patients with ischaemic heart disease, who had no evidence of neuropsychiatric disturbance in the postoperative period. In addition the results are given for tests performed on the one patient who became disorientated and confused. This patient was a 56-year-old man who was scheduled for triple coronary artery bypass grafting. At operation a small left ventricular aneurysm was resected. Postoperatively he was noted to be lethargic on day 3, but his delayed memory recall tests on days 3 and 6 did not confirm a significant degree of organic dysfunction when compared to the symptomless patients in this group. He became disorientated and mildly confused on day 7 and on day 8 a further delayed memory recall test was carried out using the test card he had seen pre-operatively. This demonstrated a marked impairment of memory function even though he had previously seen that card. In the absence of organic disturbance trans-operative recall is well preserved following open heart surgery [7]. Treatment was started with chlorpromazine 25 mg q.d.s. and dipyridamole (Persantin) 100 mg q.d.s. His confusional state cleared rapidly and repeat testing on day 10 using the card previously shown on day 4 demonstrated "normal" memory function.

The results from the 30 patients undergoing valve replacements with bubble oxygenator support demonstrated that 6 days following open heart surgery there is a slight but significant disturbance of memory function. Ninety percent of the patients had scores indicating that memory recall was not as efficient as preoperatively. Three different bubble oxygenators were used in these patients but there was no significant

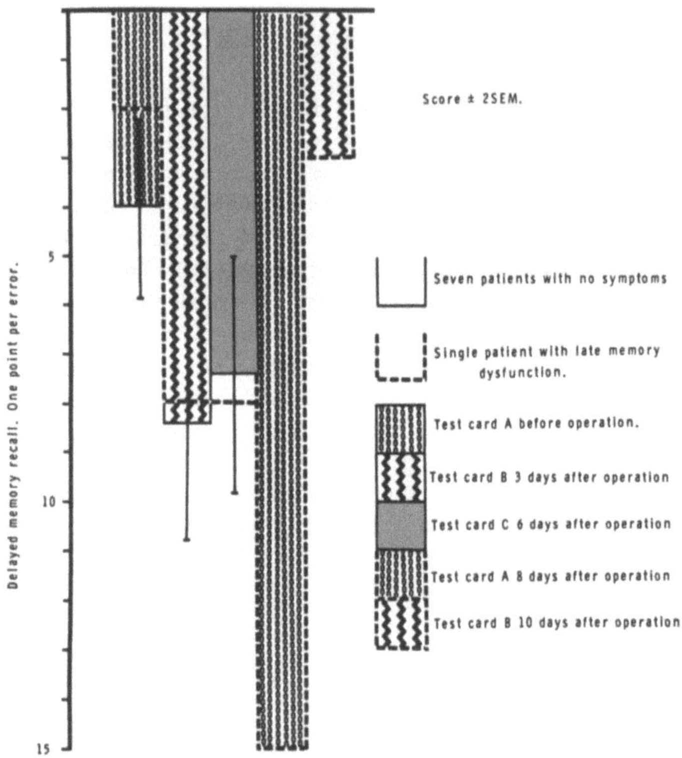

Fig. 1. Delayed recall scores following coronary artery bypass grafting. Scoring of one penalty point for each object not recalled spontaneously, with verbal or with visual prompt. Eight patients tested before operation and in days 3 and 6 after operation. Additional tests using previously used cards on days 8 and 10 in patient with memory loss and disorientation on days 7 and 8

difference in the results of delayed recall testing between the three types of oxygenator.

Postoperative evaluation by physical examination and direct questioning identified three patients with signs and symptoms of minimal early neurological dysfunction. In only one case, a patient who had diplopia for 2 days, were these signs of symptoms noted by the ward staff. In all three cases both signs and symptoms had cleared by day 4.

Nine patients had symptoms which could be taken to indicate neurological dysfunction with an onset between 3 and 8 days after operation. In the majority of these cases these referred to visual disturbance. One patient had a transient loss of vision in one eye lasting 10 min, one had two similar episodes each lasting about 20 min, five patients described more minor, but still quite definite, transient visual field disturbances, and of the final two patients in this group one had a mild transient confusional state with an associated memory loss and the other had a short period of dysphasia. It was not possible to examine any of the patients when they had symptoms but at subsequent examination nothing abnormal was detected.

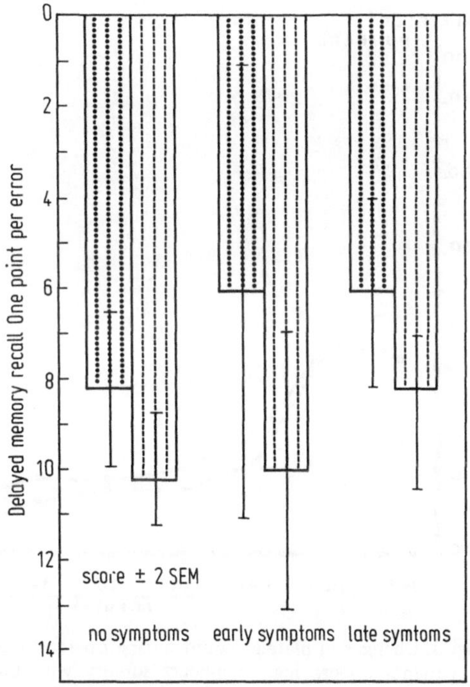

Fig. 2. Delayed recall scores following valve replacement. Change in score before operation to 6 days after operation. $t = 5.15; P > 0.001$. Scoring system as in Fig. 1

Table 1. Details of patients undergoing valve replacement

	No symptoms	Early symptoms	Late symptoms
Number	18	3	9
Valve site	8 MVR 10 AVR	1 MVR 2 AVR	6 MVR 3 AVR
Valve type	12 Bjork 2 Starr 4 Porcine xenograft	3 Bjork	8 Bjork 1 Porcine xenograft
Oxygenator			
Belco Oxibel D600	7		3
Shiley S. 100A	5	2	3
Rygg VT 5000	5	1	3
Age	60 ± 14.1[a]	49 ± 12.4	53 ± 12.3
Bypass duration	86.5 ± 20.3	75.6 ± 22.3	87.8 ± 23.1
Ischemic time	60.3 ± 14.1	50.6 ± 10.9	61.8 ± 18.6

[a]Means ± S.D.

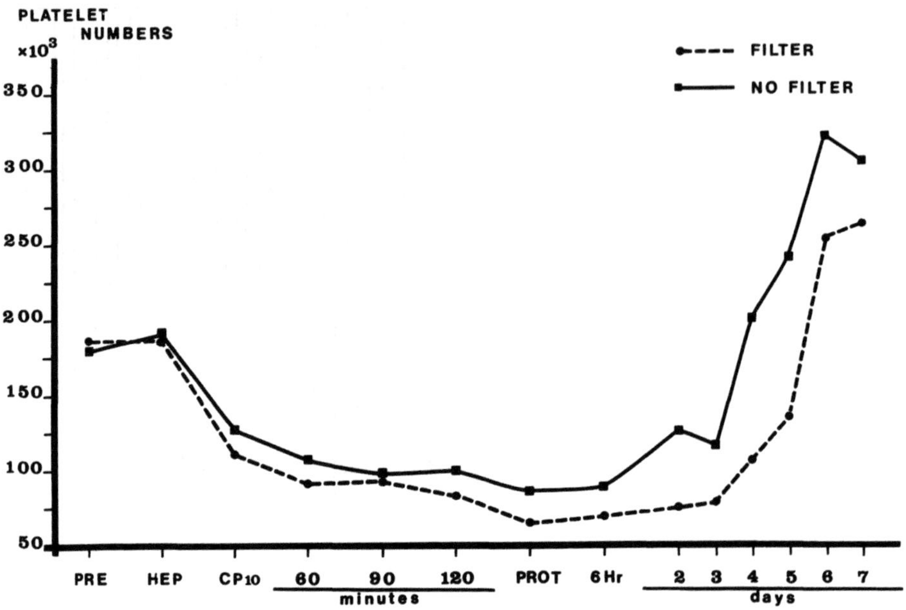

Fig. 3. Changes in platelet count during operation and during the immediate postoperative period in patients undergoing open-heart surgery with bubble oxygenators. Results from 20 patients, ten patients with arterial line filtration, ten patients without arterial line filtration

Comparison of the recall scores (Fig. 2) in these three groups of patients did not show a significant difference between them. There was no significant difference in bypass time, ischaemic time, gaseous microemboli count, cardiotomy suction or volume, platelet counts, site of surgery, type of prosthesis or anticoagulation control between the three groups (Table 1). Platelet counts fell during bypass in all patients, postoperatively the counts were depressed for the first few days and then rose rapidly and exceeded the preoperative level by the end of the first week. Typical findings for changes in platelet counts for patients undergoing cardiac surgical procedures involving the use of bubble oxygenators are shown in Fig. 3.

Discussion

The symptoms and signs observed in these patients following valve replacement would suggest an incidence of early neurological dysfunction of 10%. However, in only one case was the disability sufficient for the patient to spontaneously volunteer the symptoms, this was the patient with diplopia for 48 h following operation. It is likely that if these patients had not been part of a prospective study their symptoms would possibly have been discounted.

The incidence of late neurological dysfunction following valve replacement appears to be about 25%, but again, in only two of these nine patients was a record of the symptoms made in the patient's notes. It is interesting that the changes identified by direct questioning were insufficient to cause a significant change in memory function as assessed by delayed memory recall. This could be due to the transient nature of the disturbances as no patient in this group was actually tested when symptoms were present. In addition it is difficult to be certain that the more minor visual field disturbances do represent true organic dysfunction, but with repeat questioning the patients would give a very firm and definite history.

The period 2–8 days following implantation of a prosthetic heart valve must represent a time of risk for embolic or organic damage. The sewing ring of the valve provides an intravascular stimulus to aggregation and in addition the platelet population is rapidly increasing at this time and must consist of many young platelets which are known to be more susceptable to aggregating stimuli.

It is interesting that in the eight patients scheduled for coronary artery bypass grafting, the only patient with any neurological symptoms in the postoperative period was the patient who had a ventricular aneurysm resected. It is probable that the area adjacent to the aneurysm could have provided a focus for platelet aggregation to occur, which would not be present in the other seven patients in this group.

It is tempting to relate the occurrence of transient episodes of neuropsychiatric dysfunction in the later postoperative period to platelet aggregation and embolization. The symptomatology is similar to that described in other states where platelets are known to be hyperactive [1] and in the one case described with marked symptoms treatment with platelet suppressive drugs produced a rapid resolution of the condition.

In an extensive review of the subject of post-cardiotomy delirium Dubin et al. [8] highlighted the wide range of presentation of delirium in patients following open heart surgery. It is possible that further studies of the possible role of platelets in the causation of organic brain dysfunction following open heart surgery may provide evidence of an aetiological factor which has received little consideration up to the present time. If platelet aggregation is implicated treatment with platelet suppressive drugs will either totally prevent the dysfunction or result in a considerable clinical improvement.

Acknowledgments. The author would like to thank Ciba Laboratories, Horsham and Astra U.K. for financial support, Dr. J.M. Collis for statistical analysis, and Mrs. A. Gibbins for preparation of the typescript. The author is in receipt of a grant from the East Anglian Regional Health Authority with respect to some aspects of the work presented.

References

1. Preston FE, Martin JF, Stewart RM, Davies-Jones GAB (1979) Thrombocytosis, circulating platelet aggregates and neurological dysfunction. Br Med J 2:1561
2. Branthwaite MA (1972) Neurological damage related to open-heart surgery. A clinical survey. Thorax 27:748
3. Branthwaite MA (1973) Detection of neurological damage during open-heart surgery. Thorax 28:464
4. Heller SS, Frank KH, Malm JR, et al. (1970) Psychiatric complications to open-heart surgery. N Engl J Med 283:1015

5. William M (1953) Investigation of amnesic defects by progressive prompting. J Neurol Neurosurg Psychiatry 16:14
6. Bethune DW (to be published) Test of delayed memory recall suitable for assessing post-operative amnesia. Anaesthesia 35
7. Bethune DW (1980) The assessment of organic brain damage following open-heart surgery. In: Speidel H, Rodewald G (eds) Psychic and neurological dysfunctions after open-heart surgery. INA 19:100–106 Thieme, Stuttgart
8. Dubin WR, Field HL, Gastfriend DR (1979) Post cardiotomy delirium: A critical review. J Thorac Cardiovasc Surg 77:586

Comparison of Psychometric Findings Following Use of Bubble and Membrane Oxygenator

H.J.L. Boccalon

Introduction

Gilberstadt and Sako in 1967 [5], Kornfeld et al. in 1965 [6] established that significant disorders of the central nervous system occur with greater frequency after cardiac surgery using extracorporeal circulation (E.C.C.) than after other types of surgery. Frequency varies according to author and whether behavorial or neurological disturbances are considered. Burgess et al. [2], Egerton and Kayj [4], Rimon et al. [7], related that psychiatric complications after cardiac surgery vary from 13%–57%. Tufo et al. [8] describes 43% of behavorial disturbances and 50% of neurological complications. Now, the small number of clinically discernible neurological complications motivated the use of a protocol of psychometric tests, designed to objectify more sensitively the cerebral changes following cardiac surgery.

Study Protocol

Patient Selection

In our study with Chevalier 1976 [3] 40 patients were selected to undergo cardiac surgery using E.C.C.: valve replacement [2, 3], aortocoronary bypass [8], ventricular aneurysm resection [5], and congenital heart disease [4]. Patients' ages ranged from 16–68 years. Hemodynamical postoperative complications excluded patients from the study because such complications introduced new factors.

Surgical Procedure

Extracorporeal circulation was performed using the partial hemodilution method. The priming contained: 500 cc of 5% glucoside serum, 100 cc Ringer lactate, 100 cc human albumin, 100 cc mannitol, 4 cc 10% calcium gluconate, and 20 meq of bicarbonate, for a total volume of 1750 cc. A roller pump was used; the tubes were the Bentley type. A filter was placed between the cardiotomy reservoir and the oxygenator; i.e., on the return aspiration circuit (Bentley ref. 427). The oxygenators used in these studies were divided into two groups: bubble oxygenators for 22 patients

Psychopathological and Neurological Dysfunctions Following Open-Heart Surgery. Ed by Becker et al.

(Bentley trademark) and membrane oxygenators for 18 patients (Teflo, Travenol trademark). Supervision of the E.C.C. was rigorous, with pressure controls and a perfusion flow equal to 2400 cc/min per m^2 corporeal surface.

Control Tests

A preoperative electroencephalogram was recorded in order to evaluate possible disturbances before surgery; preoperative surveillance was performed as a postoperative control (18 patients).

The psychiatric and neurological postoperative manifestations were noted.

Psychometric tests were chosen to include the mental functions most sensitive to a change in cerebral oxygen.

This is a prospective study to evaluate the effect of oxygenation type during E.C.C. upon cerebral functions. The battery was composed of six tests with the object of centering the memory in its different aspects: the power of concentration and attention, visual/motor coordination, learning aptitude, motor rapidity, and verbal fluency, as well as general dynamism and vivacity of reaction. The evaluation of the patient was performed by the same physician, first 48 h before surgery and then 4 and 9 days after it. Patients stay no more than 2 days in the intensive care unit. The tests executed were the following, numbered from T1 to T6: immediate memory test T1 for logical memory, deferred memory test T2, visual memory test T3 (from the Benton test), test of the dim barrier T4 (Zazzo test), verbal fluency test T5 (Thurstons test), and cubes T6 (Alexander scale). For each test, the physician gives a note in between 1 and 40. In the group of 40 patients studied the repartition of membrane and bubble oxygenators is determined by the surgeons involved in this study. The physician involved with the psychometric tests is excluded from this choice until the end of the study. Twentytwo Patients underwent E.C.C. with a bubble oxygenator, the other 18 with a membrane oxygenator.

Results

Statistical Analysis

Analysis of the variables and comparison of averages pointed to the conclusion that the results obtained from the last four tests (T3, T4, T5, T6) were not statistically significant postoperatively, relative to the preoperative evaluation. However, tests T1 and T2, i.e. those evaluating immediate logical memory and deferred logical memory, permitted biological variation to be distinguished by analysis of the variations.

Qualitative Analysis

Because of the possibility of the patient learning by repetition on the third test, we allowed deterioration criteria with three possibilities:

1. either a postoperative score lower than the preoperative,
2. the postoperative score identical to the preoperative, or
3. the postoperative score higher than the preoperative score by less than 10%.

Here we are only studying tests T1 and T2, for which the precedent analysis showed that there were significant variations linked to cardiac surgery. We show total results (Table 1), excluding those of nine patients where the E.C.C. lasted longer than 115 min, since psychic disturbances were present in all cases; this is in agreement with the works of other authors: Tufo et al. [8]. We express the results in percentages of memory changes compared to the total number of patients.

We then studied the results in relation to age (Table 2) after dividing the two groups into one group younger than 50 and another 50 years or older.

Discussion

The Protocol

The entire study is performed while each patient remains within the department of cardiac surgery; the third control of each test could be too soon after surgery; it would be interesting to perform a control 1 month later, but this control could not be done systematically. We are particularly interested in the immediate post operative disturbances of cerebral functions, their influence on the behavior of patients, and on the cooperation of the patients with therapy and the postoperative course.

Table 1. Memory changes using bubble or membrane oxygenator (E.C.C. < 115 min)

	Bubble		Membrane	
	4 th day	9 th day	4 th day	9 th day
T1	67.5%	45.5%	45%	22%
T2	62%	53.5%	61.5%	16.5%

Table 2. Memory changes after E.C.C., related to the age of the patient and type of oxygenator

		Bubble		Membrane	
	age	4th day	9th day	4th day	9th day
T1	⩾ 50	75%	41%	45%	22%
	< 50	60%	50%	45%	22%
T2	⩾ 50	75%	67%	67%	22%
	< 50	50%	40%	56%	11%

Compared to the preoperative results, both postoperative controls are statistically significant for T1 and T2 only. Fiability index F equals 10.41 for T1 and 9.50 for T2. E.C.C. proved to disturb immediate and deferred memory in about one patient out of two at the fourth postoperative day. In the future we have to change tests T3, T4, T5 and T6.

The Duration of E.C.C.

In our study, we verified that a long period of E.C.C., longer than 115 min, was always accompanied by disturbances in the psychometric tests in the nine patients studied. This conclusion was previously established by Tufo et al. [8].

The Oxygenator Type

On the fourth postoperative day there was a change in the answers to the tests T1 and T2 from more than 60% of the patients, with the exception of the group who used the membrane oxygenator for immediate memory test T1 (45%). The potential of recuperation on the 9th postoperative day seemed more significant in patients submitted to the membrane oxygenator, since the percentage of disturbances was not more than 22% for T1 and 16.5% for T2, while it was 45.5% for T1 and 53.5% for T2 using the bubble oxygenator.

The Age of Patients

Finally, we verified that patients under 50 years of age showed a smaller change in the tests, above all in deferred memory (T2): 50% of patients under 50 years of age disturbed, compare to 75% of patients over 50 years, for the bubble oxygenator group; 56% of patients under 50 years disturbed compare to 67% of patients over 50 years, for the membrane oxygenator group. Recovery of cerebral functions was significant on the 9th day, especially for patients submitted to the membrane oxygenator (only 22% of patients with T1 disturbances), and for patients under 50 years of age (11% for T2).

Psychiatric and Neurological Disturbances

We verified psychiatric problems in 15% of the patients studied, which corresponds to the lowest rates previously cited by other authors as Blachly and Starr [1], Burgess et al. [2], Egerton and Kay [4], Kornfeld et al. [6]. The development has always been favorable. Answers to T1 and T2 tests were always disturbed. They include: confusion with hallucinations and four nervous breakdowns. These six psychiatric complications occurred after E.C.C. using bubble oxygenators four times and membrane oxygenators twice. One E.C.C. lasted more than 115 min (3 h 12 min, with bubble oxygenator). The age of the patients was under 50 years three times and over 50 years three times.

One neurological complication of lateral homonymous hemianopsia was noted with a normal electroencephalogram before surgery and signs of diffuse circulatory insufficiency on the tenth postoperative day (second replacement of aortic prothesis, E.C.C.: 94 min.)

Only 18 patients had a preoperative electroencephalogram with a postoperative control. Four tracings were disturbed postoperatively; of these, only two corresponded to changes in tests T1 and T2. We did not find correlations between preoperative E.E.G. and postoperative responses to tests T1 and T2.

Conclusion

The small number of clinically discernible neurological complications motivated the use of a protocol of psychometric tests, designed to objectify more sensitively the cerebral changes following cardiac surgery with E.C.C. We tend to attribute this to three factors: the duration of the E.C.C. verifying that E.C.C. longer than 115 min always alters tests responses; the age of the patients, those under 50 being more capable of preserving their memory faculties intact; and above all, the type of oxygenator used, with better results from the membrane oxygenator in terms of recovery based on test answers on the ninth postoperative day.

References

1. Blachly P, Starr A (1964) Post-cardiotomy delirium. Am J Psychiatry 121:371–375
2. Burgess GN, Kirklin JW, Steinhakber RM (1967) Some psychiatric aspects of intracardiac surgery. Mayo Clin Proc 42/1:12
3. Chevalier JP (1976) Etude des altérations des fonctions cérébrales après chirurgie cardiaque sous circulation extra-corporelle. Medical dissertation, University of Toulouse
4. Egerton N, Kay H (1964) Physiological disturbances associated with open heart surgery. Br J Psychiatry 110:433–439
5. Gilberstadt H, Sako Y (1967) Intellectual and personality changes following open-heart surgery. Arch Gen Psychiatry 16:210–214
6. Kornfeld DS, Zimberg S, Malm JR (1965) Psychiatric complications of open heart surgery. N Engl J Med 273:292–487
7. Rimon R, Lehtonen J, Scheinin TM (1967) Psychiatric disturbances after cardiovascular surgery. Acta Psychiatry Scand 203:125–130
8. Tufo HM, Adrian N, Shekelle R (1980) Central nervous system dysfunction following open-heart surgery. JAMA 21:1333–1339

Use of Prostacyclin to Prevent Postoperative Psychic and Neurological Disturbances After Open-Heart Surgery: A Clinical Study

H. Pokar, N. Bleese, H. Fischer-Düsterhoff, P. Götze, G. Huse-Kleinstoll, J. Koedijk, M-J. Polonius, K. Prüssmann, V. Tilsner

Postoperative psychiatric disturbances still occur very often after open-heart operations, and the reason for them is generally thought to lie in the extracorporeal circulation (ECC). The aggregation of thrombocytes is assumed to be one of the traumata induced by ECC, mostly brought about by contact with the large surfaces within the heart-lung machine, by mechanical alterations due to suction with the coronary suction lines, and by the blood coming in contact with collagen in the pericardium.

The introduction of microfilters in the ECC did make it possible to reduce the number of cases of postoperative organic damage, but even our figures in Hamburg still show that 50% of the open-heart patients show signs of psychopathological damage postoperatively. Substances which counteract thrombocyte aggregation, such as aspirin and dipyridamole, have also proved inadequate in solving this "thrombocyte problem".

As we know, one of the most powerful agents for counteracting thrombocyte aggregation is a prostaglandin known as prostacyclin (PGI_2). After it had been successfully synthesized in 1977 PGI_2 proved, amongst other things, to have very good protective qualities for the thrombocytes during ECC in animal experiments. Up until now little has been done to ascertain the effect of PGI_2 on humans during ECC, and so we have started a pilot study to check whether its protective effect is quite as pronounced in man as it is in animals. Our results so far show that both the total number of thrombocytes and their capacity to aggregate are positively affected. I should like to demonstrate this briefly by means of a thrombocyte-spreading test according to Breddin.

Figure 1 shows a normal preoperative thrombocyte spreading in a patient with an ASD II; Fig. 2 depicts the thrombocyte spreading from the same patient after an ECC lasting only 15 min. The damage is obvious – pronounced vacuolization, the thrombocytes containing only a few or no granulomeres whatsoever. Figure 3 shows the postoperative thrombocyte spreading in a patient after 2 h of ECC which included PGI_2. Here are young thrombocytes, rich in granulomeres, only slightly activated, with no signs of vacuolization. These forms are usually so quick to react that even after a very short ECC they can hardly be found at all.

The point of this study was to establish whether psychopathological disturbances occurred less often postoperatively if the thrombocytes are protected by PGI_2 during ECC. In all we plan to study 25 patients under treatment compared with the same number in a control group. All the patients were operated on for a valve deficiency. So far we have treated and examined 19 patients with PGI_2 and the control group

Psychopathological and Neurological Dysfunctions
Following Open-Heart Surgery Ed by Becker et al

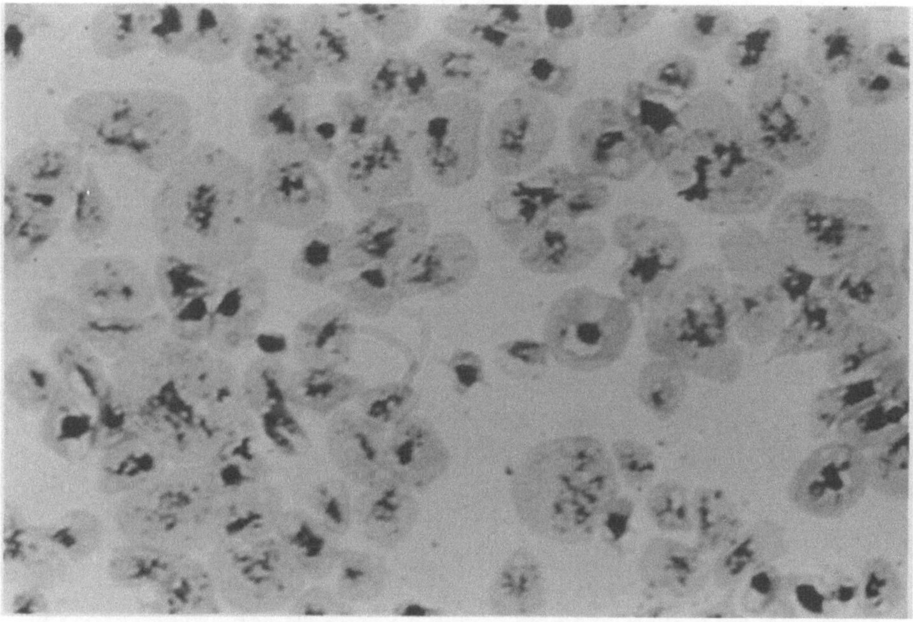

Fig. 1. Normal preoperative thrombocyte-spreading test (Breddin) in a patient with an ASD II

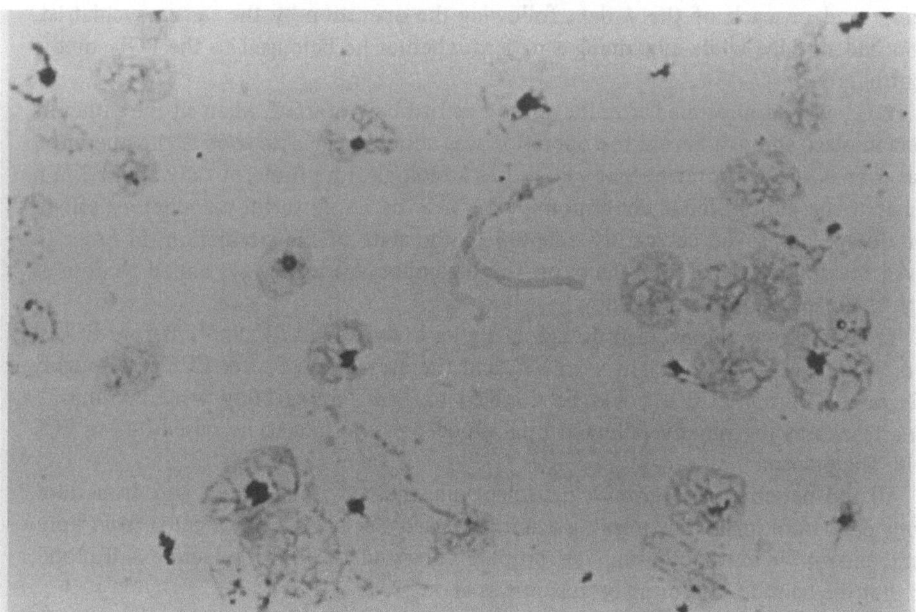

Fig. 2. Thrombocyte spreading in the same patient (Fig. 1) 15 min after ECC is started

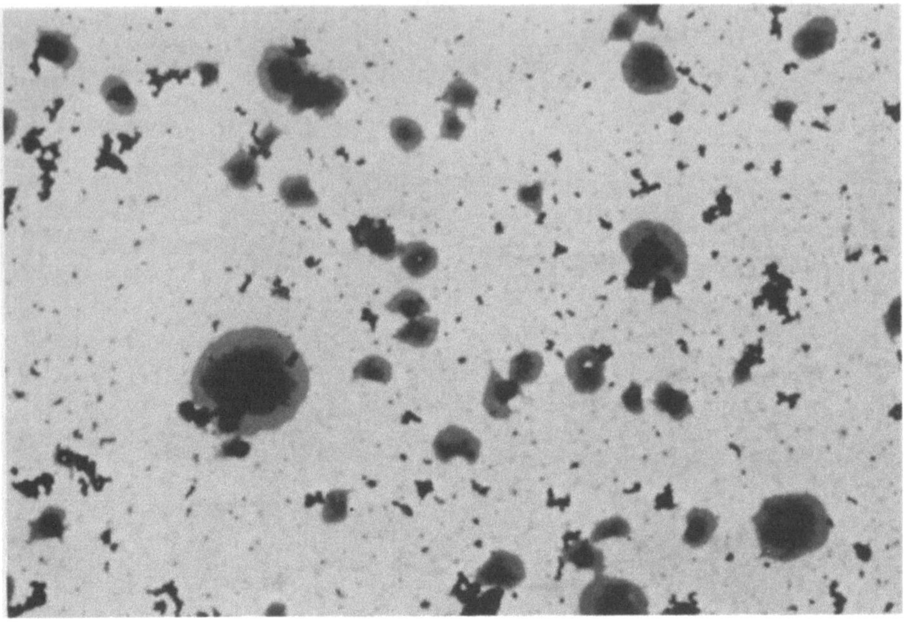

Fig. 3. Postoperative thrombocyte spreading in a patient after 2 h of ECC which included PGI_2

currently totals 15. The neurological and psychiatric examinations were carried out before and on each of the 4 days following the operation by the same psychiatrist, who had no idea while examining a patient whether he belonged to the PGI_2 or the control group.

PGI_2 [1] was administered after the anesthetic had been started, when all the catheters were in place and just before the operation was about to begin; as soon as the operation was over it was withdrawn. Since PGI_2 has a biological halftime of only about 3 min it has to be administered continuously. Because of its powerful vasodilatory effect, the dosage has to be constantly adapted to the state of the circulation. In order to make maximum use of its effects on the thrombocytes we always aimed to dose as high as the circulation would allow.

Table 1 shows the average dosage in ng/kg body weight $\times$ min^{-1}. Before ECC it was 14.07 ng/kg body weight $\times$ min^{-1}, and the average dose after ECC was roughly the same. During ECC is could be doubled to 27.95 ng/kg body weight $\times$ min^{-1}. In a few cases the rapidly falling arterial blood pressure had to be raised during ECC with angiotensin.

All the patients were given a neurolept anesthesia with fentanyl and droperidol, with pancuronium as the relaxing agent. We used the bubble oxygenator from Polystan, model UKE, venotherm. The priming consisted of Ringer's lactate and blood, so that the hematocrit during perfusion was about 25%–30%.

---

1 Prostacyclin sodium synthesized by the "Upjohn Company" and formulated by the Wellcome Foundation Ltd. was kindly supplied by Wellcome Research Laboratories. Prostacyclin is an investigational drug of both companies.

Table 1. Dosage of prostacyclin during operation (ng/kg per min)

	Pre – ECC	During ECC	Post – ECC
n	19	19	19
x	14.07	27.95	14.09
S	3.90	5.01	3.72

Table 2. Operative procedures

Operation	PGI_2 group			Control group		
	♂	♀	Σ	♂	♀	Σ
Aortic valve replacement	3[a]	1	4	3	1	4
Mitral valve replacement	4	6	10	1	3	4
Aortic and mitral valve replacement	1	4	5	3	2	5
Aortic, mitral, and tricuspid valve replacement	–	–	–	1	1[b]	2
Total	8	11	*19*	8	7	*15*

[a]1 with ACVB
[b]De Vega

Table 2 shows the operative procedures for both groups. There were four aortic valve replacements in both groups, and ten mitral valve replacements in the PGI_2 group, but only four in the control group; in both groups there were five double valve replacements plus two triple valve replacements in the control group including one De VEGA correction of the tricuspid valve. The previous "Hamburg study" showed that apart from patients with multiple valve replacement, psychoorganic disturbances occur most often in patients where the mitral valve has been replaced; the PGI_2 group with its ten mitral valve replacements could therefore be seen as a disadvantage. On the other hand, the control group includes two patients with a triple valve replacement, so that the chances of postoperative disturbances in the two groups seem about equal.

Figure 4 shows how the number of thrombocytes in each group changed. The initial value before operation in both groups was approx. 180 000/mm^3. The first check after the operation gave a value in the PGI_2 group of 145 000/mm^3, and in the control group of only 100 000/mm^3, a difference which in the one-tailed t test is statistically highly significant. By the first and second postoperative day the differences are statistically hardly measurable and by the 3rd and 4th days no differences can be detected.

The postoperative neurological findings revealed only a slight difference compared with the preoperative state: reflex anomalies, differences in the pupils or nystagmus. There were 11 positive findings in the PGI_2 group and ten in the control group, so the difference is insignificant. Since we must assume that thrombocyte

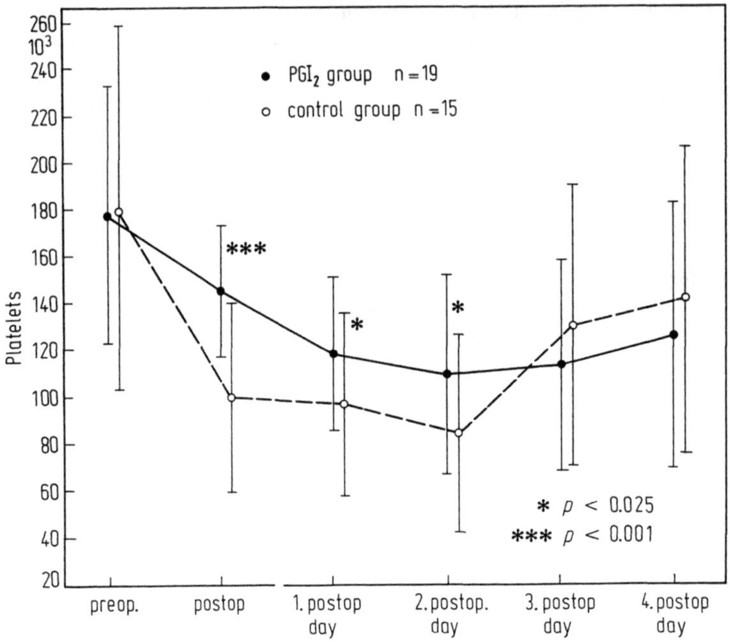

Fig. 4. Platelet behaviour with and without PGI_2

aggregates occur evenly distributed over the whole brain, circumspect damage is hardly to be expected.

Table 3 contains the preoperative psychiatric findings. In the PGI_2 group 12 patients had no symptoms and seven suffered from affective emotional syndrome, while in the control group six patients had no symptoms, eight had affective emotional syndrome, and one had a slight psychoorganic syndrome. The definitions for these syndromes are based on the criteria used by the "Hamburg group".

Table 4 shows the postoperative findings. Of the 19 patients in the PGI_2 group 12 showed no change or were "better". If the total number were not so small one could say it was 63%. In the control group only 5 of the 15 patients were unchanged,

Table 3. Preoperative Psychiatric Findings

	PGI_2 group			Control group		
	♂	♀	Σ	♂	♀	Σ
Unremarkable	5	7	12	4	2	6
Affective emotional syndrome	3	4	7	3	5	8
Slight psychoorganic	–	–	–	–	1	1
			19			15

Table 4. Postoperative psychiatric findings (1–4 postoperative day)

	PGI_2 group			Control group		
	♂	♀	Σ	♂	♀	Σ
Unchanged or "better"	5	7	12	2	3	5
Slight psychoorganic syndrome	2	–	2	–	1	1
Paranoid hallucinatory syndrome	–	–	–	2	–	2
Delirious syndrome	–	–	–	–	1	1
			14			9

or we could say 33%. Patients were described as "better" when an affective emotional syndrome which had existed before the operation was no longer apparent; this applied to two patients in the control group.

In both groups the slight psychoorganic syndrome predominated – in the PGI_2 group in five of the seven patients with symptoms, in the control group in six of ten. There were two cases of severe psychoorganic syndrome amongst the PGI_2 patients, and one case in the control group, which also included two patients with paranoid hallucinatory syndrome and one with delirious syndrome. Whilst paranoid hallucinatory syndrome is strictly speaking not a psychoorganic disturbance, it is conceivable that organic factors play a role in its development.

As far as time factors were concerned there was no basic difference between the two groups; usually the syndromes became apparent on the second postoperative day and in seven cases extended to the 4th day: five slight psychoorganic syndromes and both paranoid hallucinatory syndromes.

We naturally tried to pinpoint other factors apart from PGI_2 which could explain the marked decrease in psychiatric disturbances in this group of patients (Table 5). A comparison of the average age of the patients in both groups revealed no differences, nor was there any difference within the groups themselves between those showing symptoms and those without. The same applied to the length of anesthesia and of ECC. There was a statistically significant difference between the two groups concerning the length of time for which the patients were postoperatively respirated, but again there was no difference within the groups, regarding the average respiration time, between those with symptoms and those without. None of the patients suffered during or after the operation from hypoxia or a significant reduction in the hemodynamic parameters which might explain the cerebral disturbances.

The study of 100 patients made in Hamburg established amongst other things that fentanyl – which is the main agent in neuroleptanesthesia – has no influence on postoperative psychiatric disturbances. A comparison of the average fentanyl dosage per kg body weight $\times$ h^{-1} revealed that the fentanyl doses in the PGI_2 group were significantly lower (one-third). What this implies about the effect of PGI_2 is not yet clear (Table 6).

Table 7 shows which type of operation was related to which psychiatric disturbance. In both groups half the patients suffered from symptoms after an aortic valve replace-

Table 5. Comparison of age, duration of anesthesia, ECC, and postoperative ventilation between the PGI_2 group and the control group (PGI_2 and C)

	Age (years)		Duration of anesthesia (hours)		Duration of ECC (min)		Duration of postoperative ventilation (hours)	
	PGI_2	C	PGI_2	C	PGI_2	C	PGI_2	C
n	19	15	19	15	19	15	19	15
x	46.7	49.9	5.4	6.0	103.4	124.9	9.5	16.7 $p < 0.001$
±	14.0	8.4	0.9	1.2	33.8	38.4	4.8	5.5
Max	70	66	7.3	8.6	195	218	25	30
Min	21	36	3.8	3.4	64	60	5	8

Table 6. Dosage of fentanyl during operation (μg/kg per hour).

	PGI_2 group	Control group
n	19	15
x	6.69 **	10.25
±	2.27	4.68

** = $p < 0.01$

Table 7. Relationship between type of operation and psychic disturbances

	PGI_2		Control	
	Unremarkable	Psychic disturb.	Unremarkable	Psychic disturb.
Aortic valve replacement	2	2	2	2
Mitral valve replacement	7	3	2	2
Aortic and mitral valve replacement	3	2	–	5
Aortic, mitral, and tricuspid valve replacement	–	–	1	1
Total	12	7	5	10

ment, and in the control group after mitral valve replacement too. This corresponds with the findings in the study of the 100 patients. In the PGI_2 group ten were operated on for mitral valve replacement and only three developed symptoms; five had a double valve replacement and only two of them developed symptoms. In the control group all five double valve patients suffered from disturbances and so did one of the two triple valve patients. This high rate after multiple valve replacement tallies with the findings in the 100 patient study, so that in all one can say that symptoms were to be expected in two-thirds of all the patients in the control group.

At the moment all one can say on the basis of these findings is that the use of PGI_2 during the operation tends to reduce the number of postoperative cerebral disturbances after heart valve operations. When our study is complete we shall be in a better position to clarify this matter.

References

1. Götze P (1980) Psychopathologie der Herzoperierten. Enke, Stuttgart
2. Longmore DB, Bennett G, Gueirrara D, Smith M (1979) Prostacyclin: A solution to some problems of extracorporeal circulation. Lancet 1:1002–1005
3. Moncada S, Gryglewski RJ, Bunting S, Vane JR (1976) An enzyme isolated from arteries transforms prostaglandin endoperoxides to an unstable substance that inhibits platelet aggregation. Nature 263:663–665
4. Pokar H, Huse-Kleinstoll G (1980) Possible intraoperative influences of anesthesia and extracorporeal circulation on the postoperative psychopathological phenomena. In: Psychic and neurological dysfunctions after open-heart surgery. Thieme, Stuttgart, p 130

The Effects of Prostacyclin on Reducing Cerebral Damage Following Open-Heart Surgery

D. Longmore

Introduction

Cardiopulmonary bypass has been a routine procedure for a quarter of a century. Until the discovery of prostacyclin with its powerful inhibiting effect on the blood platelet, by Vane and his group in 1977 [1], there was no opportunity for revolutionary changes which promise to make the technique safer. Surgical results, however, have gradually improved because of small incremental refinements of technique. Better prosthetic implants and a better understanding of homograft materials have also helped. From the late 1950s to the mid-1970s, open-heart surgery was still too difficult and expensive to be undertaken outside specialized centres. It was routine only in adults with well-advanced disease and on children and infants with congenital deformities. The indications for surgery were strict. Only patients with disease so advanced that it was potentially lethal were referred for operation, and then only when cardiac failure was imminent. The possibilities of bacterial endocarditis or advancing pulmonary hypertension were also indications for surgery.

Now the indications for surgery are less stringent and consequently the patient spectrum has changed over the past 5 years. One of the most common contemporary cardiac operations is the coronary bypass vein graft. Frequently, this procedure is carried out on the apparently fit working patients who only complains of chest pain. Sometimes the procedure is done on patients with a chance finding of EKG change on routine insurance examination. This operation, because of the patient profile, is mainly done on active males in the prime of their working life (Figs. 1, 2).

Coronary artery blockage is usually part of a generalized disease. Accordingly, it may be naive to assume that any surgery which is undertaken can be anything but palliative. Figure 1 compares the incidene of coronary artery disease and cerebrovascular disease in England with their incidence in the United States of America. The incidence of these two diseases in a typical year is similar in the two countries at over 52% of all deaths. The histogram shown in Fig. 1 is further subdivided to separate the mortality of males from females and the working age group, aged 16–64 years, from deaths at all ages. This breakdown shows that the commonest cause of death in the working male is coronary artery disease. Importantly from the viewpoint of any group involved in the study of cerebral communications, the figures confirm that cerebrovascular disease is frequently associated with coronary disease.

Figure 2 shows the inexorable increase in the incidence of coronary artery deaths in the United Kingdom since 1931, when reliable figures became available for the

Psychopathological and Neurological Dysfunctions
Following Open-Heart Surgery Ed by Becker et al

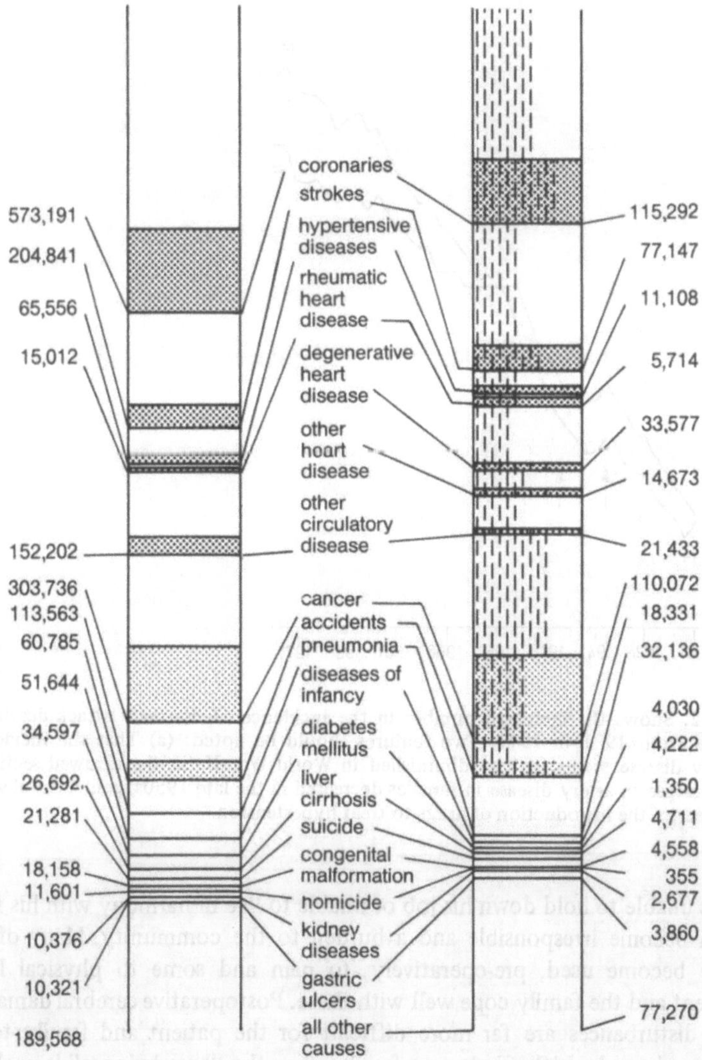

Fig. 1. **The incidence of cardiovascular disease compared in a typical year between England and Wales, and the United States. Cardiovascular disease accounts for over 50% of all deaths. It should be noted that in the working age group (*shaded*) the incidence of coronaries is greater in the male (*vertical hatching*), whereas after retirement the incidence of coronaries in males and females is approximately equal**

first time in any country. Not only is coronary artery disease now numerically the most important cause of death, but it promises to be an even sinister threat to productive life unless effective preventive measures can be introduced. Coronary artery surgery can now frequently offer an increased life span and usually elimination of pain on exertion and an increased exercise tolerance. Surgical triumphs of this kind are, however, worthless if the patient's brain is so damaged during the operation that

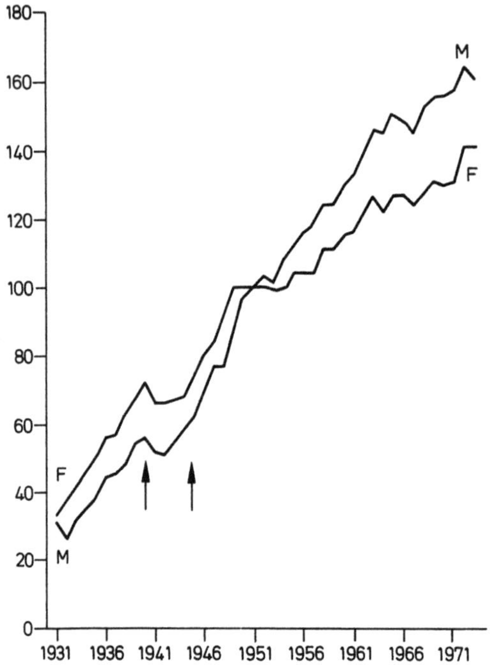

Fig. 2. Shows the increased number in the incidence of coronary attack deaths in England and Wales from 1931 to 1971. Two features should be noted: (a) That the incidence of coronary artery disease seems to have diminished in World War II (in the arrowed section). (b) The rate of increase in artery disease in females decreased in the late 1950s, coincidental with, and possibly related to, the introduction of drugs to treat hypertension

he is unable to hold down his job or unable to live in harmony with his family. He may even become irresponsible and a burden to the community. Many of these patients have become used, pre-operatively, to pain and some to physical limitations; the patient and the family cope well with these. Postoperative cerebral damage and psychiatric disturbances are far more difficult for the patient and family to manage. The economic and social effects on a family when the "breadwinner" is unable or reluctant to work postoperatively are difficult to assess. It is known that less than half of the patients apparently medically fit for work after vein grafting in the United States of America actually worked [2].

The members of the international study group are only too conscious of the unacceptably high incidence of cerebral damage and psychiatric disturbances which are the all too common complications of contemporary cardiac surgery. Our attempt as an international group in trying to detect, quantify, and classify cerebral damage for the first time must be a major step forward in solving the problem. We have a huge task to face. Even when we can demonstrate and measure the damage we have to identify the causes.

A multi-million dollar industry has built up around cardiopulmonary bypass. Physicians, surgeons and manufacturers of equipment are as conscious as this group is that something needs to be done to eliminate brain injury and psychiatric disturbance. The difficulty has always been that the causes of these injuries are manifold. The manufacturers of equipment tend to blame the surgeon for any complications which occur. The surgeon, on the other hand, has so many ancillary products and procedures to whom he can attribute any disastrous sequelae that he may overlook his own shortcomings of technique. Neither can be blamed for their point of view. The manufacturers are ethical. They cannot introduce any new applicance without satisfying the regulatory bodies and complying with rigorous test procedures laid down in regulations for devices. This is a costly and slow process which endangers patients in two ways: New real advances are held back or even lost, manufacturers attempting to produce safer cardiopulmonary devices face stiff competition from rivals with vested interests in the present generation of equipment. Existing, approved, though potentially unsafe techniques, such as ethylene oxide sterilization used in the United States, are perpetrated.

There has never before been a medical problem of such complexity with such numerical importance. In the United States in 1977 96 000 patients underwent open-heart surgery for coronary vein graft. There are two entities the manifestations of which are now easy to separate. On the one hand, a patient's decreased cerebral function may be due to organic brain damage whilst on the other, apparently similar symptoms can arise entirely from psychological damage and stress. To compound the problem, brain injury and psychological disturbance can occur progressively in the pre-operative, operative, and postoperative periods. The discovery of prostacyclin (prostaglandin I_2) by John Vane and his group in the Wellcome Research Laboratories gives us new hope for the reduction of the problem of brain injury. Its use promises to eliminate many causes of cerebral damage arising from blood damage. Some argue that it is the first major advance in cardiopulmonary bypass since the technique was introduced.

Prostacyclin is a prostaglandin. It is one of the metabolites of arachidonic acid. It is now recognized as a naturally occurring substance which prevents intravascular clotting. Arachidonic acid, its precursor, metabolizes in two ways in the vascular system: (i) in the platelet, to form thromboxane A2 which is a powerful component of the platelet-clotting cascade[1], and (ii) in the blood vessel walls, to form prostacyclin which is secreted into the plasma adjacent to the endothelium. Prostacyclin interacts with the surface of platelets to stabilize them. The effect is to prevent platelet aggregation and breakdown. The half-life of both of these substances is only a few seconds. The life of PGI_2 is longer than that of TXA_2, thus in the normal vessel a balance exists in favour of inhibition of the platelet.

Platelet loss and aggregation in open-heart surgery has always been linked with postoperative disorders, including bleeding and cerebral damage. These problems are even more pronounced when extracorporeal oxygenation is used for long-term respiratory support. Attempts to overcome platelet-related complications have included the use of less traumatic oxygenation methods, notably the use of membranes

1 The mechanism of blood clot formation is still not fully understood. Several interdependent mechanisms exist. Platelet activation and the release of granular material from platelets is an important component of the clotting diathesis caused by extra corporeal circulation.

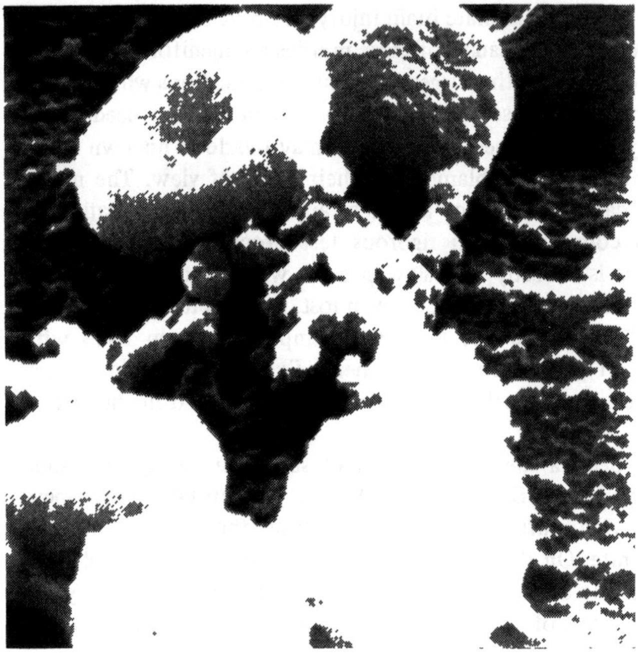

Fig. 3. Shows platelets and red cells adherent to the silicone rubber membrane after exposure to full heparinized blood

instead of bubble columns, discs, drums and screens etc., and other improvements in the extracorporeal apparatus such as less traumatic and pulsatile blood pumps. Some centres use 40-μm filters in the arterial lines, whilst an equal number ban filters from the circuit, fearful of the addition of additional surface area which may trigger the clotting mechanism. The use of weak inhibitors of platelet aggregation, including prostaglandin E, and dipyridamole (persantin) have been tried – all without measurable success.

Although the use of heparin, until recently the only practical anticoagulant for the extracorporeal circulation, prevents gross clotting of blood, the clotting systems are stimulated when blood passes over a foreign surface, such as the extracorporeal tubing. It should be remembered that during a 90-min bypass, blood passes through several miles of tubing and is exposed to over a square mile of oxygen bubbles, which in turn are dissipated by contact with polymethylsiloxane antifome. Platelet adhesion and activation occur soon after contact between blood and a foreign surface and result in formation of platelet and cellular aggregates. Figure 3 shows a typical thrombus formation 2 min after exposure of a silicone rubber membrane to heparinized blood. Heparin is thought to stimulate platelet aggregation. In addition, there is release of anti-heparin activity and pro-coagulant acitivity from platelets and leucocytes after contact with foreign surfaces not prevented by heparin. This encourages fibrin deposition despite the presence of heparin. Platelets adhere to and aggregate on any surface other than normal vascular endothelium, even if heparinization is adequate, now we know that endothelium is not inert and that it actively generates prostacyclin. The presence of prostacyclin in sufficient concentration in the blood passing through the extracorporeal apparatus should help to prevent unwarranted platelet activity. Platelet aggregates and microthrombi are always present in the blood leaving an extracorporeal circuit, and on return to the patient are known to be responsible for thrombotic occlusion of the microvasculature. Defibrination commonly leads to severe postoperative bleeding problems, sometimes requiring re-operation. The use of prostaglandin E_1, during extracorporeal circulation has been reported previously with encouraging platelet-sparing results. Prostacyclin is the most potent anti-aggregating agent yet discovered. It is probably more than 30 times as active as prostaglandin E_1. Like prostaglandin E_1, it acts by increasing platelet cyclic AMP.

The value of the addition of prostacyclin to the extracorporeal circuit to inhibit platelet activity has been previously demonstrated in animal experiments [3], in renal dialysis, and in charcoal haemoperfusion [4]. We studied the use of PGI_2 in extracorporeal circulation in dogs. In this experimental work we studied the use of prostacyclin alone, heparin alone, and a combination of both at various dose levels. We also tried to repeat the work reported by Fletcher on cardiopulmonary bypass in primates, using massive haemodilution alone without the use of any anticoagulants.

For the experiments we used a simple cardiopulmonary bypass apparatus with a Bentley Temptrol Paediatric Oxygenator; a single roller arterial pump (finely adjustable) for occlusion. We placed two arterial filters in series in the arterial line. The animals were bypassed for 1 or 2 h. Serial platelet counts, platelet aggregations, and fibrinogen levels were done in 15-min intervals. Samples of blood were also taken 5 min after bypass was started and 5 min before the end of bypass to study protein denaturation and the presence of toxic materials in the plasma, using the fetal heart toxicity test. This was done with fetal hearts which were taken from Their's (T.O.) pure strain mice which had been mated 15 days previously. Fifteen control and 15 test hearts were each cultured in 2 ml "Wellcome" 199 culture medium and 1 ml serum. Serum for the control hearts was obtained from 50 ml blood drawn from the bypass circuit proximal to the first filter after the prime was mixed with the circulating blood. This blood sample was centrifuged and 1 ml of the supernatant plasma was added to the control hearts. Plasma for the test hearts was obtained from 50 ml blood drawn from the same site just before the bypass was ended (after 1 h 50 min). The hearts were cultured in 95% O_2 and 5% CO_2 at 37 °C. They were examined under a dissecting microscope every 24 h and returned to the culture after the beating rate had been recorded.

In addition to these studies, haematocrit counts were measured, screen filtration pressure tests [5] were done to demonstrate the presence of platelet aggregates, and the pressure differential across the two arterial filters was measured. Figure 4 shows the bypass apparatus with the pressure take-off points proximal to the first filter and distal to the first and second filters. An increasing pressure gradient between these two points indicates that the filters are becoming blocked either with clot or platelet aggregates. When the pressure gradient across one or both of the filters was seen to rise slowly then fall suddenly, it was assumed that the filter had blocked and unloaded the deposits blocking its mesh into the arterial line. When this happened in the proximal filter the pressure drop was transferred to the second filter. In the one dog which was

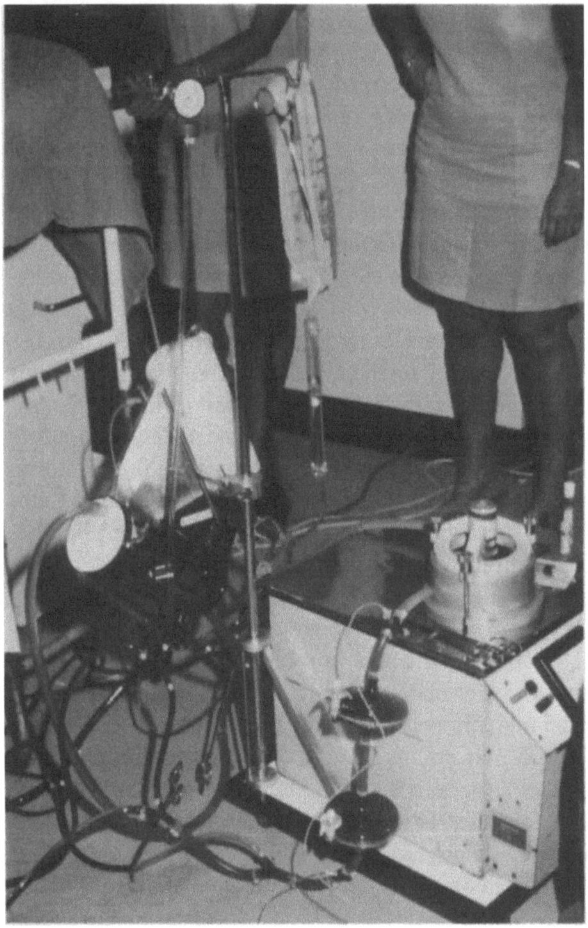

Fig. 4. Shows an experimental bypass with two filters in series in the arterial line with pressure take off points proximal to the first between the two and distal to the second filter

bypassed without heparin or prostacyclin the filter element in the second filter burst. Figure 5 shows the failed filter element and the clot present on its surface.

Scanning electron microscopy of the filters was also used to compare the first and second filters with each other in each of the series. Figure 6 is a scanning electron micrograph (at a magnification of 32125) of the second filter in the arterial line. In this case heparin was used alone as the anticoagulant. The dosage was 3 mg/kg heparin given 5 min before bypass was started. A further 3 mg was added to the priming fluid and a reinforcing dose of 1.5 mg/kg was given 1 h after the initial dose. Thrombus formation is advanced with platelets adherent to the filter mesh. The platelets have broken down. Fibrin strands enmeshing red and white blood cells can be seen. Figure 7 shows a similar filter at the same magnification when heparin, at the same dosage, was supplemented with a prostacyclin infusion of 10 ng/kg per minute starting 15 min before bypass, and being increased to 20 ng/kg during bypass.

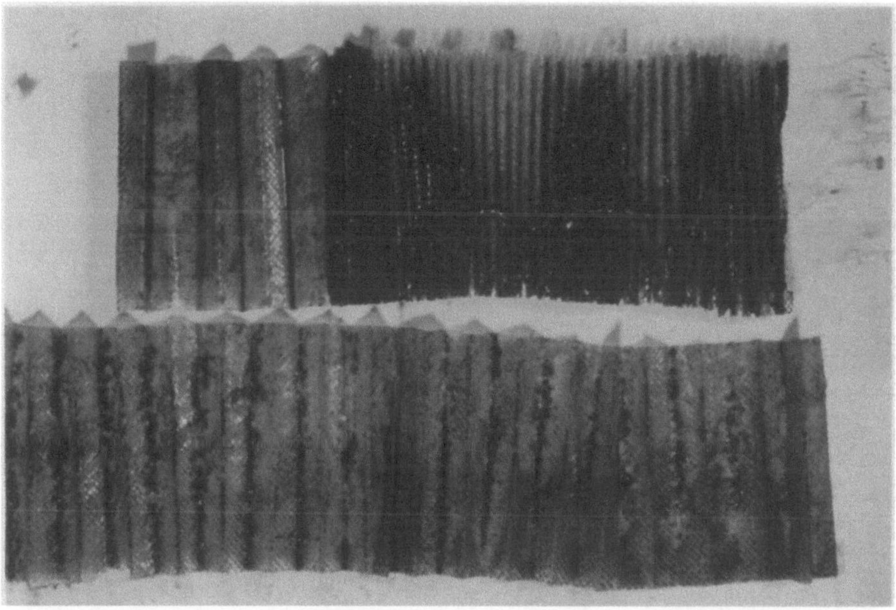

Fig. 5. Filter element showing clot taken from the arterial line of an experimental bypass when no prostacyclin and heparin were used. It is frequently said that a mass of haemodilution can be used instead of anticoagulation. Most usually clot is formed which passes into the patient, and a filter in the arterial line will fail in this situation

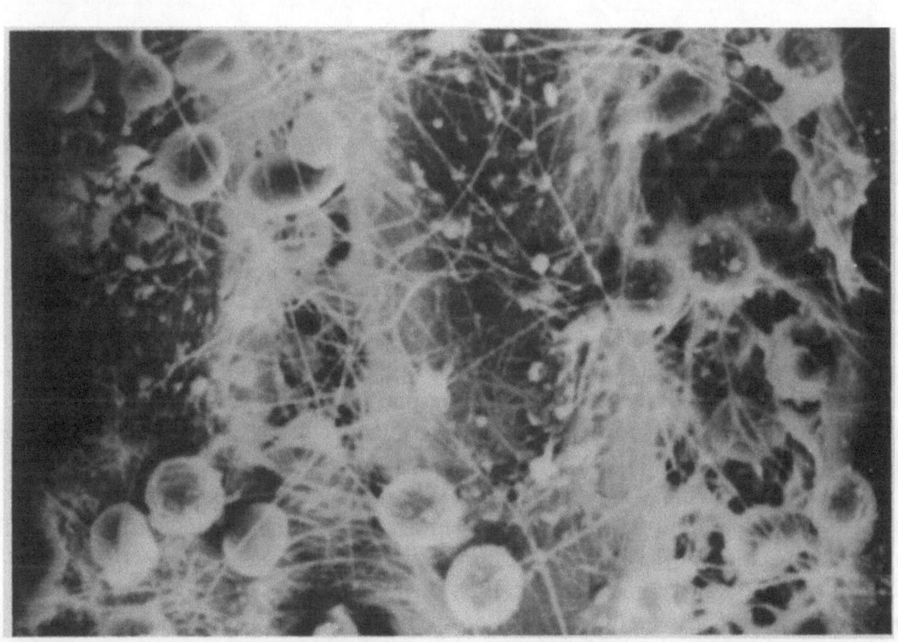

Fig. 6. The deposition of thrombus with platelet activity, fibrin strands, and enmeshed red and white cells, on a second filter placed in series in the arterial line of an experimental cardiopulmonary bypass after 2 h

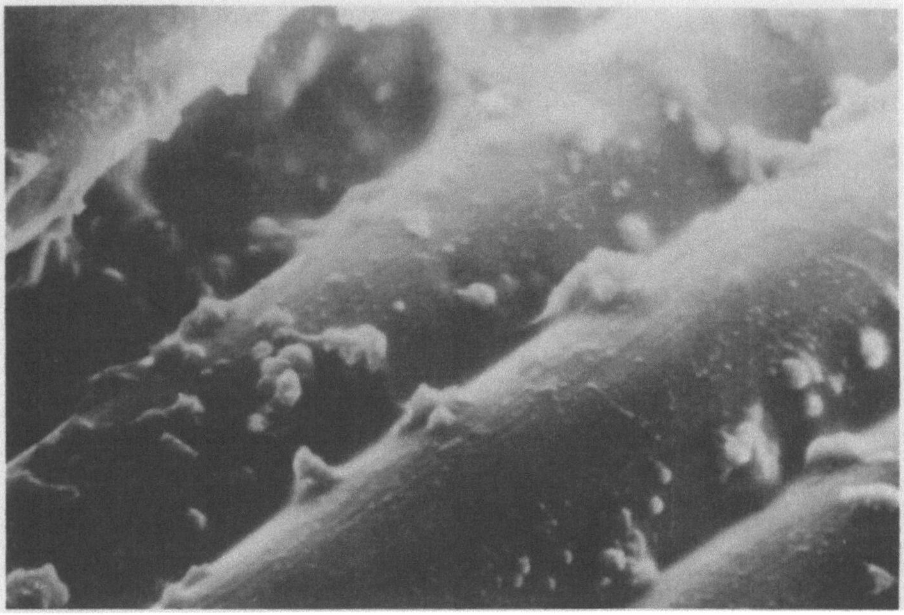

Fig. 7. Filter element identical to that in Fig. 6 with only a few adherent platelets at the end of an experimental 2-h bypass with prostacyclin added

The filter element has no obvious deposition of protein on the surface. The few platelets which have adhered to the filter mesh have not broken down. There is debate about the desirability of using filters in the arterial line. Undoubtedly they can form a valuable trap for air inadvertently admitted from the oxygenator and for particles from the apparatus, but arterial line filtration with heparin alone may be a source of embolization and platelet destruction. When prostacyclin comes into general use, arterial line filters may be mandatory.

The results of this series of experiments were clear. In the conventional "heparin alone" bypass, the platelet count fell to approximately 30% of its pre-operative figure, and after the administration of protamine to 25%. The ability of the platelets to aggregate was reduced to about 15% of their pre-operative level, thus experimentally confirming the well-known clinical observation that after bypass with heparin and neutralization of heparin with protamine, the blood clotting mechanism is severely impaired.

Figure 8 shows the comparative platelet counts with heparin plus prostacyclin, prostacyclin alone, and conventional heparinization. Figure 9 shows the return of normal aggregation in the heparin and prostacyclin bypass. There was virtual elimination of platelet activity postadministration of protamine in the conventional heparin bypass. Figure 10 shows the comparison of the beating rate and the survival time in the fetal heart test with blood taken from animals with conventional heparinization. Figure 11 compares fibrinogen levels in the three groups. The fall in plasma fibrinogen in the prostacyclin alone bypass is due to clot formation in the stagnant areas of the

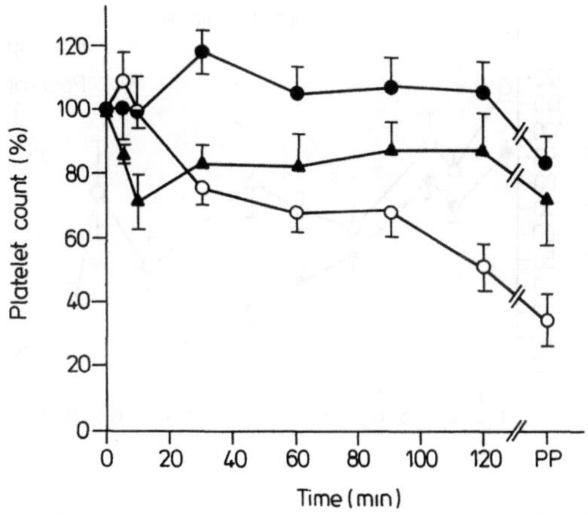

Fig. 8. Shows the platelet counts: the *upper line* with heparin and prostacyclin, the *middle line* prostacyclin alone, and the *lower line* heparin alone

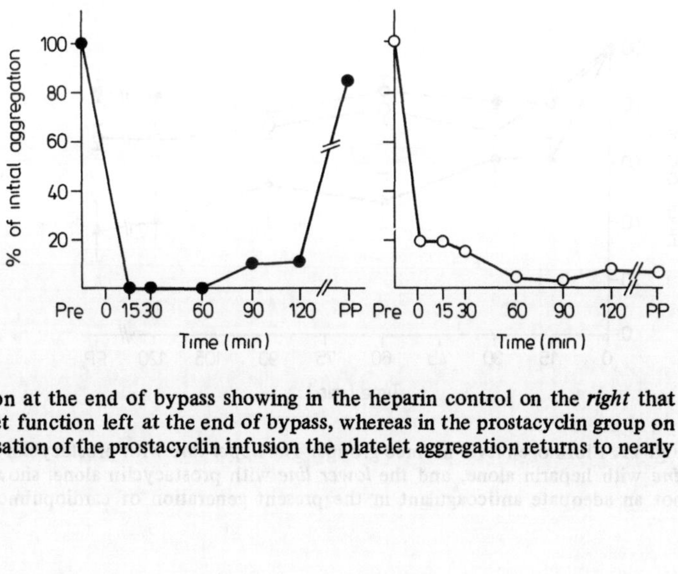

Fig. 9. Platelet aggregation at the end of bypass showing in the heparin control on the *right* that there is very little platelet function left at the end of bypass, whereas in the prostacyclin group on the *left* following the cessation of the prostacyclin infusion the platelet aggregation returns to nearly normal

oxygenator which was used. This clot formation could be prevented by gentle agitation of the oxygenator to avoid areas of stasis.

We have recently carried out a double blind clinical trial in which prostacyclin was given to 12 of 23 consecutive patients undergoing coronary artery revascularization.

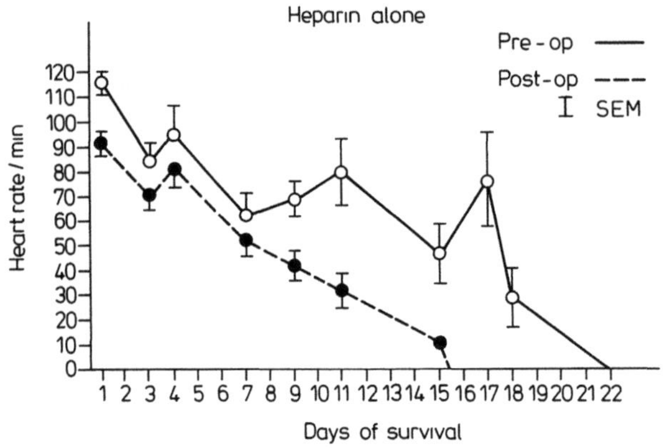

Fig. 10. Shows the diminution of beating rate and survival rate of fetal hearts exposed to plasma taken from the bypass apparatus at the beginning of operation and towards the end, before the administration of cardio-active drugs. This diminution of the performance of the fetal hearts in presumably associated with protein damage from denaturation, or the presence of toxic materials from platelet release. It does not take place when prostacyclin is used

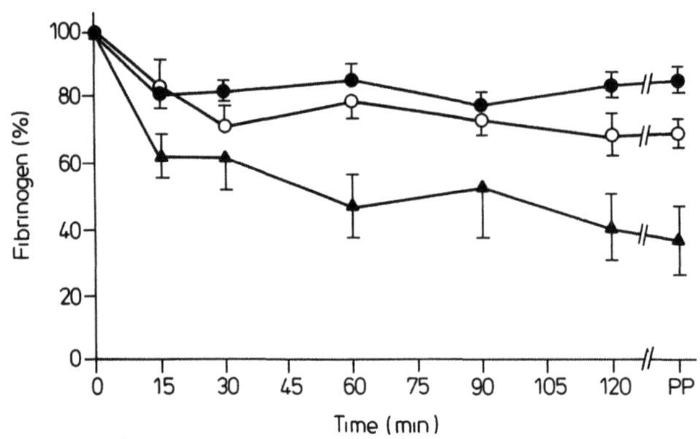

Fig. 11. Fibrinogen level in three groups: The *upper line* with prostacyclin plus heparin, the *middle line* with heparin alone, and the *lower line* with prostacyclin alone, showing that prostacyclin is not an adequate anticoagulant in the present generation of cardiopulmonary bypass equipment

The patients were studied for routine haematology biochemistry and, in addition, psychometric and neurological status and platelet function. These included:

Haematocrit
Haemoglobin
Platelet count
Corrected platelet count
Fibrinogen levels
T.C.T.
P.T.T.K.

Prothrombin time
White blood count
Platelet aggregation
% initial platelet aggregation
Haemochron time (activated clotting time)
(Antithrombin III)
Blood pressure recording before, during and after prostacyclin infusion
Perfusion pressure
Perfusion flow rates
Coulter counted platelets
C.K. total
C.K. M. B.
Heart rate
Blood loss 0–6 h, 6–12 h, 12–18 h
Blood given
Urine output
Fluids given
Rewarming time
Protein denaturation and damage test (fetal heart culture method)
Particle counts in pump washings
Particle counts in pump prime
Particle counts in any drugs which are administered

Sampling times for the majority of these parameters were as follows:

1. During the 24-h pre-operative period (psychometric and neurological tests only)
2. Immediately after induction of anaesthesia (control)
3. Thirty minutes after beginning of infusion of drug
4. Five minutes after heparin
5. Five minutes after beginning of bypass
6. a)
   b) Every 30 min on bypass
   c)
7. At the end of bypass before cardioactive drugs (fetal heart test only)
8. Fifteen minutes after protamine administration
9. Two hours after bypass
10. Six hours after bypass (CK assay only)
11. Twenty-four hours after bypass
12. Three days after bypass (CK assay and psychometric tests)
13. Six days after bypass (psychometric and neurological tests)

The psychometric test, which consisted of short- and long-term memory recall tests as conceived by Bethune [6], were done pre-operatively and 3 and 6 days postoperatively.

The values of haemoglobin, haematocrit, platelet and white cell counts were consistently higher in the prostacyclin-treated group than in the group given placebo, with times of significance usually during early bypass, when the biological results of extracorporeal circulation appear most drastic. Platelet aggregation was substantially inhibited by prostacyclin from the start of infusion to the end of bypass and function returned sharply to 70% of normal as soon as infusion ceased. This contrasted with the placebo-treated group in whom platelet function declined with the progress of bypass and fell to below 40% of the initial function in the immediate post-bypass period, and remained below mean treated group function until 24 h post-bypass. Activated clotting times were significantly longer in the prostacyclin treated group throughout heparin anticoagulation, presumably due to the so-called enhancing effect of prostacyclin, though its mechanism is not known. Synergistic effects of this increased anticoagulation have not yet been clarified, but it is expected that Platelet Factor 4, Fibrinopeptide A, $B_{\beta 1-42}$ and Antithrombin III levels may also be affected and may even be involved in prostacyclin's apparent ability to potentiate heparin anticoagulation.

The well-maintained platelet counts shown in the prostacyclin-treated group, significantly greater than the placebo group from the start of bypass onwards, obviously account for the immediate return to function in that group as soon as prostacyclin infusion stopped. Assays of β-Thromboglobulin, a protein liberated into plasma almost solely upon platelet release, ought to parallel this phenomenon. β-Thromboglobulin levels would be expected to increase proportional to platelet destruction. Platelet integrity preservation would be reflected by unchanged TG plasma levels.

Prostacyclin did not have any affect upon prothrombin and partial thromboplastic times, or upon fibrinogen levels. Thrombin times appeared to be slightly longer in the treated group. Prostacyclin did not apparently affect changes normally seen in creatine kinase levels during surgical invasion, but this result should be more thoroughly investigated. Mild and undocumented myocardial infarcts, sometimes occurring in the investigated periods, altered total C.K. and C.K.-M.B. levels in individual cases,

Table 1. Summary of clinical measurements

	Prostacyclin	Placebo
Blood use (ml)		
During operation	596 ± 226	909 ± 260
After operation (19 h)	1073 ± 200	1495 ± 331
Total across operation	1669 ± 303	2404 ± 485
Blood loss (ml)		
0– 6 h	250 ± 29	499 ± 103
6–18 h	103 ± 8	273 ± 67
18 h +	132 ± 18	138 ± 23
Total	485 ± 48	910 ± 172
Administration of other fluids (ml)		
During operation	3095 ± 357	3384 ± 471
After operation (18 h)	841 ± 46	846 ± 44
Total	3936 ± 346	4230 ± 454
Urine output (ml)		
During operation	1120 ± 108	1435 ± 229
After operation	1992 ± 337	1637 ± 115
Total	3112 ± 426	3072 ± 221

Figures are mean = SEM

masking any other affects which have been present and affecting mean'd values so that creatine kinase should not be studied in this way. C.K.-B.B. assays were negative in all but one case, but this is a false negative result as liberated enzymes resulting from organic damage may not cross the blood brain barrier and in mild cases of brain damage remain undetected in plasma. Recent work by Åberg and Ponquist show cerebrospinal fluid levels of both C.K.-B.B. and adenylate kinase to be much more sensitive indicators of mild brain damage resulting from cardiac surgery. The psychological and neurological tests which attempted to intercept symtoms of mild brain damage revealed no differences between the groups, however. We are in some doubt about the sensitivity of these tests and feel that they should perhaps be redesigned.

Clinical measurements are shown in Tables 1 and 2.

The most dramatic of these was the significant fall in blood loss in the prostacyclin group. Total postoperative blood loss was halved in the prostacyclin group, an effect linked indubitably with well-maintained platelet counts and well-preserved function. Blood pressures and perfusion pressures were lower in the prostacyclin group, as expected, but its vasodilation effects were not generally troublesome.

To understand the place of prostacyclin in cardiopulmonary bypass, and its potential of preventing brain injury, it is necessary to relate its effects to the known main

Table 2. Diastolic and perfusion pressures

	Pressure (mmHg)		
Sample	Prostacyclin	Placebo	Significance
Diastolic pressure			
2	91.3 ± 8.8 (n = 12)	84.9 ± 13.5 (n = 11)	$P < 0.05$
3	67.0 ± 16.7 (n = 12)	85.9 ± 6.7 (n = 11)	$P < 0.01$
4	54.9 ± 11.9 (n = 12)	88.4 ± 17.7 (n = 11)	$P < 0.01$
8	78.4 ± 13.5 (n = 12)	74.4 ± 11.6 (n = 11)	NS
Perfusion pressure			
5	64.6 ± 26.0 (n = 12)	62.1 ± 15.2 (n = 11)	NS
6a	58.2 ± 14.6 (n = 12)	71.2 ± 25.3 (n = 11)	NS
6b	70.4 ± 13.6 (n = 12)	74.4 ± 16.6 (n = 11)	NS
6c	79.1 ± 13.8 (n = 10)	90.6 ± 16.7 (n = 8)	NS

Table 3. The main pre-operative period causes of brain dysfunction

A. Organic
1. Cerebral emboli from clot in the left side of the heart
2. Paradoxical embolization through defects in the cardiac septa
3. Septic emboli from infection in the heart

B. Psychopathological
4. Psychological stress due to anxiety about undergoing open-heart surgery
5. Disturbances due to patient's inability to cope with being a cardiac cripple
6. Pre-existing coincidental mental illness

Table 4. Causes of brain damage during operation

1.	Air embolization
2.	Particle embolization
3.	Embolization from blood products
4.	Toxins from the extracorporeal apparatus
5.	Haemolysis
6.	Toxins due to protein denaturation caused by mechanical damage and toxic materials released from platelet granules
7.	Prolonged hypotension possibly exacerbated by non-pulsatile blood flow
8.	Biochemical disturbances, notably CA^{2+} and K^{+} abnormalities
9.	Low or very high PaO_2 and high $PaCO_2$
10.	Inadequate anaesthesia (conscious patient)

causes of cerebral injury in the pre-operative period, during operation, and post-operatively. The significance of the presence of prostacyclin is described in relation to each of the common causes of brain damage.

The use of prostacyclin does not eliminate all possible sources of brain damage across operation but many of the commoner and most of the more serious causes are partially or completely eliminated.

The surgeon who is evaluating the patient for operation and the referring physician, frequently overlook the existence of a history of previous psychiatric disturbances. The surgical team tend to concentrate only on the purely cardiac aspects of the heart on which he is planning to operate will in fact still function as an effective pump after the insult of surgery and cardiopulmonary bypass. This problem may exercise him so much that he may overlook warning features in the medical history. A history of psychiatric illness or even a transient stroke are frequently forgotten or suppressed by the patient who wants an operation. There is less justification for a surgeon failing to detect the presence of previous cerebral emboli, but it can be overlooked even in cases of mitral stenosis and left atrial myxoma where it classically occurs. It is usually overlooked in patients with previous myocardial infarcts. The reason for this is that neurological recovery is often fairly complete and the patient may appear to be normal. A really thorough neurological examination will reveal residual disabilities, but usually this is not done.

Causes of brain damage during operation are very much more important than the main ones being listed in Table 4.

Air Embolization

A distinction has to be made between air embolization derived from room air admitted to the patient and oxygen bubbles derived from the oxygen admitted to the oxygenator for the purpose of gas exchange. Air consists of 80% nitrogen which is insoluble in the already saturated patients' blood and tissue fluids. During cariopulmonary bypass some nitrogen is washed out of the patients' blood by the flow of oxygen in the oxygenator, making it possible for some nitrogen to diffuse from bubbles into the tissue fluids. Oxygen bubbles which pass into the circulation are gradually absorbed into the tissue fluids and tissues.

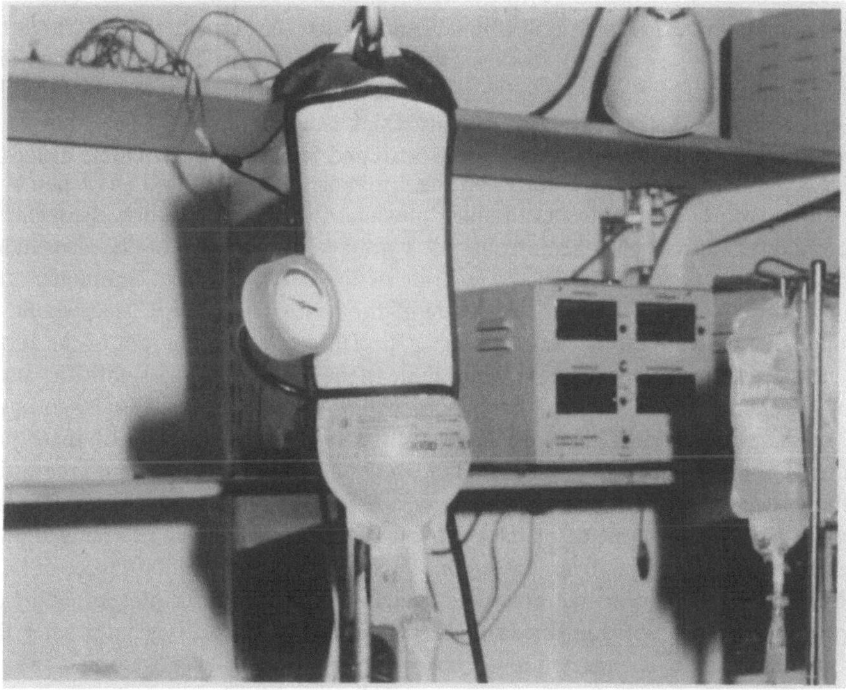

Fig. 12. Illustrates a pressurized system which is frequently used in administration of cardioplegic solution through a conventional drip chamber with the risk of admitting air

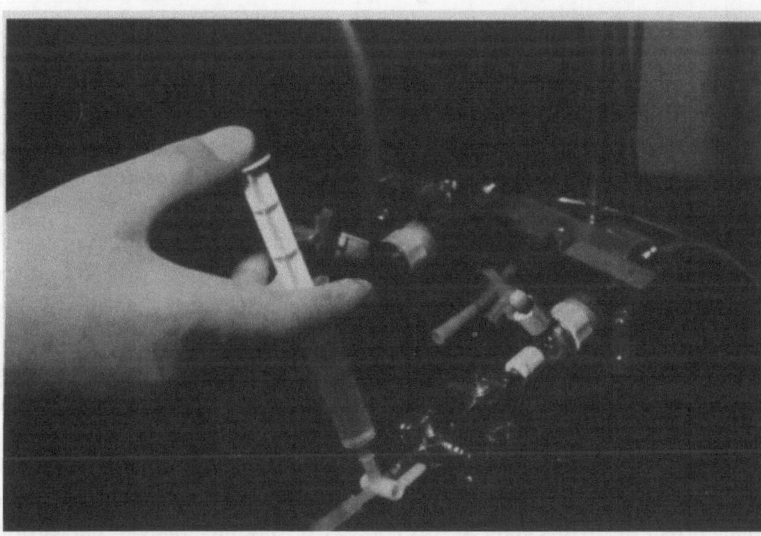

Fig. 13. Shows the danger of admitting air when flushing out pressure measuring catheters in the left atrium

The commonest cause of embolization during bypass is air, usually termed "surgical" air, which is left in, or let into, the heart during the operation. The inside of the heart is roughened and ridged with the presence of the musculi pectinati in the atria and the trabeculae carneae in the ventricles. Any air which is allowed into the heart is usually beaten into a froth by the movement of the heart and is extremely difficult to dislodge.

Air commonly enters the aorta when the aortic cannula is inserted and when cold cardioplegic solutions are introduced under pressure. Figure 12 shows how dangerously cardioplegic solutions may be introduced. Figure 13 reminds us of the dangers of taking pressure measurements on the left side of the heart. The most commonly used technique for removing air from the inside of the heart is to place a stab wound in the apex of the left ventricle and to insert a special needle into the root of the aorta. The heart is then allowed to beat while the patient is still on bypass with the aorta clamped to expel froth. An injection of isoprenaline to make the heart beat vigorously and to drive air through the coronary vessels is often used. In spite of these precautions bubbles frequently reach the brain, and small air bubbles remain on the endocardial surface for many hours and act as a focus for platelet aggregates. The air embolus may either consist of platelets surrounding the air bubble or streams of pure platelet emboli separating from the bubble surface. Another common source of large bubbles which can lodge in the brain and similarly act as a site for platelet emboli is oxygen, which is entrained in the arterialized blood leaving the oxygenator when the levels are allowed to become too low. Prostacyclin prevents platelet aggregates around these bubbles. All oxygenators pass varying numbers of microbubbles into the general circulation. Bubble oxygenators depend for their gas exchange on making a froth of blood to oxygenate it and to allow CO_2 to diffuse out. The blood is then defoamed over silicone antifoam. Streams of microbubbles pass into the patient throughout the operation. Tens of thousands of these, between 5 μm and 100 μm in size, may be counted in the arterial line during a bypass. Ultrasound equipment is used to size the bubbles. If two sensors are placed on the arterial line, one near to the oxygenator, and one near to the patient, it is seen that bubbles of less than half a micron go into solution in the blood and do not usually reach the patient. Larger bubbles not only reach the patient but can also be counted in the patient's carotid and other accessible peripheral arteries [7]. The bubbles which pass into the brain cause damage in two ways, either by blocking vital small end arteries or by forming foci on which platelet aggregates can form.

Membrane oxygenators produce fewer air bubbles properly used. Nevertheless, most contemporary membrane oxygenators use Celgard 2402 or 2502 polypropylene membranes which are made as two-ply microporous membranes, with pore sizes ranging between 200 Å and 400 Å. To work properly these membranes need a coating of protein which covers the water meniscus bridges across the micropores in the membrane. Figure 14 shows this situation schematically, approximately to scale. The deposition of the protein layer probably depends to some extent on platelet adhesion to the surface and platelet breakdown. In oxygenators with microporous membranes, the administration of prostacyclin theoretically might not be advantageous. The beneficial effect of prostacyclin in this context is to reduce platelet deposition, platelet loss, and the thickness of the protein layer which itself diminishes oxygenating capacity. The theoretically harmful effect may be to allow microbubbles to pass through

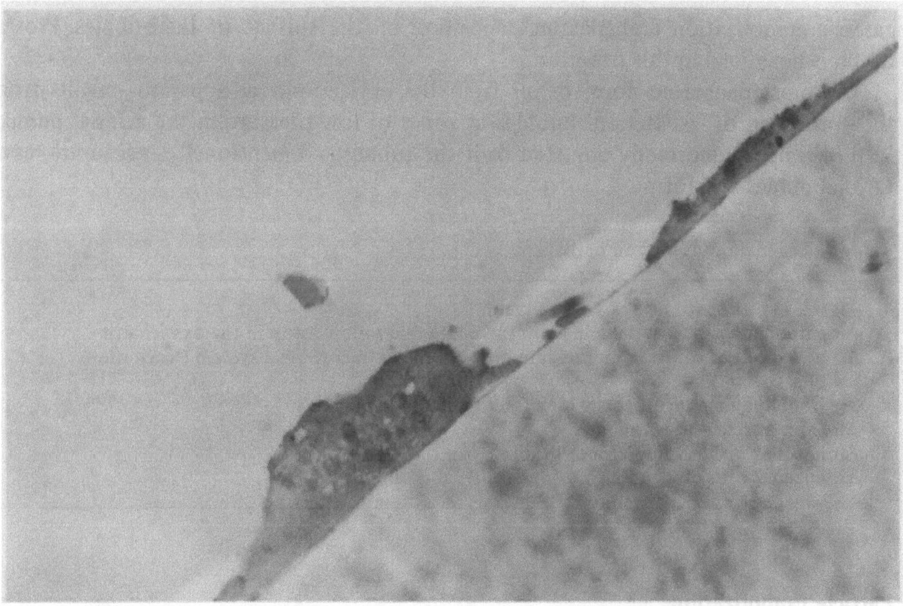

Fig. 14. Shows a deposition of protein on a microporous membrane taking place in spite of the administration of heparin and prostacyclin

the membranes because there is no protein barrier. Preliminary studies of membranes used in the presence of PGI_2 suggests that a different and thinner but still adequate protein layer is deposited on the Celgard membrane in the presence of PGI_2.

There are two other sources of micro-emboli from the extracorporeal apparatus. Figure 15 shows the changing solubility of dissolved gases in clear fluids at various temperatures. Warming the prime in the bypass apparatus is likely to produce massive

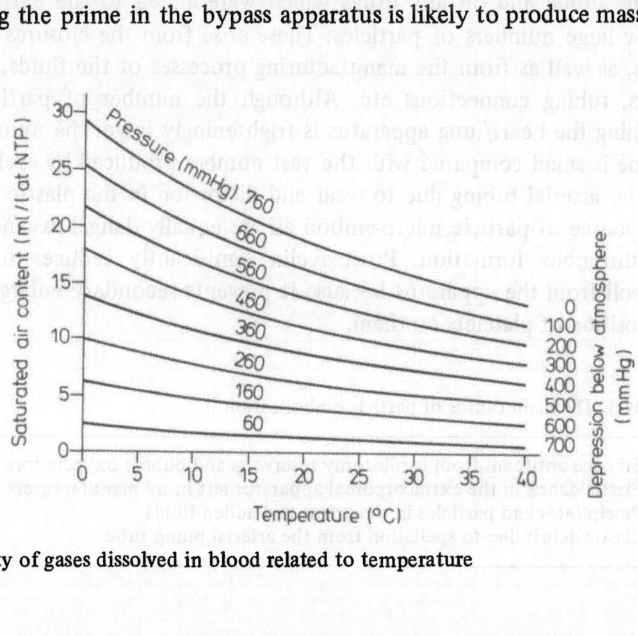

Fig. 15. Varying solubility of gases dissolved in blood related to temperature

gaseous embolization and platelet deposition on the surface of the bubbles. Prostacyclin is beneficial in this situation.

The most dangerous form of air from the extracorporeal apparatus results from the formation of 'cavitation' bubbles in zones of low pressure in the arterial pumps. If the pump is incorrectly adjusted or if the tubing is dimensionally inaccurate, cavitation bubbles will form.

Table 5. The main causes of air embolism

1. Air left in or let into heart by the surgeon
2. Air entrained in the arterial line from the pump due to low levels in the oxygenator
3. Air pulled out of solution by pressure drops in the extracorporeal system ('cavitation bubbles')
4. Air from bubble oxygenators which fail to defoam completely
5. Air from warmed clear fluids
6. Air injected with cardioplegia solutions
7. Air injected with pressure-measuring needles and cannulae

Particle Embolization

There are many sources of particles which pass into the patient during bypass. When bubble oxygenators are used up to 7 g silicone antifoam may pass into the patient. This usually enters the patient as a coating on red cells, white cells, and platelets. The fate of this silicone in the patient's central nervous system is unknown; rarely can it be identified in the sectioned brain of patients who have succumbed after operation.

Particle counts done on the fluids used for washing the extracorporeal apparatus, in the prime and on any drugs which were added to the extracorporeal apparatus, show large numbers of particles. These arise from the closures and rubber aspirating sites, as well as from the manufacturing processes of the fluids, the oxygenator reservoirs, tubing connections etc. Although the number of particles found even after flushing the heart/lung apparatus is frighteningly large, the number of particles in the prime is small compared with the vast number produced by spellation from the inside of the arterial tubing due to wear and distortion in the plastic pump tube. Whatever the source of particle micro-emboli all are equally dangerous and all can be the centre of thrombus formation. Prostacyclin significantly reduces the danger of particle emboli from the apparatus because it prevents secondary enlargement of these due to deposition of platelets on them.

Table 6. The main causes of particle embolization

1. Silicone antifoam from cardiotomy reservoirs and bubble oxygenators
2. Plastic debris in the extracorporeal apparatus left in by manufacturers
3. Precipitates and particles in the prime and added fluids
4. Plastic debris due to spellation from the arterial pump tube

Embolization From Blood Products

The prevention of embolization from blood products during bypass is the most obvious area in which prostacyclin would be expected to be beneficial. Prostacyclin, with its effect on platelet aggregates, removes a major source of embolization from the extracorporeal apparatus. This alone should significantly reduce the incidence of brain damage. Furthermore, prostacyclin, in preventing the formation of platelet aggregates on filters in the arterial line, makes it possible and safe to place filters in this site to remove other potential emboli.

During conventional bypass operations, even with adequate heparinization, intravascular clotting takes place in parts of the vascular system which are underperfused, this possibly being made worse by the lack of pulsatility. Clotting also takes place in areas where any vortex or eddy formation is present. In this situation platelets aggregate and liberate an anti-heparin agent causing a clot to form. This clot will propagate as more platelets adhere and eventually block important vessels. Prostacyclin eliminates this dangerous complication when heparin is used as an anticoagulant.

Prostacyclin reduces the dose of heparin required, causing "the heparin sparing effect". Heparin itself is prepared from several biological sources (animal lung, gut and liver). Heparin is not a single molecular species. Some constituents of commercial heparin, particularly the higher molecular weight fractions, actually stimulate the formation of platelet aggregates and micro-emboli. The reduction of the dose level of heparin also reduces the requirements of protamine, in turn diminishing the likelihood of the formation of heparin-protamine macromolecules.

Table 7. The sources of embolization from blood

1. **Platelet aggregates in the patient**
2. **Platelet aggregates from the extracorporeal apparatus passing into the arterial line**
3. **Whole blood clots from extracorporeal apparatus**
4. **Intravascular clotting (disseminated intravascular clotting)**
5. **Heparin – protamine macromolecules**
6. **Heparin – induced platelet aggregates**

Toxins Liberated from the Extracorporeal Apparatus

The effects of toxins from the extracorporeal apparatus listed in Table 8 are not influenced by the presence of prostacyclin. This should not detract from consideration of their dangers. Many deaths have been caused by residual ethylene oxide and freons and plasticisers from the extracorporeal apparatus. When red blood cells are haemolysed, the products are toxic, but prostacyclin has no contribution to make in reducing the harmful effects of haemolysis.

Table 8. Toxins from the extracorporeal apparatus during bypass

1. Residual ethylene oxide and freons from sterilization procedures
2. Plasticisers (phthalates etc.) leached from tubing
3. Drugs administered via the arterial line (penicillin fits, etc.)
4. Changes in tonicity when non-isotonic substances are added to the arterial blood
5. Haemolysis

Protein Denaturation

In the animal experiments we noted that the protein fraction of the blood contained less toxic material, as measured by the very sensitive fetal heart toxicity test. In previous studies, without the use of prostacyclin, we have always shown depression of beating rate and survival time in fetal hearts when they were exposed to plasma taken at the end of bypass [8]. In this study the corresponding plasma from prostacyclin patients was comparable in its effects with that from a normal healthy volunteer. It is not known whether the depression of the fetal hearts which ordinarily follows bypass is associated with mechanical damage to proteins, or with protein damage due to release of platelet granules. The beneficial effects of prostacyclin suggest the latter mechanism.

Hypotension During Bypass

Prostacyclin is a potent naturally occurring substance. A high level of circulating prostacyclin can be dangerous. A dose rate of up to 8 ng/kg body weight per minute has an anti-platelet effect without causing hypotension, while higher concentrations cause a drop in the blood pressure. In the conscious subject headache and colic sometimes occur when a dose rate of 9 ng/kg prostacyclin per minute is exceeded. In the clinical trail we used a dose level of 8 ng/kg per minute before bypass and doubled this dose when bypass commenced. Hypotension was not a problem and vasopressors were not required.

Table 9. The causes of hypotension during bypass

1. Possible hypotensive effect of prostacyclin
2. Low pressures due to anaesthetic and other drugs
3. Low pressures due to inadequate flow
4. Relative hypotension (when patient was hypertensive before operation)
5. Low pressures due to cannulae blocking vessels and reducing cardiac output before going on bypass
6. Non-pulsatile flow causing organ underperfusion

One other cause of brain damage during operation is inadequate anaesthesia during bypass. Anaesthetic agents are diluted when the patient goes on bypass. A patient may be paralysed and awake during substantial periods of the operation with consequential psychiatric trauma. Brain damage which occurs during operation may be enhanced by postoperative complications which can by themselves cause brain damage.

Table 10. The biochemical disturbances which occur during bypass

1. Disturbances due to dilution of blood reducing enzyme and trace element levels
2. Relative biochemical abnormalities due to distortion by hypothermia of CO_2 levels and selective enzyme inhibition by hypothermia
3. Metabolic or respiratory acidosis

Table 11. The causes of brain damage after operation

1. Hypotension
2. Air released from inside the heart
3. Excessive drug therapy (hypnotics, diuretics)
4. Sleep deprivation, pain, and fear in intensive care
5. Embolization from clot on a cardiac implant or disintegration of an implant

Postoperative hypotension due to bleeding, sometimes leading to re-operation, is a distressingly frequent occurrence when heparin is used. Many surgeons legislate for up to 2 h to be spent obtaining haemostasis before closing the chest after bypass is finished. This is because the few remaining platelets have lost the power to coagulate. When prostacyclin is present the platelets are protected. Prostacyclin has no influence on the other postoperative causes of brain damage.

Because we have the potential for eliminating, with the use of prostacyclin, so many of the known causes of brain damage, it is now necessary for us to refine our techniques for logging causes of brain damage. By doing this we should be able to detect early any single new cause which appears.

An international register of postoperative cerebral sequelae will be of immense value in monitoring the advances which must follow the introduction of prostacyclin into general usage to make cardiopulmonary bypass safer.

Conclusion

We hope now to enter a new era of cardiac surgery. Dry operative fields, no postoperative bleeding, better extracorporeal apparatus which will not fill the patient with emboli, all promise to virtually eliminate organic brain damage, renal failure – which is already uncommon – and other organ damage. International co-operation in the collection of data about the remaining psychopathological complications will enable us to detect any flaws in design of extracorporeal apparatus and operations.

Any lapses in manufacturing or sterilizing techniques will become immediately apparent; it is now up to us to continue to seek co-operation and to maintain a multidisciplinary approach. A pusillanimous approach to the huge problem of complications of cardiopulmonary bypass will not suffice in the last 2 decades of the twentieth century. A new generation of apparatus must be designed to take advantage of prostacyclin. Apparatus which does not require heparinization of the patient will make heart surgery with prostacyclin as complication-free as conventional general surgery.

References

1. Moncada S, Vane JR (1977) The discovery of prostacyclin – A fresh insight into arachidonic acid metabolism. In: Kharasch N (ed) Biochemical aspects of prostaglandins and thromboxanes. Academic Press, New York pp 155–177
2. Fashionable Surgery. World Med 16:57–60
3. Longmore DB, Bennett JG, Guerreiro D, Smith M, Bunting S, Moncada S, Reed P, Read NG, Vane JR (1979) Prostacyclin: a solution to some problems of extracorporeal circulation. Lancet 1:1002–1005
4. Bunting S, Moncada S, Vane JR, Woods HF, Weston MT (1979) Prostacyclin improves haemocompatibility during charcoal haemoperfusion. In: Vane JR, Bergstrom S (eds) Prostacyclin. Raven, New York p 361
5. Swank R, Roth JG, Jansen J (1964) Screen filtration pressure method and adhesiveness and aggregation of blood cells. J Appl Physiol 19/2:340–346
6. Bethune DW (1981) Psychometric testing in the evaluation of the post-operative cardiac patient. In: Longmore DB (ed) Towards safer cardiac surgery. Medical Technical Press, Lancaster, pp 613–619
7. Pearson DT, Carter RF, Hammo MB, Waterhouse PS (1981) Gaseous microemboli during open heart surgery. In: Longmore DB (ed) Towards safer cardiac surgery. Medical Technical Press, Lancaster, pp 325–355
8. Longmore DB, Smith MA (1981) Toxins in open heart surgery. In: Longmore BD (ed) Towards safer cardiac surgery. Medical Technical Press, Lancaster, pp 447–475

Improved Cerebral Protection during Open-Heart Surgery. A Psychometric Investigation on 339 Patients

T. Åberg, M. Kihlgren, L. Jonsson, K. Stjernlöf, U. Lönn, T. Rystedt, H. Tydén, C.-J. Westerholm, A. Taube

Introduction

During recent years the incidence of cerebral complications after open-heart surgery has gratifyingly diminished. However, these complications do still occur. Furthermore, using psychometric methods, with the patient as his own control, we have shown that even in patients who have been thought to have undergone a totally uncomplicated open-heart procedure, there are signs of cerebral injuries, sometimes permanent [1].

In an analysis of the factors predisposing to decreased psychometric scores after operation, it was found that the picture was compatible with the microembolism theory. There were two possible sources of microemboli – the heart-lung machine and the operative field.

Working along the lines of the microembolism theory, and trying to eliminate emboli at the source, several changes in the routines of extracorporeal circulation were instituted. The effects of these changes were investigated with the same psychometric tests in a new group of patients [2].

The frequency of clinically obvious cerebral complications decreased from 14.5% to 3.5%. At the same time the psychometric scores improved markedly. However, they did not reach the level of those in a similarly tested control group.

Further refinements in the handling of the extracorporeal circulation were then made. The purpose of this communication is to present the results of a third psychometric investigation, to define the current rate of cerebral complications, to critically scrutinize psychometric testing as a method of measuring subclinical brain injury, and to describe the principles we have used in the management of extracorporeal circulation.

Material and Methods

Altogether 339 patients with a cerebrally normal postoperative course were tested pre- and postoperatively. Four different groups of patients were compared, three of which have been presented in detail earlier [1, 2].

Control group: 46 patients operated upon for general thoracic surgical (GTS) diseases, mostly lung tumors.

Psychopathological and Neurological Dysfunctions Following Open-Heart Surgery Ed by Becker et al

ECC group I: 99 patients operated upon with extracorporeal circulation in 1972–1973 [1], with no apparent cerebral complications postoperatively. The Björk-AGA heart-lung machine was used with a disc oxygenator, moderate hemodilution (Htkr ≈ 32), and 30 °C hypothermia. Coronary suction was avoided outside the heart, and the pericardial blood was discarded. The left ventricular drainage cannula was inserted as a rule, though the apex.

ECC group II: 124 patients operated upon in 1974–1976 [2], also without signs of cerebral complications. In most of them a bubble oxygenator was employed. Clear fluid prime was used. Coronary suction was allowed outside the heart. A micropore filter was always used in the coronary return line, but not consistently in the arterial line. A new system for drainage of the left ventricle and de-airing of the heart was introduced [3].

ECC group III: 70 patients operated upon in 1978–1979. Clear fluid prime was used (Htkr ≈ 20–25). Blood transfusions were avoided during cardiopulmonary bypass. Modern bubble oxygenators were employed (see below). pO_2 was monitored routinely in the arterial line so that the oxygen blood flow ratio could be kept as low as possible.

Protocol. For details, see [1]. Three psychometric tests were used: Synonyms (Syn), a test of verbal comprehension; figure rotation (F.rot), a test of visuospatial ability, and figure identification test (F.iden), a test of perceptual speed. The results of the combined series of tests are expressed as the sum of the scores in the subtests (SS_3).

The tests were given on the days immediately preceding surgery and then again postoperatively as soon as the patient was fit to be tested (i.e., up and about, no drains, only weak analgetics needed, and oral nutrition). This proved to be at about 7 days after operation in all investigations (SD 2.1 days).

The distribution of diagnoses in the ECC groups is given in Table 1. The results are expressed as the individual differences between pre- and postoperative scores. Student's *t*-test was used. Unless otherwise stated, one-tailed tests were applied. Correlation coefficients were obtained between continuous variables and individual differences in test scores.

Table 1. Number of patients in different diagnostic groups

	ECC group I		ECC group II		ECC group III	
Diagnosis	No.	%	No.	%	No.	%
Congenital heart disease	15	15	9	8	4	6
Coronary heart disease	19	19	35	28	38	54
Mitral valve disease	22	22	28	23	7	10
Aortic valve disease	35	35	45	36	15	21
Aortic and mitral disease	7	7	7	6	6	9
Total	99	100	124	100	70	100

Results

Mortality. In the ECC group I investigation, there were four patients dying with or from cerebral complications (3%). During the time course of the ECC group II investigation, there was one patient dying from a cerebral complication (0.5%), and the corresponding figures for ECC group III, were one and 0.3%.

Cerebral Complications. In ECC group III, 71 patients were tested preoperatively. One of them suffered from obvious confusion postoperatively, given a frequency of clinically obvious cerebral complications of 1.4%. This low frequency was corroborated in an analysis of 350 adult patients, operated on between 1978 and 1979, where six patients (1.8%) exhibited some kind of cerebral complication. (One of them died.)

Thus, a progressive decrease in the incidence of cerebral complications occurred from ECC group I (14.5%) to ECC groups II (3.5%) and III (< 2%).

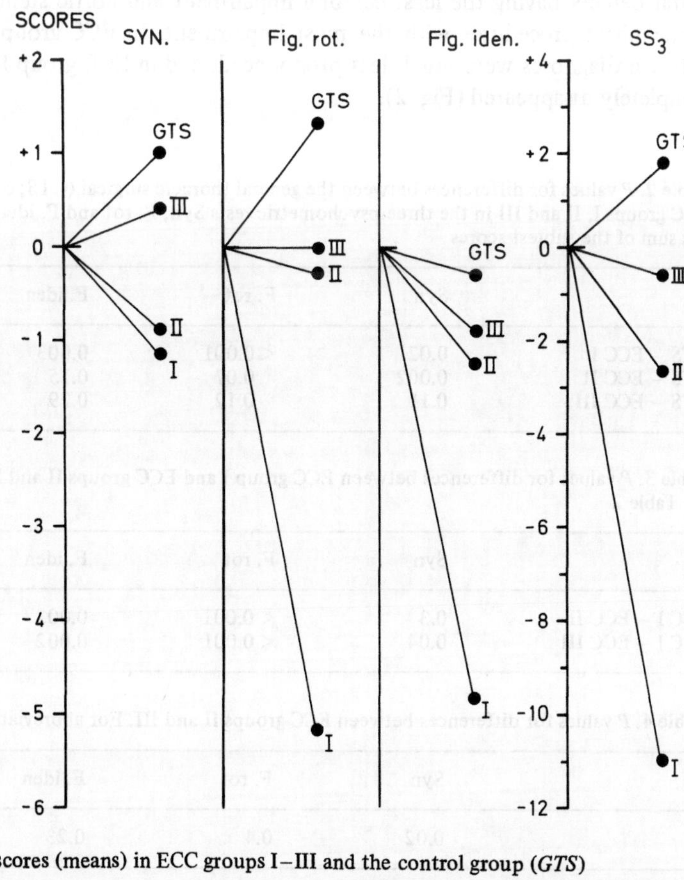

Fig. 1. Psychometric scores (means) in ECC groups I–III and the control group (*GTS*)

Psychometric Scores. There was less decrease in the test scores in ECC group III than in ECC groups I and II. Compared with the control group, however, ECC group III still showed signs of depression of cerebral function (Fig. 1).

Means and standard deviations for different tests, and 95% confidence intervals, are given in Table 2 for all four groups. A further improvement in test scores in the more recent investigations is evident from the fact that the mean values are approaching those of the control group. Furthermore, the standard deviations had decreased considerably and were now at the level of the controls.

t-Test values for differences between the control group and ECC groups I–III are given in Table 2. The *P* values of SS_3, which were extremely low in ECC group I, were considerably higher in ECC group II and where about 0.09 in ECC group III. *t*-Test values for the difference between ECC groups I and II, and between ECC groups I and III (i.e., the improvement in the quality of the open-heart procedure since the first investigation), are given in Table 3.

t-Test values for the difference between ECC groups II and III (i.e., the improvement between the two most recent investigations) are given in Table 4. The statistical interpretation of these data will be discussed further below. In ECC group I, the diagnosis had a marked influence upon the test results, patients with simple atrial septal defects having the least cerebral impairment and aortic stenosis and combined aortic-mitral procedures with the most impairment. In ECC group II the differences between diagnoses were much less pronounced, and in ECC group III they had almost completely disappeared (Fig. 2).

Table 2. *P* values for differences between the general thoracic surgical (GTS; control) group and ECC groups I, II and III in the three psychometric tests Syn, F. rot and F. iden (see p. 344). SS_3 in the sum of the subtest scores

	Syn	F. rot	F. iden	SS_3
GTS – ECC I	0.02	< 0.001	0.003	0.002
GTS – ECC II	0.002	0.07	0.15	0.02
GTS – ECC III	0.11	0.12	0.29	0.09

Table 3. *P* values for differences between ECC group I and ECC groups II and III. For abbrevations, see Table 2

	Syn	F. rot	F. iden	SS_3
ECC I – ECC II	0.3	< 0.001	0.002	0.001
ECC I – ECC III	0.04	< 0.001	0.002	< 0.001

Table 4. *P* values for differences between ECC groups II and III. For abbreviations, see Table 2

Syn	F. rot	F. iden	SS_3
0.02	0.4	0.23	0.17

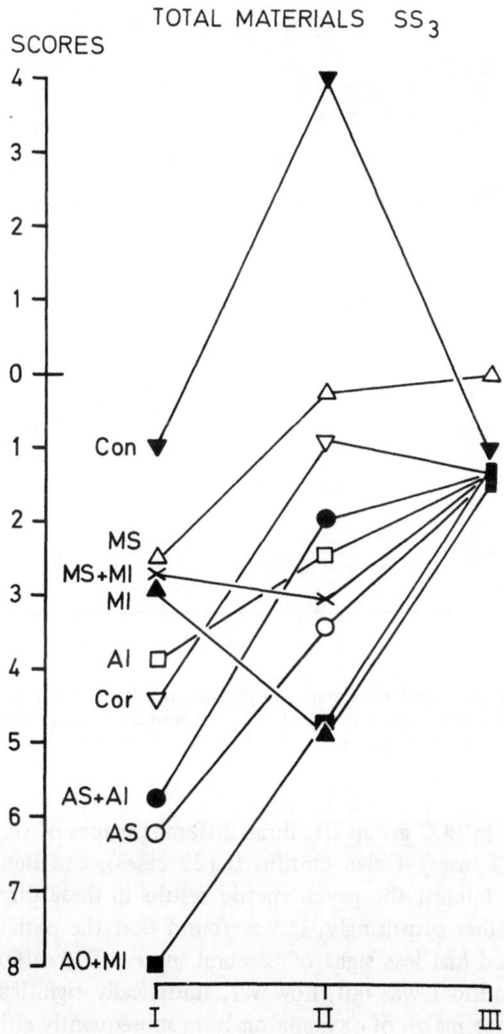

Fig. 2. Psychometric scores (means) in ECC groups I–III distributed by diagnoses. *Con*, congenital heart disease; *MS*, mitral stenosis; MI, mitral incompetence; *AS*, aortic stenosis; *AI*, aortic insufficiency; *AI + MI*, combined aortic and mitral operations; *Cor*, coronary artery bypass operations

One of the findings in ECC group I was that the test scores were markedly lower in patients with valvular calcifications than in those without. This difference disappeared in ECC group II and neither was it evident in ECC group III.

In ECC group I there was a statistically significant correlation between perfusion time and decrease in test scores. As seen in Fig. 3, the correlation became weaker in ECC group II. Furthermore, the curve shifted upwards, toward less impairment in test scores, and the slope of the curve became less steep. In ECC group III there was no longer a significant correlation between perfusion time and test scores, and the resulting curve was almost horizontal.

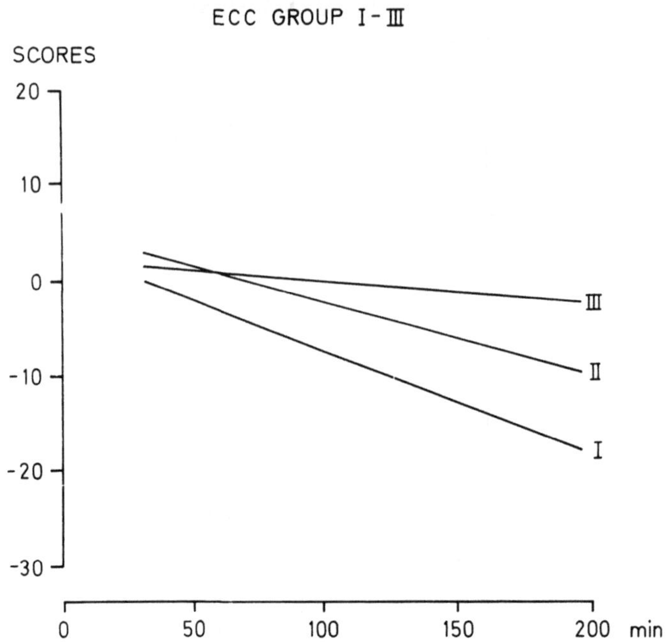

Fig. 3. Correlations between individual differences in pre- and postoperative psychometric scores (sum of the three subtests) and perfusion time. Curve equations: ECC group I: *Y*, −0.11 X + 3.36; *r*, −0.44; ECC group II: *Y*, −0.07 X + 5.26; *r*, 0.28; ECC group III: *Y*, −0.026 X + 2.43; *r*, 0.13

In ECC group III, three different makes of oxygenators were used, Galen Optiflo I (17 cases), Galen Optiflo II (29 cases), and Bentley Bos 10 (24 cases). As a matter of interest the psychometric results in these three groups of patients were analyzed. Rather surprisingly, it was found that the patients in whom a Bentley Bos 10 was used had less signs of cerebral injury. The differences between Bentley Bos 10 and Optiflo I was not, however, statistically significant (P = 0.20, two-tailed t-test). All three makes of oxygenators have subsequently either been withdrawn from the market or substantially revised.

Table 5. Some clinical parameters (means)

	ECC I	ECC II	ECC III
Age (years)	50	55	49
Perfusion time (min)	128	94	117
Blood given (units)	24	15	7.6
Intensive care unit time (days)	6.5	3.8	3.1

The length of time in the intensive care unit no longer reflects the severity of the postoperative course, but rather the fact that we have a large ICU, but few ordinary beds

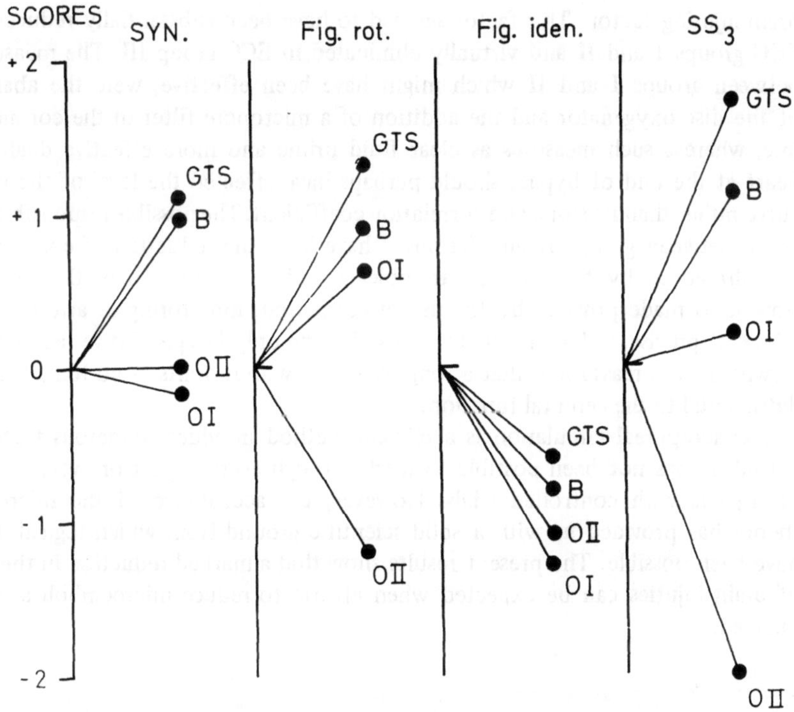

Fig. 4. Psychometric scores (means) in ECC group III, divided according to make of oxygenator. *OI*, Galen Optiflo I; OII, Cobe Optiflo II; *B*, Bentley Bos 10; *GTS*, Control group

Discussion

The main finding of these investigations is that the quality of open-heart surgery has markedly improved as regards cerebral protection. However, there are still signs of cerebral injuries: Firstly, occasional deaths or occur from cerebral causes, secondly, there is still an incidence of clinically obvious nonfatal complications from the brain. Thirdly, there are psychometric signs of continued threat to the brain. Thus it is necessary to further develop open-heart surgery in this respect.

The principle followed when trying to reduce cerebral injuries has been to reduce or eliminate emboli at the source. From the findings in ECC group I it was concluded that there were two sources for embolic matter, the operative field and the pump oxygenator. The operative field may be made less prone to create emboli by a meticulate surgical technique, awareness and care, and by using a system for prolonged drainage of the left ventricle before discontinuing bypass [3]. A prolonged drainage of the left ventricle will help to mobilize and remove intracavitary debris from the operative site as well as any remaining air.

In ECC group I and II there was a significant correlation between duration of perfusion and test scores. This correlation no longer exists in ECC group III. The earlier correlation suggested that the open-heart procedure produced a continuing brain-injuring factor. This factor seemed to have been substantially reduced between ECC groups I and II and virtually eliminated in ECC group III. The measures taken between groups I and II which might have been effective, were the abandonment of the disc oxygenator and the addition of a micropore filter in the coronary return line, whereas such measures as clear fluid prime and more effective deairing of the heart at the end of bypass should perhaps have affected the level of the correlation curve rather than its slope and correlation coefficient. The possible responsible measures taken between groups II and III might have been the reduction of coronary suction brought about by the use of cardioplegia and the reduction of the oxygen-blood flow ratio made possible by the use of continuous monitoring of arterial pO_2. With a lack of precise, well-controlled studies, this can only be speculative. From a practical viewpoint it is reassuring, that a long bypass – within limits – no longer seems to be detrimental to the cerebral function.

Extracorporeal circulation is a clinical method in which numerous factors are involved. It has not been possible to work through every aspect or every combination of aspects with controlled trials. However, the acceptance of the microembolism theory has provided us with a solid scientific ground from which logical deductions have been possible. The present results show that a marked reduction in the incidence of brain injuries can be expected when efforts to reduce microemboli at source are pursued.

Summary

In a psychometric investigation in 1973 (ECC group I), where patients undergoing open-heart surgery were studied before and after operation, it was found that patients without clinical cerebral complications still exhibited psychometric signs of cerebral injury. An analysis of that material pointed to the relevance of the microembolism theory. There were two sources of microemboli, the heart-lung machine and the operative field. Several changes in the routines of the open-heart procedure were instituted, all aiming at reduction or elimination of microemboli at the source. Two further psychometric investigations have subsequently been performed (ECC groups II and III). Altogether 339 patients have been studied. The changes instituted were: Between ECC group I and II: Abandonment of the disc oxygenator in preference to the bubble oxygenator. Switch from moderate hemodilution to clear fluid prime. Introduction of prolonged drainage of the left ventricle at the end of bypass. Micropore filter in the coronary suction line. Between ECC group II and III: Modern bubble oxygenators. Avoidance of blood transfusions during bypass. Routine monitoring of arterial pO_2 and keeping the oxygen-blood flow ratio as low as possible.

Cerebral mortality decreased from 3% to 0.3%. Incidence of clinically obvious cerebral complications decreased from 14.5% to less than 2%. Psychometric scores after operation were markedly decreased in ECC group I but there was a consecutively smaller decrease in ECC groups II and III. The differences were statistically significant. In ECC group III there are still signs of cerebral injuries, and it is concluded that open-heart surgery at the present time places the patient's brain in jeopardy. Thus, further efforts to improve the quality of open-heart surgery are needed. The acceptance of the microembolism theory has provided us with a solid scientific ground, from which logical deductions have been possible. The present results show that a reduction in the incidence of brain injuries can be expected when efforts to reduce microemboli at source are persued.

References

1. Åberg T, Kihlgren M (1974) Effect of open-heart surgery on intellectual function. Scand J Thorac Cardiovasc Surg [Suppl 15]
2. Åberg T, Kihlgren M (1977) Cerebral protection during open-heart surgery. Thorax 32:525
3. Åberg T, Hallén A, Dubiel WT, Johansson L (to be published) A versatile system for drainage of the left heart during open-heart surgery.

Microembolization Due to Microbubbles Released from the Oxygenator

H.J. Krebber, G. Lutz, M.-J. Polonius, G. Rodewald

Introduction

Microemboli originating from various sources within the extracorporeal circulation unit may cause structural and functional damage of all organs [3, 4]. However, neurological and psychopathological disturbances following open-heart surgery in particular have to be related to microembolization [1, 8]. Generally we have to distinguish between gaseous and particulate emboli. Hill and co-workers found an incidence of particulate emboli of 19% in the brains of patients who died following open-heart procedures. After introduction of filters for blood transfusion and coronary suction the incidence was lowered to 6%, but the incidence of fat emboli remained unchanged [3].

Though mortality and morbidity after open-heart procedures decreased considerably over the past few years there still remained a high incidence of psychopathological disturbances after such procedures [1, 2, 11]. The clinical features, and the often short duration of symptoms and their reversibility suggest the presence of gas emboli in many cases. The distribution of size and number of microbubbles released from oxygenators were investigated and the results will be presented. Conditions that enhance the production of bubbles will be outlined and measures demonstrated that are suitable to reduce bubble activity in the arterial line of extracorporeal circulation units.

Methods

Microbubbles were analyzed during regular open-heart procedures and in experimental bypass circuits. Two different methods for bubble detection were used:

1. An ultrasonic, narrow beam bubble detector, TM 8[1] which functions by ultrasonic reflection (not a Doppler method) was used in experimental circuits and clinically for size and population analysis.
2. In experimental circuits an additional bubble chamber was used that allowed volumetric measurements of the bubbles collected, and made it possible to draw samples of gas for qualitative analysis which was performed by mass spectrometry.

[1] Technical laboratories, 1 High Street, Hartley Wintney, England

Psychopathological and Neurological Dysfunctions
Following Open-Heart Surgery Ed by Becker et al

With the ultrasonic device we were able to detect bubbles as small as 10 μ theoretically, but the noise disturbances were very high and measurements unreliable in this range. We therefore confined ourselves to a spectrum ranging from 30 μ upward.

The bubble chamber (Fig. 1) is a modification of the one developed by Eberhard and co-workers at PMC.[2] For volumetric measurements we used the change of compressibility with the amount of gas added to a known volume of fluid. With regular calibration we were able to achieve a high reliability of the measurement.

The experimental circuit consisted of an oxygenator, a deoxygenator, the bubble chamber, and roller pumps P_1, P_2 and P_3 (Fig. 2). Pump P_3 was used to allow a defined and constant volume to flow through the chamber. In some experimental

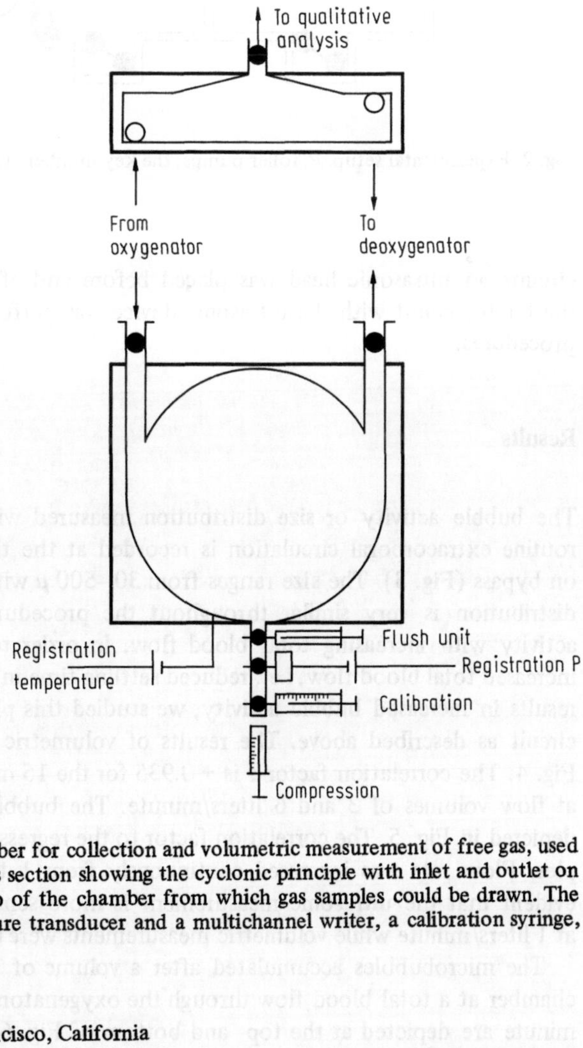

Fig. 1. Diagram of the bubble chamber for collection and volumetric measurement of free gas, used at Hamburg University. *Top*, a cross section showing the cyclonic principle with inlet and outlet on different levels and a dome-like top of the chamber from which gas samples could be drawn. The recording unit consisted of a pressure transducer and a multichannel writer, a calibration syringe, and a compression syringe

---

[2] Pacific Medical Center, San Francisco, California

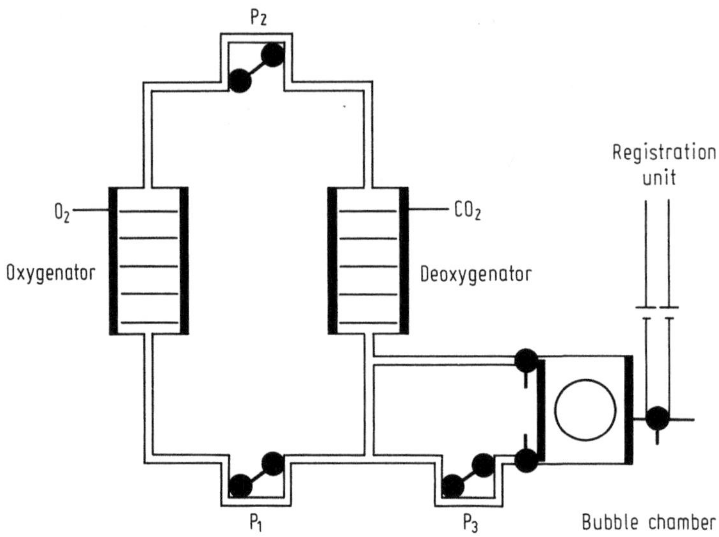

Fig. 2. Experimental setup. *P*, roller pumps; the key-numbers indicate the position

circuits an ultrasonic head was placed before and after the bubble chamber. Later the bubble count with the ultrasonic device was performed during routine open-heart procedures.

Results

The bubble activity or size distribution measured with an ultrasonic device during routine extracorporal circulation is recorded at the times 5, 10, 15, 30 and 60 min on bypass (Fig. 3). The size ranges from 30–500 μ with a maximum of 30 μ. The size distribution is very similar throughout the procedure with an increase in bubble activity with increasing total blood flow. In order to confirm our impression that increased total blood flow, i.e., reduced settling time in the reservoir of the oxygenator results in increased bubble activity, we studied this phenomenon in an experimental circuit as described above. The results of volumetric measurements are depicted in Fig. 4. The correlation factor r is + 0.935 for the 15 measurements, which were taken at flow volumes of 3 and 6 liters/minute. The bubble activity for the size 30 μ is depicted in Fig. 5. The correlation factor to the regression slope is + 0.928 for 20 samples. Flow rate was increased continuously from 1 to 6.5 liters/minute. It became evident that the ultrasonic measurement is more sensitive, registering activities even at 1 liters/minute while volumetric measurements were unreliable below 3 liters/minute.

The microbubbles accumulated after a volume of 30 liters has flown through the chamber at a total blood flow through the oxygenators of 4 liters/minute and 6 liters/minute are depicted at the top and bottom of Fig. 6 respectively. The gas to blood

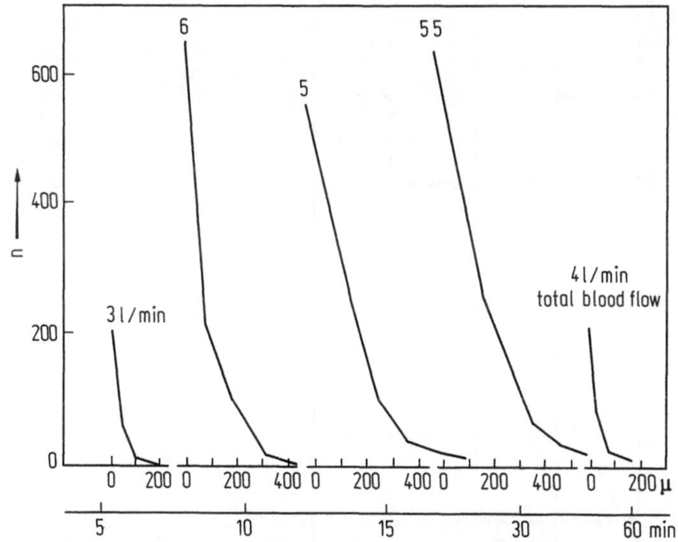

Fig. 3. Size distribution of bubbles during routine ECC, on *y axis* the mean bubble count of a certain size; on *x axis* the size and the time of the analysis

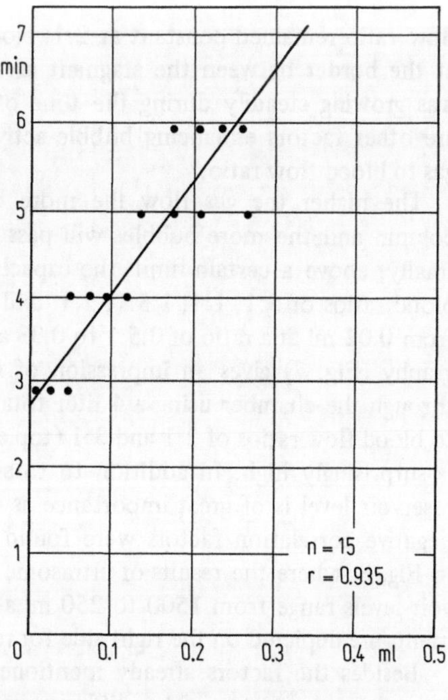

Fig. 4. Volumetric measurements. Correlation between total blood flow and volume of free gas

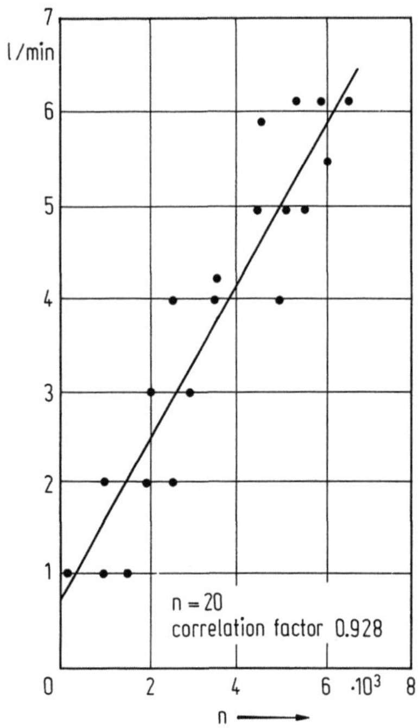

Fig. 5. Results of ultrasonic bubble detection with the TM 8, correlation between total blood flow and bubble activity in the arterial line

flow ratio remained constant at 2:1. Note the circular collection of fine foam found at the border between the stagnant area and the flow zone of the chamber, which was growing steadily during the time of the experiment. As mentioned above there are other factors enhancing bubble activity and release of free gas: for example, the gas to blood flow ratio.

The higher the gas flow the more bubbles are passed through the oxygenating column and the more bubbles will pass through the defoamer and the reservoir, and finally, above a certain limit, the capacity of the defoamer will be reached. (For gas blood ratios of 5:1, 1:1, 1.5:1, 2:1, and 3:1 our study revealed an increase in free gas from 0.02 ml at a ratio of 0.5:1 to 0.33 at 2:1, and 0.54 ml at a 3:1 ratio). The photography (Fig. 7) gives an impression of what it looks like when 30 liters have flown through the chamber using a 4 liter total blood flow through the oxygenator and gas to blood flow ratios of 2:1 and 3:1 (top and bottom). The amount of free air collected is surprisingly high. In addition to total blood flow and gas to blood flow ratio the reservoir level is of great importance as it limits the settling time as well. Fairly high negative correlation factors were found for bubble activity and volume as depicted in Fig. 8, where the results of ultrasonic detection are depicted on the left side. Reservoir levels range from 1500 to 250 ml above minimum level. The volumetric measurements are depicted on the right side for reservoir levels of 1000 and 250 ml.

Besides the factors already mentioned we found some differences among various types of oxygenators. The differences have been quite remarkable, but sometimes

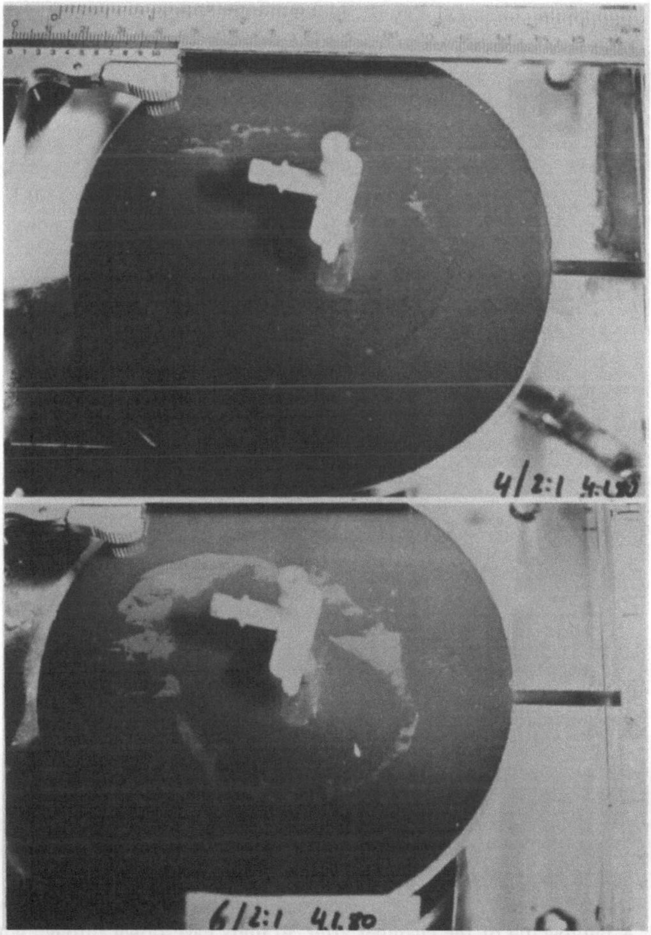

Fig. 6. Photograph of the bubble chamber. *Above* for a total blood flow of 4 liters/minute, *below* for 6 liters/minute. Gas to blood flow ratio was 2:1 and a total of 30 liters has been flown through the chamber

there were even differences between oxygenators of the same make, probably due to incomplete coating with antifoam. While gross failures of defoaming are easily detected, defoaming will be difficult to note in minor cases during clinical use, except when a gas detector is connected to the arterial line.

Microemboli, especially microbubbles, can be avoided as follows: By keeping the gas to blood flow ratio as low as possible, which means adjusting the actual pO_2 to approximately 100 mmHg by frequent control of blood gas analysis. By observing the reservoir level closely and keeping a safe level above the minimum which helps to reduce bubble activity. Especially when high total blood flow is required it is important not to run low reservoir levels. In addition filters in the arterial line may be of beneficial effect as shown in Fig. 9. Here again the bubble distribution is shown, the number n on the y axis, and the size at various times on the x axis, ranging from

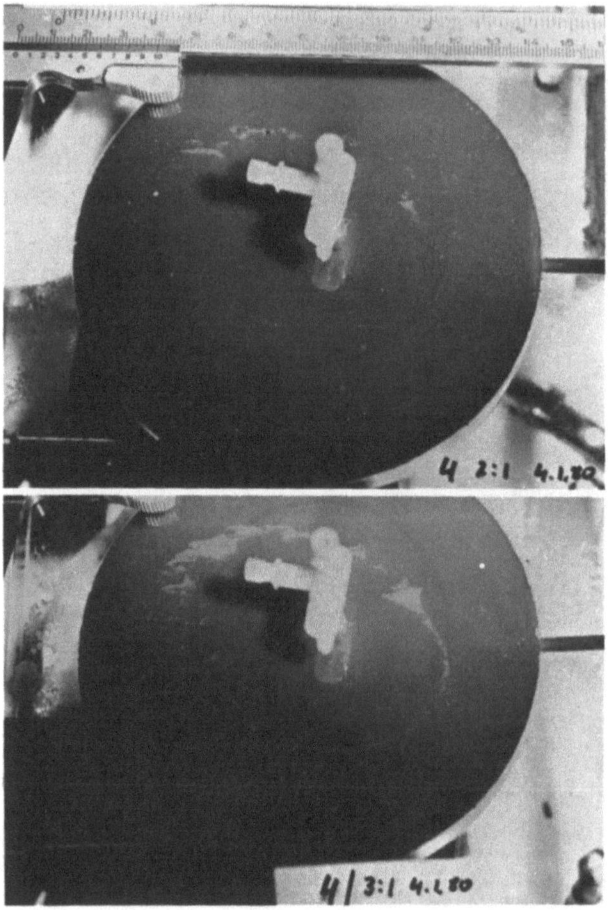

Fig. 7. A photograph of the chamber after 30 liters have flown through with a gas to blood flow ratio of 2:1 *above* and 3:1 *below*

30 μ to 500 μ for each slope seen from the left to the right. The small segments represent the number of microbubbles that passed through the filter. The function of the filter is widely constant over the time of the whole experiment. Figure 10 represents the findings of a case where the filter lost its effectiveness due to the development of microchannels through the Dacron wool. Through these channels the bubbles passed easily. The channel effect increases with time. Again the narrow lines represent the bubble activity before the filter and the small segments below represent the microbubbles that have passed through the filter.

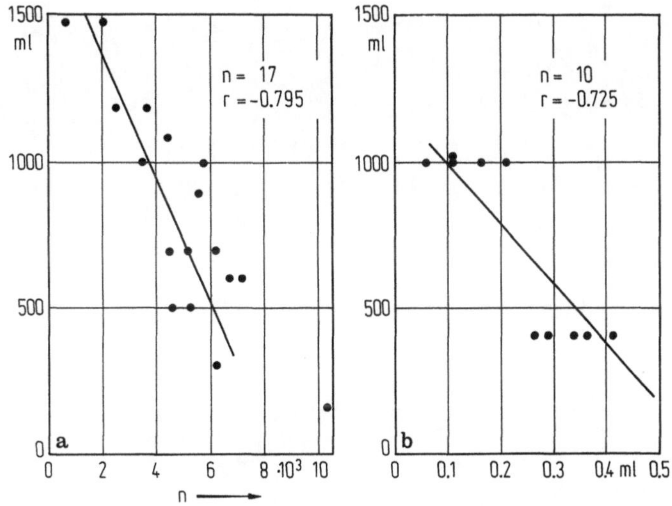

Fig. 8. Bubble activity assessed with the TM 8 *on the left* and results of volumetric measurements *on the right* demonstrating the correlation between oxygenator level and free gas in the arterial line. (*Ordinate*, oxygenator volume; *abscissa*, number of bubbles or volume of free gas)

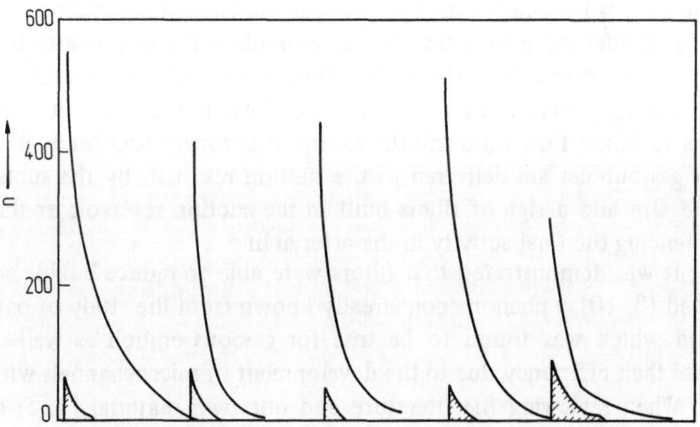

Fig. 9. Bubble activity in the arterial line recorded proximally and distally of an arterial line filter. The *black triangle* represent the number of bubbles distal to the filter

Discussion

Microbubbles were found equally distributed during ECC. The study was designed to evaluate various conditions that were likely to increase bubble activity in the arterial line of ECC units. As bubbles are likely to produce cerebral damage and neurological deficiency [1] measures against bubble activity were investigated. Besides special additional equipment as filters on settling chambers emphasis was laid on the way in which

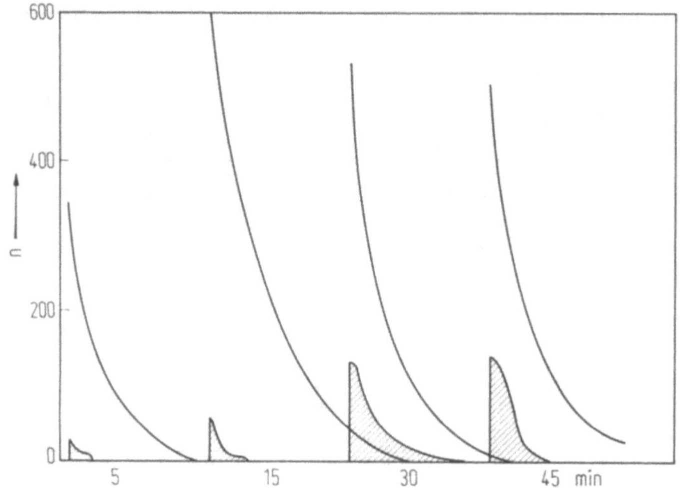

Fig. 10. Recording of a case with filter failure due to increasing inefficiency of the filter. There is an increase in bubble activity distal to the filter

the ECC was managed in experimental and clinical procedures. It became evident that, in particular the settling time in the reservoir of the oxygenator influences bubble activity in the arterial line. The settling time is dependent on total blood flow, total volume of the oxygenator, and the actual blood level in the reservoir. Further factors were the gas to blood flow ratio and the extent of coronary suction in clinical circuits as plenty of gas bubbles are delivered to the suction reservoir by the suction return. Therefore the size and design of filters built in the suction reservoir or the return line were influencing the final activity in the arterial line.

It was demonstrated that filters were able to reduce bubble activity when properly used [8, 10], a phenomenon already known from the study of particulate microemboli and which was found to be true for gaseous emboli as well. Some filters tend to lose their efficiency due to the development of microchannels within the filter.

When reviewing the literature and our own material [1, 5, 6, 9, 10] it becomes evident that a huge amount of material has already been collected that proves the presence of microbubbles in the arterial line during routine ECC. However, the gap between the number of bubbles detected in the arterial line or even in the carotid artery [10], and neurological or psychopathological disturbances [11] is still to be closed.

Acknowledgment. We would like to thank A. Jatridis and J.J. Osborn of Pacific Medical Center in San Francisco for introducing us to the methology of this subject. Our now extensive work in this field is based on the work they started.

References

1. Bass RM, Longmore DB (1969) Cerebral damage during open-heart surgery. Nature 222:30
2. Goetze P (1980) Psychopathologie der Herzoperierten. Enke, Stuttgart
3. Hill JD, Aquillar MJ, Baranco A, De Lanerole P, Gerbode F (1969) Neuropathological manifestation of cardiac surgery. Ann Thorac Surg 7:562
4. Lee WH, Millon W Jr, Rowe J, Harrison P, Bradiston MP (1969) Effects of extracorporeal circulation on personality and cerebration. Ann Thorac Surg 7:562
5. Lichti EL, Simmons EM, Almond CA (1972) Detection of microemboli during cardiopulmonary bypass. Surg Gynecol Obstet 134:977
6. Loop FD, Szabo J, Rowlinson RD, Urbanek K (1976) Events related to microembolism during extracorporeal perfusion in man. Effectiveness of in-line filtration recorded by ultrasound. Ann Thorac Surg 21:413
7. Kessler J, Patterson LH (1970) The production of microemboli by various blood oxygenators. Ann Thorac Surg 9:22
8. Krebber HJ, Hill JD, Osborn JJ, Jatridis A (1980) Microemboli during extracorporeal circulation. Thorac Cardiovasc Surg 28
9. Miller SS, Mandl JP (1977) Comparison of the effectiveness of various extracorporeal filters at reducing gaseous emboli. Am Sect Proc 55
10. Pearson DT, Watson BG, Waterhouse PS (1978) An ultrasonic analysis of the comparative efficiency of various cardiotomy reservoirs and microporous blood filters. Thorax 33:352
11. Speidel H, Dahme B, Flemming B, Götze P, Huse-Kleinstoll G, Meffert HJ, Rodewald G (1979) Psychische Störungen nach offenen Herzoperationen. Nervenarzt 50:85

Effect of Pulsatile Flow and Arterial Line Filtration on Cerebral Cellular Damage During Open-Heart Surgery

K.M. Taylor

Introduction

The incidence of neurological dysfunction following cardiac surgical procedures using cardiopulmonary bypass [1–3] has been variously estimated at between 15% and 44%. Despite many improvements in bypass technology in recent years, neurological dysfunction remains a significant complication of open-heart procedures. Many research workers have begun to document the clinical characteristics and psychological patterns associated with this neurological damage; other workers have attempted to investigate major etiological factors involved in the pathogenesis of the neurological dysfunction.

There is, however, a continuing problem for the investigator, i.e., the current lack of an acceptably reliable, objective and sensitive investigative model. Psychometric [1, 2] testing has been used widely, with excellent results, and the use of electroencephalography [4] and cerebral function monitoring [5] continues to be refined. These methods are not, however, apparently sensitive enough to allow quantification of cerebral damage, except in the most expert hands. There is, therefore, an obvious need for a sensitive and quantifiable index of cerebral damage in order to assess the neurological effects of various perfusion regimes, and hence study etiological factors and lines of therapy.

This paper describes initial research with a new technique for assessing cerebral cellular damage associated with cardiopulmonary bypass procedures. Though the technique is presently based on a dog model, we shall indicate possible future developments which may allow clinical application.

The technique is based on the direct measurement in samples of dog cerebrospinal fluid (CSF) of the enzyme creatine phosphokinase (CPK) and its isoenzyme CPK'B'.

CPK and CPK'B' Content in Brain Tissue

Cerebral tissue content of CPK enzyme is low when compared with other tissues (Table 1). However, over 80% of this CPK total is made up of the 'B' isoenzyme of CPK. Release of CPK from damaged brain cells into the cerebrospinal fluid may easily be detected by measurement of total CPK and CPK'B' isoenzyme levels in

Psychopathological and Neurological Dysfunctions
Following Open-Heart Surgery Ed by Becker et al

Table 1. Distribution of creatine phosphokinase and 'B' isoenzyme in dog tissue, expressed in units per gram of tissue

Tissue	Total CPK (U/g)	CPK 'B' (U/g)	'B' % of total
Left ventricular muscle	480	92	19
Skeletal muscle	1030	176	17
Brain	85	70	82

the CSF which normally contains very low levels of these substances [6, 7]. Release of CPK and CPK'B' into the CSF has previously been described in conditions of cerebral hemorrhage, infarct, infection, and trauma [8–12]. Previous studies have also indicated that the relative content of CPK and CPK'B' are identical in human, baboon, and dog brain tissue [12–14].

Design of Study

Previous workers have suggested that among other factors the following may be of major significance in the pathogenesis of neurological dysfunction following open-heart procedures:

1. *The use of nonpulsatile perfusion* during cardiopulmonary bypass, with associated reduction in the perfusion of the cerebral microcirculation [15–20].
2. *The production of microemboli* (e.g., gaseous, particulate matter, blood cell aggregates) during the perfusion, with consequent microembolic cerebral damage [21–27].

It was decided to test the dog model in relation to these possible etiological factors, assessing cerebral cellular damage by the quantitative rise in CSF levels of CPK and CPK 'B' during and after periods of cardiopulmonary bypass.

Materials and Methods

Adult mongrel dogs were studied. Anesthesia was induced with sodium thiopentone and maintained with nitrous oxide, oxygen, and intravenous morphine. A right lateral thoracotomy was performed and after heparinization (500 IU/kg) the heart was cannulated for atrioaortic cardiopulmonary bypass (CPB) using two caval cannulae and a 14G aortic return cannula. The dogs were submitted to a 60-min period of total bypass at normothermia, maintaining mean arterial pressure during perfusion at 60 mmHg. A conventional bubble oxygenator (Optiflo) was used in all cases, and the bypass circuit was primed with 1.5 liters Ringers lactate solution. After the 60-min period of CPB the heart was decannulated and protamine sulphate (5 ml) given to reverse heparinization. The residual blood in the bypass circuit was returned to the dog in the postoperative period. No drugs were administered during or after operation with the exception of sodium bicarbonate, potassium chloride, and morphine. After ensuring hemostasis, the chest was closed with underwater-seal drainage. The drain was then removed and the dog extubated and transferred to a recovery area until 24 h postoperation. Throughout the operative procedure serial arterial blood gas and plasma potassium estimations were obtained.

Study Groups

Three groups of dogs were studied, using the above operative, anesthetic, and biochemical techniques for each dog.

Control Group (n = 10)
These dogs were submitted to 60 min of nonpulsatile CPB with no arterial line filter.

Filtered Group (n = 10)
These dogs were submitted to 60 min of nonpulsatile CPB with a 40-μ screen filter (Ultipor, Pall Biomedical Corp. Glen Cove, New York, USA) inserted in the arterial line.

Pulsatile Group (n = 10)
These dogs were submitted to 60 min of pulsatile CPB, using a modified roller pump system (Cobe-Stockert, Cobe Labs. Inc., Lakewood, Colorado, USA) with no arterial line filter.

The preoperative and operative characteristics of the three groups are shown in Table 2. There were no significant differences between the groups.

Technique for Obtaining CSF Samples

Cerebrospinal fluid samples were obtained by direct puncture of the Cisterna Magna, using an 18G Abbocath cannula (Fig. 1). The cannula is passed through the dorsal atlantooccipital membrane, and advanced through the dura mater and subarachnoid space. The cannula was inserted before the onset of CPB and left in place until the

Table 2. Preoperative and operative parameters – control, filter, and pulsatile groups. (mean ± SEM)

Parameter	Control	Filter	Pulsatile
Weight (kg)	22.89 ± 1.6	23.16 ± 1.8	22.3 ± 3.5
Bypass Details			
Core temp (Co)	37.5 ± 1.0	37.3 ± 0.96	37.3 ± 0.52
Mean arterial BP (mmHg)	61.6 ± 0.88	60.8 ± 0.93	63.0 ± 2.81
Pump flow (liters/minute)	1.38 ± 0.42	1.41 ± 0.36	1.96 ± 0.59
pO_2 (mmHg)	186 ± 13.9	195 ± 12.0	169 ± 21.3
pH	7.34 ± 0.06	7.38 ± 0.08	7.45 ± 0.03

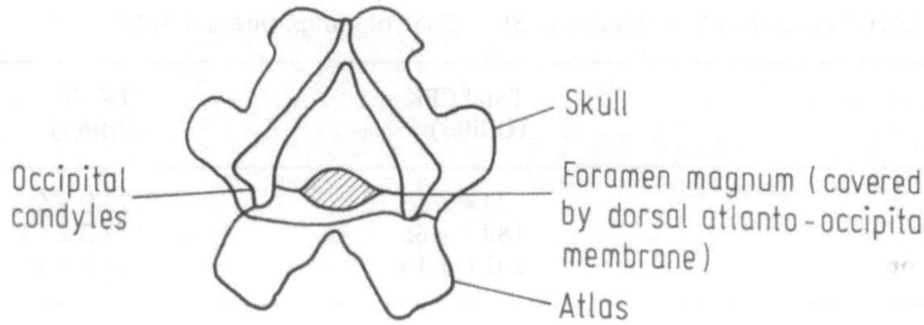

Fig. 1. Cisterna magna puncture technique in the dog. The cisterna magna, in the subarachnoid layer, lies in the angle between the cerebellum and the medulla oblongata. Structures passed during cisterna magna puncture: 1) skin and subcutaneous tissues; 2) dorsal neck muscles; 3) dorsal atlanto-occipital membrane; 4) dura mater; 5) arachnoid membrane

end of CPB. The cannula was then removed. At 24 h postoperatively the dog was again anesthetised with sodium thiopentone and the cisterna magna again cannulated for the final CSF specimen. CSF samples for assessment of total CPK and CPK'B' were obtained:

Pre-CPB – 2 min before the onset of CPB
End-CPB – 2 min before the end of CPB
24 h – 24 h postoperation.

Technique for CPK and CPK'B' Determinations

Total CPK and CPK'B' activities were measured using the Merck-l-Test CK (No. 3381) and the Merck-l-Test Ck-B (No. 14300) kits respectively, as described by Neumeier et al. [28]. Accurate measurements may be made down to a level of 5 U/liter. Each sample was processed in duplicate. The spectrophotometer used was the CKB 2086 and the data processed by the LKB 2082 data processor.

Statistical analyses were performed using Student's *t*-test.

Results

Control Group (Nonpulsatile: no filter) (Table 3)
Total CPK levels rose in all dogs during the period of CPB (Fig. 2). The mean end-CPB level was 188.7 U/liter ± 65 SEM, representing a ten-fold increase over pre-CPB levels. At 24 h postoperatively despite apparent full clinical recovery of the dogs, total CPK levels were still markedly elevated at 101.8 U/liter ± 16 SEM. The pattern of change in CPK'B' levels was identical, with a mean end-CPK level of 157.3 U/liter ± 64 SEM. Levels were still elevated at 24 h postoperatively at 49.6 U/liter ± 13 SEM.

Filter Group (Nonpulsatile: Filter inserted) (Table 4)
The rise in total CPK in these dogs was substantially smaller than the control group,

Table 3. Total CPK and CPK 'B' levels in CSF – Control group. (mean ± SEM)

Sample	Total CPK (U/liter)	CPK 'B' (U/liter)
Pre-CPB	23.4 ± 13	22.0 ± 5
End-CPB	188.7 ± 65	157.3 ± 64
24 h postop.	101.8 ± 16	49.6 ± 13

Table 4. Total CPK and CPK 'B' levels in CSF – filtered group. (mean ± SEM)

Sample	Total CPK (U/liter)	CPK 'B' (U/liter)
Pre-CPB	14.1 ± 8	11.3 ± 5
End-CPB	47.6 ± 12	29.1 ± 19
24 h postop.	27.9 ± 2.8	19.7 ± 1.5

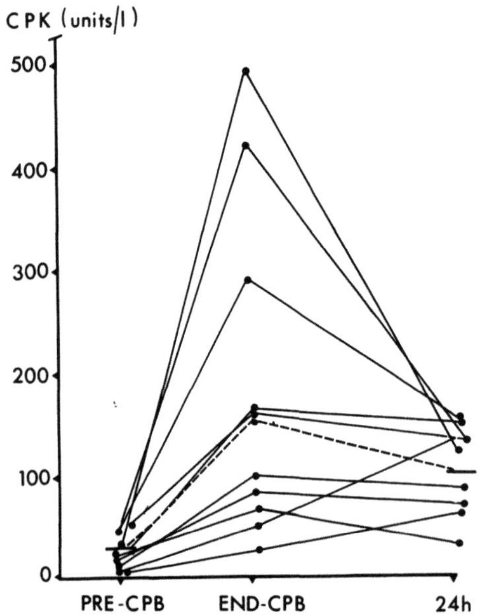

Fig. 2. Total CPK levels in ten dogs submitted to 60 min nonpulsatile cardiopulmonary bypass with no arterial line filter

the mean end CPB-level being 47.6 U/liter ± SEM. At 24 h postoperatively total CPK levels had fallen to just above preoperative levels at 27.9 U/liter ± 2.8 SEM.

Similarly, CPK'B' levels rose to a mean end-CPB level of 29.11 U/liter ± 18.6 SEM, with 24 h postoperative levels of 19.7 U/liter ± 1.5 SEM.

Table 5. Total CPK and CPK 'B' levels in CSF – pulsatile group. (mean ± SEM)

Sample	Total CPK (U/liter)	CPK 'B' (U/liter)
Pre-CPB	25.4 ± 11.0	20.2 ± 2.8
End-CPB	53.5 ± 13.6	27.86 ± 13.0
24 h postop.	26.8 ± 3.4	20.6 ± 3.5

The rise in total CPK and CPK'B' levels during bypass was significantly lower than the control group ($P < 0.01$).

Pulsatile Group (Pulsatile Flow: No filter) (Table 5)
Total CPK levels rose to a small extent during CPB, to a mean end-CPB level of 53.5 U/liter ± 13.6 SEM. At 24 h postoperatively levels had returned to just above preoperative values, i.e., 26.8 U/liter ± 3.4. CPK'B' levels reached a mean end-CPB level of 27.86 U/liter ± 13 SEM and at 24 h postoperatively had returned to approximately preoperative values.

The rise in total CPK and CPK'B' levels during CPB was significantly lower than in the control group ($P < 0.005$).

Discussion

This study in dogs has clearly demonstrated that very considerable rises occur in CSF levels of total CPK and CPK'B' isoenzyme during conventional cardiopulmonary bypass. In addition, we have shown that significantly lower CPK and CPK'B' levels are encountered when either arterial line filtration ($P < 0.01$) or pulsatile perfusion ($P < 0.005$) are employed.

Results obtained with the control group showed a satisfactory consistency in the pattern of change in both total CPK and CPK'B' levels in the CSF during the study period. In all ten dogs, enzyme levels rose substantially during perfusion and remained significantly elevated at 24 h postoperation. No dogs in the control group exhibited any gross evidence of focal neurological disturbance in the postoperative period. All resumed spontaneous ventilation within 1 h postbypass, and at 24 h all were sufficiently recovered to walk, eat, and drink unaided. This suggests that the CSF enzyme model is a sensitive index of cerebral cellular damage. It might be thought that dog brain reacts differently in terms of CPK release compared to primates. Previous studies have, however, indicated that both CPK and CPK'B' contact are identical in man, baboon, and the dog [7, 13, 14].

In the present study, the model was used in comparative studies of the effects of arterial line filtration and pulsatile perfusion. Microembolism during CPB is generally regarded as a significant etiological factor in post-bypass cerebral dysfunction due to the presence of air [21, 22], silicone particles [23], fat [24, 25], platelet aggregates [26], and fibrin [27]. Previous studies have indicated that incorporation of a micropore filter in the arterial return line not only reduces particle counts in the arterial line downstream of the filter [29–31], but is also associated with a reduction in cerebral dysfunction. Improvement in visual motor test scores [30], increased cerebral metabolic uptake for oxygen and glucose [32], reduced electrophysiological abnormality [5], and reduced intellectual impairment [1] have all been reported in association with arterial line filtration.

The possibility that nonpulsatile perfusion might produce a degree of cerebral damage has also received considerable support from the results of previous studies. Cerebral capillaries have been shown to constrict during nonpulsatile perfusion [18, 20] and Wright and Sanderson [19] have shown preservation of cerebral histology with pulsatile perfusion. The author has indicated that pulsatile flow preserves normal patterns of hypothalamo-pituitary axis stress responses [33–35] in contrast to the abnormal responses seen during nonpulsatile perfusion [17, 36].

The present study has shown that pulsatile perfusion, at the same levels of mean flow and pressure, is associated with significant reduction in the CSF levels of CPK and CPK'B', and is thus entirely in keeping with the concept of the physiological superiority of pulsatile cardiopulmonary bypass.

The principal purpose in these studies has, however, been in relation to the evaluation of CSF levels of CPK and CPK'B' in the quantitative assessment of cerebral damage during cardiac surgery. Initial experience has been most encouraging. The model has proved to be sensitive, and to exhibit a pleasing consistency of enzyme-release patterns in the groups of dogs studied. It has clearly shown that substantial amounts of cerebral tissue enzyme are released into the CSF during conventional CPB and that the use of arterial line screen filtration and pulsatile perfusion appear to be of significant benefit.

We believe that this new experimental model may be of value in the assessment of cerebral damage related to cardiopulmonary bypass, particularly in the evaluation and development of improved perfusion techniques.

Future development of this technique is currently focussed on the possible use of the brain amines β-endorphin and encephalin. These substances, also thought to be liberated from damaged brain cells, may produce a corresponding rise in blood levels, and might offer a possible clinical model for direct assessment of cerebral damage in patients, as opposed to animal models. Correlation studies using β-endorphin and encephalin rises in CSF and blood are currently in progress.

References

1. Åberg T (1974) Effect of open-heart surgery on intellectual function. Scand J Thorac Cardiovasc Surg [Suppl 15]
2. Lee WH, Brady MP, Rowe JM, Miller WC (1971) Effects of extracorporeal circulation upon behaviour, personality and brain function. Ann Surg 173:1013–1023
3. Tufo HM, Ostfeld AM, Shekelle R (1970) Central nervous system dysfunction following open-heart surgery. JAMA 212:1333
4. Wright JS, Lethlean AK, Hicks RG, Torda TA, Stacey R (1972) Electroencephalographic studies during open-heart surgery. J Thorac Cardiovasc Surg 63/4:631
5. Branthwaite MA (1972) Neurological damage related to open-heart surgery. Thorax 27:748
6. Taylor KM, Brannan JJ, Mittra SM, Gillan JG, McKenna JM (1979) Use of CSF enzyme levels in assessment of brain damage during cardiopulmonary bypass. Proc Debakey Internat Cardiovasc Soc, Houston

7. Taylor KM, Devlin BJ, Mittra SM, Gillan JG, Brannan JJ, McKenna JM (1980) Assessment of cerebral damage during open-heart surgery. A new experimental model. Scand J Thorac Cardiovasc Surg 14(2):197–203
8. Drummond MB, Belton NR (1972) Creatine phosphokinas (CPK) in the CSF; its value in the management of children with myelomeningocele and hydrocephalus. Arch Dis Child 47:672
9. Martin WA, Garey RE, Heath RG (1972) Cerebrospinal fluid creatine kinase in acutely psychotic patients. J Neurol Neurosurg Psychiatry 35:726
10. Vale S, Espejel MA, Calcaneo F (1974) Creatine phosphokinase. Increased activity of the spinal fluid in psychotic patients. Arch Neurol 30:103
11. Wolnitz AH, Jacobs LD, Christoff N (1969) Serum and cerebrospinal fluid enzymes in cerebrovascular disease. Creatine phosphokinase, aldolase, and lactic dehydrogenase. Arch Neurol 20:54
12. Sherwin A, Norris JW, Bulcke JA (1969) Spinal fluid creatine kinase in neurological disease. Neurology (Minneap) 19:993–9
13. Yasmineh WG, Hanson NW (1975) Electrophoresis on cellulose acetate and chromatography on DEAE – Sephadex A-50 compared in the estimation of creatine kinase isoenzymes. Clin Chem 21:381
14. Yasmineh WG, Pyle RB, Hanson NO, Hultman BK (1976) Creatine kinase isoenzymes in baboon tissues and organs. Clin Chem 22:63
15. Taylor KM, Jones JV, Walker MS, Rao LGS, Gray CE (1975) Plasma levels of cortisol, free cortisol and corticotrophin during cardiopulmonary bypass. J Endocrinol 67:29
16. Taylor KM (1978) Hypothalamic and pituitary changes in relation to injury. Ann R Coll Surg Engl 60:229
17. Taylor KM, Wright GS, Bremner WF, Brain WH, Caves PK, Beastall GH (1978) Anterior pituitary response to thyrotrophin-releasing hormone during open-heart surgery. Cardiovasc Res 12/2:114
18. Matsumoto T, Wolferth CC, Perlman MH (1971) Effects of pulsatile and non-pulsatile perfusion upon cerebral and conjunctival micro-circulation in dogs. Am Surg 37:61
19. Wright G, Sanderson JM (1972) Brain damage and mortality in dogs following pulsatile and non-pulsatile blood flows in extracorporeal circulation. Thorax 27:738
20. De Paepe J, Pomerantzeff PMA, Nakiri K, Armelin E, Verginelli G, Zerbini EJ (1979) Observation of the microcirculation of the cerebral cortex of dogs subjected to pulsatile and non-pulsatile flow during extracorporeal circulation. In: A propos du debit pulse. Cobe, Paris
21. Arfel G, Casanova C, Naquet R, Passelecq J, Dubost C (1967) Etude electro-clinique de l'embolie gazeuse cerebrale en chirurgie cardiaque. Electronecephalogr Clin Neurophysiol 23:101
22. Ehrenhaft JL, Claman MA, Layton JM, Zimmerman GR (1961) Cerebral complications of open-heart surgery: further observations. J Thorac Cardiovasc Surg 42:514
23. Lindberg DAB, Lucas FV, Sheagren J, Malm JR (1961) Silicone embolization during clinical and experimental heart surgery employing a bubble oxygenator. Am J Pathol 39:129
24. Miller JA, Fonkalsrud EW, Latta HL, Maloney JV (1962) Fat embolism associated with extracorporeal circulation and blood transfusion. Surgery 51:448
25. Caguin F, Carter MG (1963) Fat embolism with cardiotomy with the use of cardiopulmonary bypass. J Thorac Cardiovasc Surg 46:665
26. Guidoin RG, Anad JA, Laperche Y, Morin PJ, Haggis GH (1975) Nature of deposits in a tubular membrane oxygenator after prolonged extracorporeal circulation: a scanning electron microscopy study. J Thorac Cardiovasc Surg 69:479
27. Hill JD, Aquilar MJ, Baranco A, de Lanerolle P, Gerbode F (1969) Neuropathological manifestations of cardiac surgery. Ann Thorac Surg 7:409
28. Neumeier D, Prellwitz W, Wurzburg U, Brundobler M, Ollbermann M, Just HJ, Knedel M, Lang H (1976) Determination of creatine kinase isoenzyme – MB activity in serum using immunological inhibition of creatine kinase M-subunit activity: Activity kinetics and diagnostic significance in myocardial infarction. Clin Chem Acta 73:445
29. Osborn JJ, Swank RL, Hill JD, Aguilar MJ, Gerbode F (1970) Clinical use of dacron wool filter during perfusion for open-heart surgery. J Thorac Cardiovasc Surg 60:575
30. Carlson RG, Lande AJ, Landis B, Rogoz B, Baxter J. Patterson RH, Stenzel K, Lillehei CW (1973) The Landé-Edwards membrane oxygenator during heart surgery. J Thorac Cardiovasc Surg 66:894
31. Loop FD, Szabo J, Rowlinson RD, Urbanek K (1976) Events related to microembolism during extracorporeal perfusion in man: effectiveness of in-line filtration recorded by ultrasound. Ann Thorac Surg 21:412

32. Brennan RW, Patterson RH, Kessler J (1971) Cerebral blood flow and metabolism during cardiopulmonary bypass: Evidence of microembolic encephalopathy. Neurology (Minneap) 21:665
33. Taylor KM, Wright GS, Reid JS, Bain WH, Caves PK, Walker MS, Grant JK (1978) Comparative studies of pulsatile and non-pulsatile flow during cardiopulmonary bypass II – The effects on adrenal secretion of cortisol. J Thorac Cardiovasc Surg 75/4:574
34. Taylor KM, Wright GS, Bain WH, Caves PK, Beastall GH (1978) Comparative studies of pulsatile and non-pulsatile flow during cardiopulmonary bypass. III – Anterior pituitary response to thyrotrophin-releasing-hormone. J Thorac Cardiovasc Surg 75/4:579
35. Taylor KM, McIntyre HB, Grant JK, Ratcliffe JG (1979) Pituitary-adrenal response patterns during open-heart surgery. J Endocrinol 81:127
36. Taylor KM, Jones JV, Walker MS, Rao LGS, Bain WH (1976) The cortisol response during open-heart surgery. Circulation 54/1:20

Discussion of Session VIII

Willner commented on Dr. Åberg's paper:

I think that his paper is extremely important and illuminates a number of areas that have been confused before. What is especially illuminating is that there have been quite a number of papers concerned with relationships between duration of pump time and cognitive functioning. About half the papers seem to show a relationship and the other half don't with no obvious reason for the difference. I think Dr. Åberg's paper suggests that the difference between the papers showing such a correlation and others that don't may have something to do with the technique used and, for example, the possibility of the microemboli being filtered out. In three studies of his own he found a correlation at first, and one that disappears with an easily understandable rationale. I think that is quite a contribution because that issue has been a mystery until now.

A second issue that comes up is that one wonders about issues of cerebral mortality and morbidity. It would seem that the generation of microemboli would certainly put quite a stress on the patient. But you could also wonder why the patient's level of brain function before surgery might vary. Some people might be much more resistant to it. I think that issue could be investigated in one simple way. If you have someone whose performance is magnificant and then drops to only superb, you get the same difference as someone whose performance is quite poor and then becomes terrible. I would think it might be very interesting for Dr. Åberg to go back to the original data, the scores before the surgery, and see if the absolute scores on the tests before the surgery were related to the incidence of mortality and morbidity.

Bethune added to his presentation:

When I originally started on this study I had active collaboration from the psychologist involved. Myra Williams, and from the psychiatrists as well. I had a fairly passive role in the original design of the test format that we used. Having found something that was reasonably sensitive we carried on using it. The Weiss Block test, which we have used, has been very insensitive to the sort of damage that we are looking at, or rather the sort of change that we are seeing. We are getting marked changes in memory function, and if people could make zig-zag patterns with the Weiss Block before the operation they would do it afterwards. We never found the reverse, though.

Following Boccalon's paper Dahme commented on psychometric testing:

I would like to put a quotient to you to use psychometric testing, and it is a difficult matter. There is a large dispersal, the standard deviation is high, you have to have a large series, the smallest number that you can rely upon in subdividing your material is around 16 to 20, and you have to look at the statistical significances very critically because of the multiple calculations necessary in the evaluation. As I pointed out the days before yesterday, if you make 100 statistical calculations you are bound to end up with highly significant differences, even if there are not really any. So, being the proponent of the use of psychometric tests, I would like to say a real word of caution in using them: Really know your statistics and really have additional medical evidence of what you are finding with psychometrics.

Final Panel Discussion

Dr. Polonius:

Ladies and gentlemen, it is an honor to head, together with Dr. Spiro, the final panel discussion. It has forced us to self-discipline in ourselves attending all of the papers presented in the last 3 days. We have put three questions to ourselves. The first is: What can we do to improve the difficulties in the language barrier. In other words, how can we overcome the difficulty of the different words we use for the same symptoms. Very simply stated, how can we find a conversion table to that people in Hamburg, Milwaukee, and London always mean the same thing when they use different words. The second question is: What can we take home from these meetings? Is there anything we learned which can improve what we do at home? And the third question is: How can we introduce all the many things we have learned from the analytical papers over the last few days to improve the treatment of our patients' psychic problems?

Dr. Stanton:

With regard to the first question, I think it is quite a difficult task to approach any language problems with the use of certain terminology that some of us might or might not have felt that we thoroughly understood. The only possible solution that I can think of on the spur of the moment is that we could perhaps try to develop an abbreviated lexicon of some of the most common terminology, categorized perhaps as a starting point in the different areas: for instance, the psychiatric area where the terminology could perhaps be defined in several languages, then going through the more physiological and the psychological areas. The surgical areas are perhaps not quite so much of a problem since the basis of medicine in most languages is the Latin and the Greek derivations. However, in German there are many differences. I can see that there might be a need for such a lexicon, and that perhaps we could circulate it and try to come to some kind of agreement on some of the most common diagnostic terms. I noticed myself that even 2 days ago when some of the psychiatrically oriented presentations were being presented, the word "psychic" was generally used in the papers presented by most of the German guests, and as I was listening to that word "psychic" I was saying to myself, is it the same as psychological or is it psychiatric, or is it different, because in English, psychic has a totally different connotation?

The second question is, what have we learned? I think some of us have learned so very much (I, for one, have) that it will take weeks to literally digest it, to write for some more papers, to examine some of these things in greater detail, and to really think about a lot of the findings that have been presented, such as the comments that have been made on the way in which care is practiced vis-à-vis humanity or pediatric patients. I think that the most outstanding thing we have learned is the multitude of different approaches to solving the same problem, be it something like microemboli and how one approaches looking at the effects of that on brain dysfunction, or be it how to assess cognitive disorders and neurological problems in the postoperative period. I think we have learned that there is a lot we can share between us and that we should probably continue while we are apart to communicate with each other informally in the interim of the different congresses and other meetings where we might meet, and in between reading each other's publications in the various professional journals.

The third question is, where can we go and which directions can we go in: Dr. Katz is going to discuss the international study so I am going to assume that where we go means what can we do with what we have learned right now. There are several things, simple things, that come to mind immediately. One is that we certainly must do all we can in our sites, in our own hospitals, and in our own associations with people we work with, to try to encourage providers of care to provide patients with the most information that they possibly can; to prepare them ahead of time for some of the reactions that all of the different people here have observed. In other words, patients can be prepared to accept that after surgery there are some emotional and psychological changes that may occur. There are feelings that may occur that are normal in many patients following surgery. One thing I am going to do when I get home is to try to find out why there are no windows in intensive care units. I really have no idea.

Dr. Kimball:

The questions are simple, the answers are hard. I think if we stick with direct observation without too rapidly translating our observations into particular conceptual approaches we would be more on the same level. If we explain, we use simple words rather than complex words. After all, symptoms are the words that come from the patient, and if we stick to the words that come from the patient and then try to break them down in terms of what the patient means by them, we should all be on the same wavelength. In other words, call a spade a spade and stick to short and simple words. Sometimes we will need to break these down into simpler components, and I think that is very much the task of those of us who work in these units along with the surgeons and the nurses, instead of substituting more complex language and formulations that may have some pertinence in our own particular speciality.

They do not need to have pertinence in terms of our communication with other people who are not in the same field. After all, our basic methodology is one of hearing and listening and looking and describing exactly what is there. If we are going to use terms like "emotion" of "affect" spell out which it is and why you think it is anger, why you think it is anxiety, or why you think it is depression. Everyone would have a common set of things he or she would look at if he or she was going to call something a depression. You have to back that up with more simple description. If you are going to go so far as to talk about a defense, do not leave it at a defense rationalization or intellectualization or projection or something like that. You can say exactly what you think the patient is defending against and how he is defending against it. He is denying it and he refuses to see it. Then we can all use the common meaning of those terms.

What can we take home from the meeting? What can we do differently? Where do we go from here? I think mostly what meetings, particularly a meeting like this, are about is communication, an attempt to get on the same wavelength, an attempt to share or to develop a more common language that is interdisciplinary. Getting together does not only mean getting together in meetings, it means getting together in coronary care units and the intensive care units. We do not do that very well in our hospital. It is hard enough for nurses to get together with nurses working on other shifts. They do it better than doctors, but it is a very hasty meeting which nurses usually do not get paid for, or involves overlapping of time in many hospitals. It is just the bare essentials such as getting together in a relaxed way and listening and hearing rather than pushing through with the mechanics of the job. Here I think there is a place for more liaison people, people who really work at effecting relationships. I think that nurses are moving more and more toward being good liaison people between patients and physicians. I think there is a place for the nurse-clinician in these very busy units. A nurse will get things down to bare tacks faster than many of us. I think there are some specific things to study in this area. One thing came up which I hope we will get to tomorrow, namely, the study concerning the effect of informed consent. Is informed consent dangerous to one's health, as a recent editorial in *Science* suggested, partly with tongue-in-cheek?

I think we need to look at our own reactions because that will clue us in, those are our feelers, regarding what we think is going on with a patient, and what we feel is going on with a patient. We first have to see how we are reacting to that. Again, we need to focus on a smaller part rather than the global. When we identify something we have to define it in much more simple and specific terminology.

How can we use what we learn from psychological papers? Again, the most important thing is to listen and let patients talk. A rule of thumb is that the more you listen the more you may find out, but if you listen you also have to hear. It is a different hearing than just listening; you have to focus on what the message from the patient really is. Let the patients talk, and this means taking time. None of us have much time in this world, so we get into too many things, and we are all dashing from one meeting to another, from one patient to another, and from one operating room to another. It takes time, and we have to make that time. We do know some very concrete things. There are characteristic patterns of response, and thinking about them in terms of the stages of illness, the environment of illness, what are the tasks for the patient in those situations and what are the tasks for the staff. We know that in coronary care units and intensive care units anxiety, depression, and delirium are frequent factors with patients. I know each patient should be assessed for these daily, even if we have to break these down. How do you look at delirium and how do you detect it? How do you look for manifestations of anxiety and what are you looking for in depression? We know that in convalescence a major task of the patient is grieving, but in order for a patient to grieve the patient has to be given permission to grieve, to cry, to get angry, to show anxiety. We do not know very much about rehabilitation, because most of us only study what comes into the hospital; I am taking now about psychological aspects of rehabilitation. We do not know what makes for good coping and adaptation. We have these nice global words, but we do not know what hope is; we do not know what the ingredients of good coping and adaptation are. I think with the cardiac patients, that the morbidity, and perhaps to some extent the mortality that occurs in these groups of patients in the long run, applies mainly to patients who have reactions that we do not know anything about after they leave the hospital.

We need to study these patients in their homes and their places of work. The vague variables of how much sex you are having, or whether or not you are working, or whether you feel good or bad about your job, are simply not enough. They are just rough indices of how someone is coping.

Dr. Spiro:

Your questions about language bring to mind a comment contributed to Plato, that some day the philosopher, the scientist, and the artist will speak the same language, and then a true science of medicine will emerge. And in the 2300 years that have passed, I do not think we speak the same language yet. One of the problems really is not seeking a level of such precision of language that we cease to describe the phenomena that we want to know about. Therefore, if we are going to understand the feelings, the emotions, the hopes, and the fears of the human being we are going to be using language that means different things to different cultures, and that lacks precision.

I think we get into our biggest trouble when we invent technical language in an effort to pseudo-quantify something that is not quantifiable. You know, words like pseudo-quantify, for instance. That means you can not count it. What it really means is that I am confused about that quantification and understanding human emotions is extraordinarily difficult. When one pushes for high precision where it really does not exist I think we wind up dreaming up phrases. Then everybody nods sagely within that given subspeciality of psychiatry but none of us really knows what we are talking about. I would agree with comments made by several other panelists that a healthy dose of common sense is the best bet, that the language of emotion and feeling will remain difficult, that the true technical language is probably going to be much more on the medical and surgical side, but that with many of the issues we want to understand we are going to be struggling with language issues. I would urge that we do not cover up the struggle, but in essence that we will continue to have troubles.

What does one take home? Well, one thing that has been most striking to me is the cross-cultural issue, which is really not what the conference was called to discuss, but is one that I am constantly finding myself curious about. What is the strange design of this thing that we call the human being? And how astounding it is that people from so many different cultures, and from so many different parts of the world, describe similar phenomonena given a similar stress. As we become more and more precise in such descriptions we reach the point where we can really tease out what the cross-cultural dissimilarities are. For instance, I think that the discussion of the work ethic, and the specific issues in one of the papers today, probably make a great deal of sense in Milwaukee, but would probably make virtually no sense in some of the Middle-

Eastern cultures that I have studied, where the work ethic is quite different. We have here a model which not only helps us to understand the nature of heart surgery but, because it holds one thing constant or relatively constant, the nature of the stress, may shed light on additional issues.

That leads me perhaps to what I take home. That is closest to Sir William Osler, who once remarked that if you understand syphillis you understand all of medicine. I am beginning to think that if you really understand the full somata, psychosomata you know, back and forth, from psychi to soma, that is involved in this particular model, one may have a very basic grasp of not only psychosomatic medicine but some fundamental issues of interaction between disease states, somatic intervention, and how people react. As a psychiatrist I find this incredibly exciting. This is really what I take home; it is curiosity about applying the model and what I have learned from this conference; it is oncology, bone tumors, for instance, to the nephrology unit, and to schizophrenia, which to me is another disease that involves a series of somatic-psychosomatic interaction; the whole understanding of what stress really means and how it manifests itself in people.

Finally, the third question: how do we introduce all that we have learned? While attending the conference I have had a strong feeling that people discover the truth every 30 years or so, forget it, rediscover it, re-rediscover it. The ancient Greeks actually had a fairly good idea of how to establish a psychiatric hospital. The Arabs were geniuses at it in the fourteenth century. You know, every 50 years or so we come along and we rediscover what everyone knows, because somehow it does not get institutionalized, or else the people who really can make use of the wisdom never come into contact with it, like administrators or politicians appropriating money. That leaves me with a strong sense that the application here has to be with people who can carry it out, not with superspecialists, because superspecialists, as I think many of us here are, in the sense of wanting to take on the research problem, try to understand it, and move on to the next one, are not necessarily the best people at institutionalizing procedures. The analogy came up in my mind that once the germs theory was fairly well established, and once the basic understanding of aseptic surgery was understood, we really did not ask the surgical specialists to go into the operating room and scrub it down first. In fact, we did not even ask them to design the operating room. Instead, that knowledge really involves administrators, housekeeping service, architects, and nurses who supervise to make sure that it is done properly; and the surgeon then arrives in full splendor to carry on his art. I think for the psychiatrist it is very similar in that by the time we arrive it is too late. So I think the back home application really means to me: how do we take the information that has come out of this conference and translate it for administrators, directors of nursing, and hospital architects. I emphasize nursing over and over again because I believe that nurses are actually the group who generally carries the culture whithin a hospital. That would be my response to the back home application.

Finally, I just want to comment that I think the conference has been awfully good for psychiatry. I hope its intent is good for surgery. Part of it is that there is something about nurses, psychiatrists, psychologists, and surgeons sitting in one room and trying to force themselves to talk in common sense language enough to understand each other. It forces one to simplify one's concepts to they are sparer, leaner, and perhaps better for that interaction. It makes me think that I got to too many psychiatric meetings. We do not have enough meetings like this.

Dr. Blacher:

I was prepared to pull out my crystal ball, which might have had a greater effect. I think that we suffer constantly intradisciplinarily with the language barrier. It is hard enough when you get two psychiatrists in a room trying to communicate with each other. Usually you do not get a conversation, you get two monologues. If we get into a room with other people and other disciplines, our problems are really compounded. But I think that in general the value of a meeting like this is that we really get a total emersion in each other's point of view. I have been known to repeat myself and so I can repeat myself now and say that we all come to such a meeting knowing that we know the truth and that the other disciplines are really missing most of it. We usually end up after such meetings with a feeling that there is much more that we had not thought of. I know in the last meeting that we had 2 years ago, and I suspect it will happen again, we left with a sense of having overdosed on information, and it takes us a while to digest things. I think that one of the things that happens is that the more we know about what other people are doing in other disciplines as well as our own, the less anxious we become. Knowledge has a beautiful way of making us feel more comfortable and giving us the freedom to look at the other person's work and the other person's language as well. I have a terrible confession that I find myself excited this afternoon listening to the surgical presentations and finding a keen sense of interest and excitement and wondering how I can integrate that with my psychological information. The nurses, I am glad Dr. Spiro pointed out, are on the front line. They are the ones who have the difficulties because we leave them in the ICUs with the patients. We go in, we talk to the patients for a bit, and we may be lucky enough in some specialities to go in and write a quick note and sidle out. The nurses are there for a long period of time, taking care of the patients. They need our help a great deal, and I think that the more knowledge they have the greater help they get.

Now, what do we really take home? I, for one, am constantly finding myself after such a meeting wondering in a very strange way, with all the information we have got, whether we ask ourselves the right questions. I think we have to think about that. I will use the small segment for instance, the deliria we are concerned about. I do not advocate bubbling peoples' brains, I do not think that is such a good idea. However, we have to ask ourselves whether delirium is so bad. Whether psychosis is so terrible, under certain circumstances. For instance, I think for many of our patients the mild postoperative delirium may act as an anesthetic. I think the problem for them is what it means later, and we find that we always discuss with them how this is. If you tell the patient that this is a normal piece of behavior then his whole view of what is happening to him changes. We have to ask ourselves really, what do we want to know and where are we going to go? I think the answer to the question, where do we go from here, would have to be forward, always forward. The question is whether or not we can. If we know more – and I feel this very strongly – the more we know the treatment of the patient is going to take care of itself. Our problem is twofold: we may not know what we do or we may be too uncomfortable in the information we do have. I think that these meetings bring us together so that we become less anxious, we become more knowledgable, and I think our patients will benefit from this.

Dr. Longmore:

Mr. Chairman, ladies and gentlemen, I have been under what you psychiatrists call a stress situation today, chairing a session and reading a paper which I was not quite sure about, and because of that I have got what I think you psychiatrists call a cognitive disorder. I chose the word advisably because I heard it 142 times in one session. I counted, because I did not know what it meant, and because of this cognitive disorder I cannot actually remember the three questions which were asked, and I am reminded of our patients when we ask them what is on Dr. Bethune's little cards and they say, what cards? Because of that I propose to tell you a story. It is of two surgeons meeting each other, and one goes to the other and says, "John, that's an interesting operation you're doing there. How many of those have you done?" And the answer is "less than a hundred", which being translated means six. Then he says, "Well, John, that's very good, what sort of results are you getting?" And the answer is, "I don't think I've lost any yet". The true translation of that is that three are dead and three are in delirium. Now, that deals with the world's business.

Now, what have we learned? I think we have learned something terribly important, and something for which we should be extremely grateful. That is that there are many scientific studies of things which are almost impossible to sort out any other way. So we should be very thankful that there are so many people who come into medicine and have made the effort to be scientific about it. I think that is perhaps one of the most exciting things that I have learned.

Now what have we got to do. Well, this may be the most important thing. We have to go from here as disciples of this meeting and actually do something so that we do less damage to our patients' brains. Well, obviously we have learned that we have got to look at our patients better preoperatively and try to pinpoint any neurological problems and any other problems they have before we assault them with surgery, bubbles, microparticles, silicone tubes, plastic bands, and so on and so on. And before we give them all the stress of the operation, whatever stress is, then we must learn to hurry to apply important new discoveries like prostacyclin, which at a stroke should remove at least half of the causes of cerebral damage. Having listened to Dr. Taylor this afternoon, perhaps we should apply pulsatile flow to our patients. And having heard the filter experts, presumably we ought to filter very carefully what goes back into our patients. We should apply the membrane oxygenator rather than bubble oxygenator, and try to make the bypass equipment safer and more sophisticated. Then we should set up a cooperative effort. Now, we are very fortunate in that Jeremy Katz has demonstrated that he is a great organizer, hence my suggestion that we should appoint him to organize the international study. Now I think I want to come to the two most important observations I have made, and that is that I think we should visit each other more often. I was horrified to find that a fellow, who is only a few miles from me, was doing work which I was not aware of and on a subject which we have always needed. We do not communicate about this until we come halfway across the world and upset our time clocks so that we are talking in the middle of the night instead of the middle of the day. We have also had the opportunity of meeting people in other fields of medicine which is terribly important. So I want us to visit each other, not only to communicate about medicine, but about other matters. I think if we are going to have peace in our time, then we have got to visit each other and overcome these crazy differences we have between us. Also we have got to have international cooperation in medicine which will pave the way for cooperation in other fields.

The International Study: A Course for the Future

J.M. Katz

Introduction

In 1980, an international study concerning incidence and factors affecting the occurrence of cerebral and psychopathological reactions to cardiac surgery was preposed at the *Second International Symposium* on this subject. Since that time great progress has been made toward its implementation. The original presentation has thus been rewritten to keep the reader informed of major developments in the international study.

Background

In March 1978, the need to carry out an international study on psychological and neurological problems after heart surgery was recognized at the *First International Symposium on Psychopathological and Neurological Dysfunctions Following Cardiac Surgery*. The meeting, attended by 36 representatives from five countries, was held in Hamburg, West Germany. At that time, it was unknown whether sufficient world support existed to carry out such a study.

In March 1980, such support was demonstrated at the *Second International Symposium* on this subject in Milwaukee, Wisconsin, USA. The meeting was attended by over 200 persons representing 18 countries and 24 US States. Following the conference, it was resolved that interested meeting participants would work together toward implementation of the study.

In April 1981, the International Consortium on Cerebral and Psychopathological Dysfunctions Following Cardiac Surgery was formally established at an organizational/planning meeting in Milwaukee. The purpose of the organization is to serve as the vehicle within which the study would be carried out and within which change would be facilitated based on findings of the study.

At the meeting, an outline of a study protocol was reviewed and a preliminary Consortium organizational structure established, including necessary committees to develop the study further.

The organization is sponsored by the Medical College of Wisconsin and the Milwaukee Country Mental Health Complex, Milwaukee, and the University Hospital Hamburg-Eppendorf, Hamburg, West Germany. Currently 17 countries are represented in the Consortium.

In May 1982, the first draft of the International Study Protocol was reviewed at Working Meeting I. At the meeting, held in Milwaukee, consensus was also reached to establish a Consortium Board of Directors.

In November 1982, at Working Meeting II in Milwaukee, the second draft of the project was reviewed and data collection forms brought into near final form. Members for the Consortium Board of Directors were selected and committees established to facilitate the actual carrying out of the study.

Beginning of the Study

At the present time the study is planned to begin at selected world heart surgery centers in spring, 1983.

In Memoriam: Professor Robin D. Becker*

R.J. Flemma

It is my sad duty to inform those of you who might be unaware of the fact, that Robin Becker, our friend, associate, and collaborator in this project, died on Thursday, February 19, 1981. Many of you knew of Robin and his prodigious works prior to his coming to Milwaukee.

I, fortunately, met Robin last March at the Second International Symposium. My first impression of him was similar to that of a charismatic. He seemed to think as I did, but he expressed himself, his fervor, his concern, his compassion so eloquently and fluently that I knew I was in the presence of a most unique individual. After a party held at our home for the faculty of the symposium, my children and my wife were equally impressed by Robin. It was as though in a few moments he had joined the Flemma family. It was a very unusual experience.

We were fortunate to have Robin come to Milwaukee as a Distinguished Visiting Professor at the Medical College of Wisconsin, but even more fortunate to have him work with us personally at St. Luke's Hospital in attacking the problems that concern this group today.

Robin arrived in August of 1980. Within moments he had made his imprint. He rallied to the cause of the surgeons, cardiologists, psychologists, nurses, psychiatrists, physicians assistants and anyone else who, seeing him in action, did not want to miss the boat. I can say that there has never been such unanimity in action at our hospital, or amongst such a diverse group of people, and Robin was definitely the catalyst.

He was immediately the father confessor to every person at St. Luke's Hospital, including the coffee shop personnel. He had what we call compassion, concern, "simpatico" or any other term you might use to indicate understanding and caring. He shook hands with two hands, looked everyone in the eye directly and conveyed to all a real concern for their problems. It is no wonder that not only the patients, but the physicians, the nurses and everyone easily related their problems to Robin. His was a brief time in Milwaukee, but it was a significant time in terms of people helped.

In Israel Robin cared for the children, and I can remember the saying of the great bard, "Each tear wiped from a child's eye is like lighting a star in heaven." In Mil-

---

* This eulogy was given at the Organization/Planning Meeting for the International Consortium on Cerebral and Psychopathological Dysfunctions following Cardiac Surgery. The meeting was held April 3–5, 1981 in Milwaukee at which time the International Consortium was formally established and planning for the International Study was begun.

waukee Robin allayed the anxieties of adults undergoing cardiac surgery. If I can paraphrase the previous saying, "Each fear erased from a person's mind is like lighting a star in heaven."

Robin stimulated all of us to greater sensitivity of our roles in healing, to greater understanding of our patients; their fears, their hopes, and aspirations. He enabled us to be better physicians because our roles and the patient's aspirations became confluent when Robin was around.

We shall miss Robin greatly. Even if we knew him but shortly, I can say, "A brief light flashed across the sky of human understanding that illuminated the souls of patients and physicians." Although Robin is no longer with us, may that light continue to illuminate our path here today, as we try to bring to fruition his project that was so dear to him.

MIX
Papier aus verantwortungsvollen Quellen
Paper from responsible sources
FSC® C105338

If you have any concerns about our products,
you can contact us on
ProductSafety@springernature.com

In case Publisher is established outside the EU,
the EU authorized representative is:
Springer Nature Customer Service Center GmbH
Europaplatz 3, 69115 Heidelberg, Germany

Printed by Libri Plureos GmbH
in Hamburg, Germany